Human Genetics and Genomics

Dedication
To Shelley, Jessica, and Katie – Bruce Korf
To Mallory Lynn and David Nicholas – Mira Irons

This new edition is also available as an e-book.
For more details, please see
www.wiley.com/buy/9780470654477
or scan this QR code:

Human Genetics and Genomics

Bruce R. Korf

MD, PhD

Wayne H. and Sara Crews Finley Chair in Medical Genetics
Professor and Chair, Department of Genetics
Director, Heflin Center for Genomic Sciences
University of Alabama at Birmingham

Mira B. Irons

MD

Park Gerald Chair in Genetics
Associate Chief, Division of Genetics
Children's Hospital Boston
Associate Professor of Pediatrics
Harvard Medical School

Fourth edition

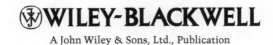

A John Wiley & Sons, Ltd., Publication

Library of Congress Cataloging-in-Publication Data
Korf, Bruce R.
    Human genetics and genomics / Bruce R. Korf, Mira B. Irons. – 4th ed.
        p. ; cm.
    Includes bibliographical references and index.
    ISBN 978-0-470-65447-7 (pbk. : alk. paper)
    I. Irons, Mira B.   II. Title.
    [DNLM: 1. Genetics, Medical–Problems and Exercises.   2. Genetic Diseases, Inborn–Problems and Exercises.   3. Genomics–Problems and Exercises.   4. Problem-Based Learning–Problems and Exercises.
QZ 18.2]

    616'.042–dc23

                                            2012024773

A catalogue record for this book is available from the British Library.

Wiley also publishes its books in a variety of electronic formats. Some content that appears in print may not be available in electronic books.

Cover image and design by Fortiori design

Set in 10/12 pt Adobe Garamond Pro by Toppan Best-set Premedia Limited

Contents

Preface

Sixteen years have passed since the first edition of this book was published, and this has been a time of enormously rapid change and advancement in the field of genetics and genomics. The increasing prominence of genomics was recognized in the last edition, when the name was changed to *Human Genetics and Genomics*. That edition also launched a reorganization of the book, first presenting basic concepts and then using a problem-based approach to illustrate clinical applications. That pattern has been retained in this new edition.

A major change in this fourth edition is the addition of a co-author, Dr. Mira Irons. This reflects the reality that the scope and pace of change in our field have expanded to the point where it is difficult for any one individual to keep up. Dr. Irons has rewritten or updated several of the chapters and case studies. Another change is the addition of a section called "Sources of Information" to each chapter. Genetics and genomics are intensively information-based sciences, and therefore are heavily dependent on access to continuously updated sources of information. We hope that this will help to guide students to reliable data sources that will assist in their future clinical or research activities.

In the previous edition of this book, it was noted that genomic approaches were beginning to inform our understanding of common as well as rare disorders. This trend has continued, with the advent of genome-wide association studies, and has spawned clinical applications, including direct-to-consumer genetic risk assessment. This edition has been updated to highlight these developments. There has also been remarkable progress in the approach to rare "single-gene" disorders. The list of conditions for which genetic testing is available has expanded dramatically, and recently whole-exome or whole-genome sequencing has been applied to solving diagnostic challenges. Most notably, many rare genetic conditions previously thought to be untreatable are now the target of clinical trials for new therapeutic approaches. We have also highlighted this development, along with the need to appreciate the process of performing clinical trials for genetic disorders.

As with previous editions, we have benefited greatly from comments and suggestions from both reviewers and readers. "Mutations" inevitably are found within the text, and we are most grateful to those who point these out so that they can be corrected. Likewise, we greatly appreciate suggestions for new content or better ways to explain some of the more challenging concepts.

As genomic approaches pervade all of medicine, one of the most common concerns expressed is that health providers cannot keep up with this new discipline. We remain optimistic that a new generation of students will embrace the new opportunities afforded by genetics and genomics to transform our approach to both rare and common conditions as they begin a process of learning that will span their entire careers.

Bruce R. Korf
Mira B. Irons

How to get the best out of your textbook

Welcome to the new edition of *Human Genetics and Genomics*. Over the next two pages you will be shown how to make the most of the learning features included in the textbook.

The Anytime, Anywhere Textbook ▶

For the first time, your textbook comes with free access to a **Wiley E-Text: Powered by VitalSource** – a digital, interactive version of this textbook which you own as soon as you download it.

Your **Wiley E-Text: Powered by VitalSource** allows you to:
Search: Save time by finding terms and topics instantly in your book, your notes, even your whole library (once you've downloaded more textbooks)
Note and Highlight: Colour code, highlight and make digital notes right in the text so you can find them quickly and easily
Organize: Keep books, notes and class materials organized in folders inside the application
Share: Exchange notes and highlights with friends, classmates and study groups
Upgrade: Your textbook can be transferred when you need to change or upgrade computers
Link: Link directly from the page of your interactive textbook to all of the material contained on the companion website

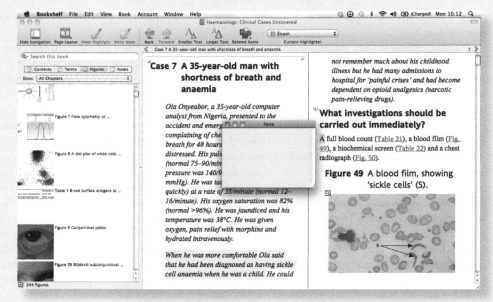

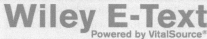

To access your Wiley E-Text: Powered by VitalSource:

- Find the redemption code on the inside front cover of this book and carefully scratch away the top coating of the label.
- Visit **www.vitalsource.com/software/bookshelf/downloads** to download the Bookshelf application.
- If you have puchased this title as an e-book, access to your **Wiley E-Text: Powered by VitalSource** is available with proof of purchase within 90 days. Visit **http://support.wiley.com** to request a redemption code via the "Live Chat" or "Ask A Question" tabs.
- Open the Bookshelf application on your computer and register for an account.
- Follow the registration process and enter your redemption code to download your digital book.
- For full access instructions, visit **www.korfgenetics.com**.

CourseSmart gives you instant access (via computer or mobile device) to this Wiley-Blackwell eTextbook and its extra electronic functionality, at 40% off the recommended retail print price. See all the benefits at **www. coursesmart.com/students**.

Instructors . . . receive your own digital desk copies!

It also offers instructors an immediate, efficient, and environmentally-friendly way to review this textbook for your course.

For more information visit **www.coursesmart. com/instructors**.

With CourseSmart, you can create lecture notes quickly with copy and paste, and share pages and notes with your students. Access your Wiley CourseSmart digital textbook from your computer or mobile device instantly for evaluation, class preparation, and as a teaching tool in the classroom.

Simply sign in at **http://instructors. coursesmart.com/bookshelf** to download your Bookshelf and get started. To request your desk copy, hit "Request Online Copy" on your search results or book product page.

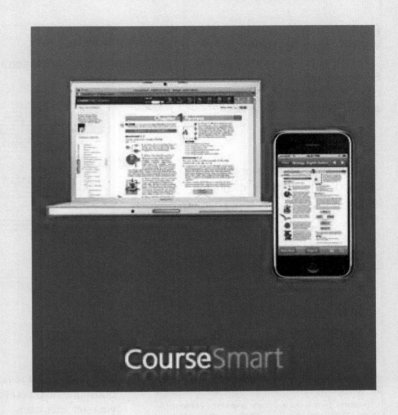

A companion website

Your textbook is also accompanied by a FREE companion website that contains:
- Figures from the book in PowerPoint format
- Interactive self-assessment MCQ tests
- Further online reading list
- Interactive problem-based learning cases
- Factsheets on basic conditions

Log on to **www.korfgenetics.com** to find out more.

Features contained within your textbook

Every chapter begins with a list of key points contained within the chapter and an introduction to of the topic.

'Ethical implications', 'Hot topic' and other boxes give further insight into topics.

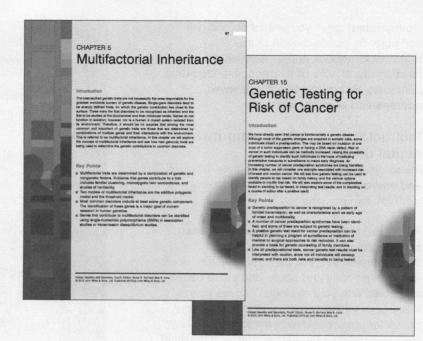

Ethical Implications 3.1 Family Ties

One of the unique aspects of genetics as compared with other areas of medicine is that information about one family member may have an impact on other relatives. This has many implications that are

important to consider when discussing family history with patients. Firstly, relevant information may not be widely known within the family. It may be necessary to ask specific

Hot Topic 5.1 Large-Cohort Studies

The ability to carry out a case–control study is dependent on access to a large cohort affected with

the phenotype of interest. Ideally, the genes will come from a single homogeneous population, thus

Self-assessment review questions help you test yourself after each chapter.

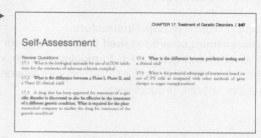

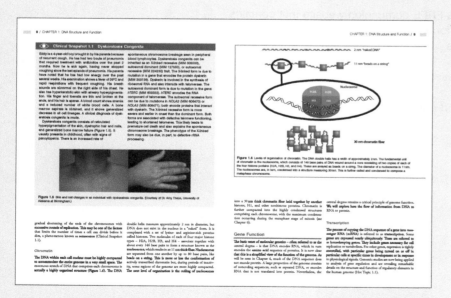

Your textbook is full of clinical photographs, method notes, cases illustrations and tables. The **Wiley E-Text: Powered by VitalSource** version of your textbook will allow you to copy and paste any photograph or illustration into assignments, presentations and your own notes.

We hope you enjoy using your new textbook. Good luck with your studies!

Part One
Basic Principles of
Human Genetics

CHAPTER 1
DNA Structure and Function

Introduction

The 20th century will likely be remembered by historians of biological science for the discovery of the structure of DNA and the mechanisms by which information coded in DNA is translated into the amino acid sequence of proteins. Although the story of modern human genetics begins about 50 years before the structure of DNA was elucidated, we will start our exploration here. We do so because everything we know about inheritance must now be viewed in the light of the underlying molecular mechanisms. We will see here how the structure of DNA sets the stage both for its replication and for its ability to direct the synthesis of proteins. We will also see that the function of the system is tightly regulated, and how variations in the structure of DNA can alter function. The story of human genetics did not begin with molecular biology, and it will not end there, as knowledge is now being integrated to explain the behavior of complex biological systems. Molecular biology, however, remains a key engine of progress in biological understanding, so it is fitting that we begin our journey here.

Key Points

■ DNA consists of a double-helical sugar–phosphate structure with the two strands held together by hydrogen bonding between adenine and thymine or cytosine and guanine bases.

■ DNA replication involves local unwinding of the double helix and copying a new strand from the base sequence of each parental strand. Replication proceeds bidirectionally from multiple start sites in the genome.

■ DNA is complexed with proteins to form a highly compacted chromatin fiber in the nucleus.

■ Genetic information is copied from DNA into messenger RNA (mRNA) in a highly regulated process that involves activation or repression of individual genes.

■ mRNA molecules are extensively processed in the nucleus, including removal of introns and splicing together of exons, prior to export to the cytoplasm for translation into protein.

■ The base sequence of mRNA is read in triplet codons to direct the assembly of amino acids into protein on ribosomes.

■ Some genes are permanently repressed by epigenetic marks such as methylation of cytosine bases. These include most genes on one of two X chromosomes in cells in females and one of the two copies of imprinted genes.

Human Genetics and Genomics, Fourth Edition. Bruce R. Korf and Mira B. Irons.
© 2013 John Wiley & Sons, Ltd. Published 2013 by John Wiley & Sons, Ltd.

Deoxyribonucleic Acid

Mendel described dominant and recessive inheritance before the concept of the gene was introduced and long before the chemical basis of inheritance was known. Cell biologists during the late 19th and early 20th centuries had established that genetic material resides in the cell nucleus and **DNA** was known to be a major chemical constituent. As the chemistry of DNA came to be understood, for a long time it was considered to be too simple a molecule – consisting of just four chemical building blocks, the bases **adenine**, **guanine**, **thymine**, and **cytosine**, along with sugar and phosphate – to account for the complexity of genetic transmission. Credit for recognition of the role of DNA in inheritance goes to the landmark experiments by Oswald Avery and his colleagues, who demonstrated that a phenotype of smooth or rough colonies of the bacterium *Pneumococcus* could be transmitted from cell to cell through DNA alone. Elucidation of the structure of DNA by James Watson and Francis Crick in 1953 opened the door to understanding the mechanisms whereby this molecule functions as the agent of inheritance (Sources of Information 1.1).

Sources of Information 1.1
Mendelian Inheritance in Man

Dr. Victor McKusick and his colleagues at Johns Hopkins School of Medicine began to catalog genes and human genetic traits in the 1960s. The first edition of the catalog *Mendelian Inheritance in Man* was published in 1966. Multiple print editions subsequently appeared, and now the catalog is maintained on the Internet as "Online Mendelian Inheritance in Man" (OMIM), located at www.omim.org.

OMIM is recognized as the authoritative source of information about human genes and genetic traits. The catalog can be searched by gene, phenotype, gene locus, and many other features. The catalog provides a synopsis of the gene or trait, including a summary of clinical features associated with mutations. There are links to other databases, providing access to gene and amino acid sequences, mutations, and so on. Each entry has a unique six-digit number, the MIM number. Autosomal dominant traits have entries beginning with 1, recessive traits with 2, X linked with 3, and mitochondrial with 5. Specific genes have MIM numbers that start with 6.

Throughout this book, genes or genetic traits will be annotated with their corresponding MIM number to remind the reader that more information is available on OMIM and to facilitate access to the site.

DNA Structure

DNA consists of a pair of strands of a sugar–phosphate backbone attached to a set of **pyrimidine** and **purine** bases (Figure 1.1). The sugar is deoxyribose – ribose missing an oxygen atom at its 2′ position. Each DNA strand consists of alternating deoxyribose molecules connected by phosphodiester bonds from the 5′ position of one deoxyribose to the 3′ position of the next. The strands are bound together by hydrogen bonds between adenine and thymine bases and between guanine and cytosine bases. Together these strands form a right-handed double helix. The two strands run in opposite (antiparallel) directions, so that one extends from 5′ to 3′ while the other goes from 3′ to 5′.

The key feature of DNA, wherein resides its ability to encode information, is in the sequence of the four bases (Methods 1.1).

✓ Methods 1.1   Isolation of DNA

DNA, or in some cases RNA, is the starting point for most experiments aimed at studying gene structure or function. DNA can be isolated from any cell that contains a nucleus. The most commonly used tissue for human DNA isolation is peripheral blood, where white blood cells provide a readily accessible source of nucleated cells. Other commonly used tissues include cultured skin fibroblasts, epithelial cells scraped from the inner lining of the cheek, and fetal cells obtained by amniocentesis or chorionic villus biopsy. Peripheral blood lymphocytes can be transformed with Epstein–Barr virus into immortalized cell lines, providing permanent access to growing cells from an individual.

Nuclear DNA is complexed with proteins, which must be removed in order for the DNA to be analyzed. For some experiments it is necessary to obtain highly purified DNA, which involves digestion or removal of the proteins. In other cases, relatively crude preparations suffice. This is the case, for example, with DNA isolated from cheek scrapings. The small amount of DNA isolated from this source is usually released from cells with minimal effort to remove proteins. This preparation is adequate for limited analysis of specific gene sequences. DNA preparations can be obtained from very minute biological specimens, such as drops of dried blood, skin cells, or hair samples isolated from crime scenes for forensic analysis.

Isolation of RNA involves purification of nucleic acid from the nucleus and/or cytoplasm. This RNA can be used to study the patterns of gene expression in a particular tissue. RNA tends to be less stable than DNA, requiring special care during isolation to avoid degradation.

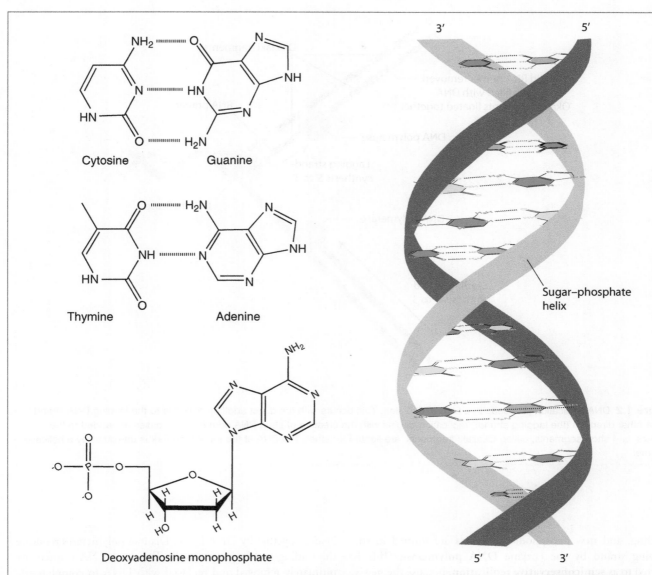

Figure 1.1 Double helical structure of DNA. The double helix is on the right-hand side. The sugar–phosphate helices are held together by hydrogen bonding between adenine and thymine (A–T) bases, or guanine and cytosine (G–C) bases. Deoxyadenosine monophosphate is shown at the bottom left.

The number of adenine bases (A) always equals the number of thymines (T), and the number of cytosines (C) always equals the number of guanines (G). This is because A on one strand is always paired with T on the other, and C is always paired with G. The pairing is noncovalent, due to hydrogen bonding between complementary bases. G–C base pairs form three hydrogen bonds, whereas A–T pairs form two, making the G–C pairs slightly more thermodynamically stable. Because the pairs always include one purine base (A or G) and one pyrimidine base (C or T), the distance across the helix remains constant.

DNA Replication

The complementarity of A to T and G to C provides the basis for DNA replication, a point that was recognized by Watson and Crick in their paper describing the structure of DNA. DNA replication proceeds by a localized unwinding of the double helix, with each strand serving as a template for replication of a new sister strand (Figure 1.2). Wherever a G base is found on one strand, a C will be placed on the growing strand; wherever a T is found, an A will be placed; and so on. Bases are positioned in the newly synthesized strand by hydrogen

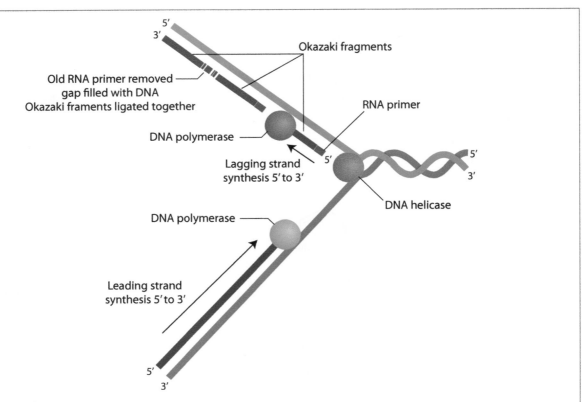

Old RNA primer removed
gap filled with DNA
Okazaki framents ligated together

Okazaki fragments

DNA polymerase

RNA primer

Lagging strand
synthesis 5' to 3'

DNA helicase

DNA polymerase

Leading strand
synthesis 5' to 3'

Figure 1.2 DNA replication proceeds in a 5' to 3' direction. This occurs with the direct addition of bases to the leading DNA strand. In the other direction (the lagging strand), replication begins with the creation of short RNA primers. DNA bases are added to the primers, and short segments, called Okazaki fragments, are ligated together. The DNA at the replication fork is unwound by a helicase enzyme.

bonding, and new phosphodiester bonds are formed in the growing strand by the enzyme **DNA polymerase**. This is referred to as **semiconservative replication**, because the newly synthesized DNA double helices are hybrid molecules that consist of one parental strand and one new daughter strand. Unwinding of the double helix is accomplished by another enzyme system, **helicase**.

DNA replication requires growth of a strand from a preexisting primer sequence. Primer sequences are provided by transcription of short RNA molecules from the DNA template. **RNA** is a single-stranded nucleic acid, similar to DNA except that the sugar molecules are ribose rather than deoxyribose and uracil substitutes for thymine (and pairs with adenine). During DNA replication, short RNA primers are transcribed and then extended by DNA polymerase. DNA is synthesized in a 5' (exposed phosphate on the 5' carbon of the ribose molecule) to 3' (exposed hydroxyl on the 3' carbon) direction. For one strand, referred to as the **leading strand**, this can be accomplished continuously as the DNA unwinds. The other strand, called the **lagging strand**, is replicated in short segments, called **Okazaki fragments**, which are then enzymatically

ligated together by DNA ligase. Distinct polymerases replicate the leading and lagging strands. The short RNA primers are ultimately removed and replaced with DNA to complete the replication process.

The human genome consists of over 3 billion base pairs of DNA packaged into 23 pairs of chromosomes. Each chromosome consists of a single, continuous DNA molecule, encompassing tens to hundreds of millions of base pairs. If the DNA on each chromosome were to be replicated in a linear manner from one end to another, the process would go on interminably – certainly too long to sustain the rates of cell division that must occur. In fact, the entire genome can be replicated in a matter of hours because replication occurs simultaneously at multiple sites along a chromosome. These origins of replication are bubble-like structures from which DNA replication proceeds bidirectionally until an adjacent bubble is reached (Figure 1.3).

One special case in DNA replication is the replication of the ends of chromosomes. Removal of the terminal RNA primer from the lagging strand at the end of a chromosome would result in shortening of the end, since there is no upstream

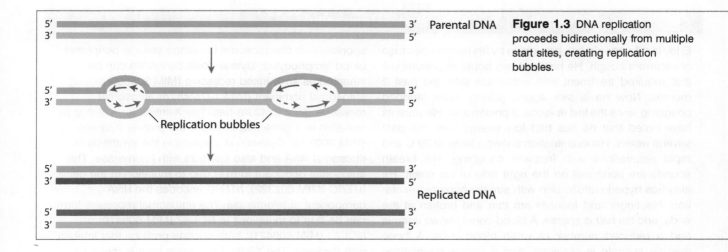

Figure 1.3 DNA replication proceeds bidirectionally from multiple start sites, creating replication bubbles.

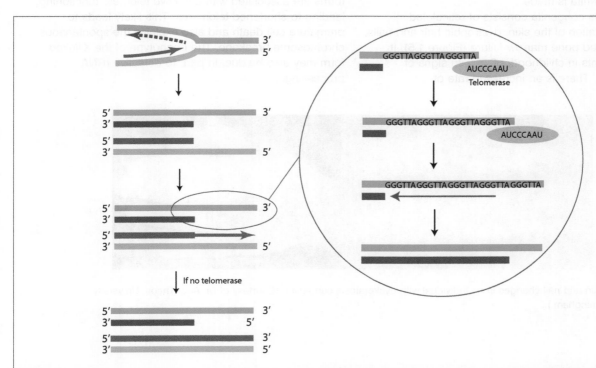

Figure 1.4 The lagging strand cannot replicate the end of the chromosome, since there is no site at which the RNA polymerase can bind (as it would be off the end of the chromosome). This is shown to the left, where the replicated chromosome has a shortened 5′ end on one strand. If telomerase is present (right), the 3′ end is extended, using an RNA template intrinsic to the enzyme. The lagging strand is then replicated using a DNA polymerase. Extension of the telomere by telomerase prevents erosion of the end of the chromosome during replication.

primer for DNA polymerase to replace the short RNA primer. This problem is circumvented by action of an enzyme called telomerase, which uses an RNA template intrinsic to the enzyme to add a stretch of DNA onto the 3′ end of the lagging strand (Figure 1.4). The DNA sequence of the **tel-** **omere** is determined by the RNA sequence in the enzyme; for humans the sequence is GGGTTA. Each chromosome end has a tandem repeat of thousands of copies of the telomere sequence that is replicated during early development. Somatic cells may replicate without telomerase activity, resulting in a

👁 Clinical Snapshot 1.1   Dyskeratosis Congenita

Eddy is a 4-year-old boy brought in by his parents because of recurrent cough. He has had two bouts of pneumonia that required treatment with antibiotics over the past 2 months. Now he is sick again, having never stopped coughing since the last episode of pneumonia. His parents have noted that he has had low energy over the past several weeks. His examination shows a fever of 39°C and rapid respirations with frequent coughing. His breath sounds are abnormal on the right side of his chest. He also has hyperkeratotic skin with streaky hyperpigmentation. His finger and toenails are thin and broken at the ends, and his hair is sparse. A blood count shows anemia and a reduced number of white blood cells. A bone marrow aspirate is obtained, and it shows generalized decrease in all cell lineages. A clinical diagnosis of dyskeratosis congenita is made.

Dyskeratosis congenita consists of reticulated hyperpigmentation of the skin, dystrophic hair and nails, and generalized bone marrow failure (Figure 1.5). It usually presents in childhood, often with signs of pancytopenia. There is an increased rate of

spontaneous chromosome breakage seen in peripheral blood lymphocytes. Dyskeratosis congenita can be inherited as an X-linked recessive (MIM 305000), autosomal dominant (MIM 127550), or autosomal recessive (MIM 224230) trait. The X-linked form is due to mutation in a gene that encodes the protein dyskerin (MIM 300126). Dyskerin is involved in the synthesis of ribosomal RNA and also interacts with telomerase. The autosomal dominant form is due to mutation in the gene *hTERC* (MIM 602322). *hTERC* encodes the RNA component of telomerase. The autosomal recessive form can be due to mutations in *NOLA2* (MIM 606470) or *NOLA3* (MIM 606471); both encode proteins that interact with dyskerin. The X-linked recessive form is more severe and earlier in onset than the dominant form. Both forms are associated with defective telomere functioning, leading to shortened telomeres. This likely leads to premature cell death and also explains the spontaneous chromosome breakage. The phenotype of the X-linked form may also be due, in part, to defective rRNA processing.

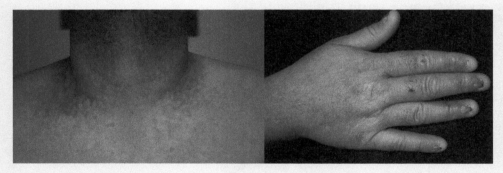

Figure 1.5 Skin and nail changes in an individual with dyskeratosis congenita. (Courtesy of Dr. Amy Theos, University of Alabama at Birmingham.)

gradual shortening of the ends of the chromosomes with successive rounds of replication. This may be one of the factors that limits the number of times a cell can divide before it dies, a phenomenon known as **senescence** (Clinical Snapshot 1.1).

Chromatin

The DNA within each cell nucleus must be highly compacted to accommodate the entire genome in a very small space. The enormous stretch of DNA that comprises each chromosome is actually a highly organized structure (Figure 1.6). The DNA

double helix measures approximately 2 nm in diameter, but DNA does not exist in the nucleus in a "naked" form. It is complexed with a set of lysine- and arginine-rich proteins called histones. Two molecules of each of four major histone types – H2A, H2B, H3, and H4 – associate together with about every 146 base pairs to form a structure known as the **nucleosome**, which results in an 11 nm thick fiber. Nucleosomes are separated from one another by up to 80 base pairs, like beads on a string. This is more or less the conformation of actively transcribed chromatin but, during periods of inactivity, some regions of the genome are more highly compacted. The next level of organization is the coiling of nucleosomes

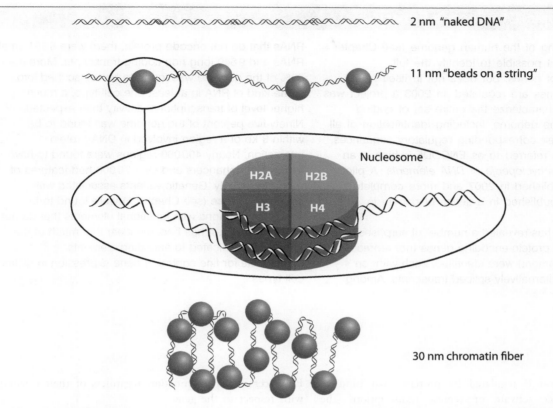

Figure 1.6 Levels of organization of chromatin. The DNA double helix has a width of approximately 2 nm. The fundamental unit of chromatin is the nucleosome, which consists of 146 base pairs of DNA wound around a core consisting of two copies of each of the four histone proteins (H2A, H2B, H3, and H4). These are arrayed as beads on a string. The diameter of a nucleosome is 11 nm. The nucleosomes are, in turn, condensed into a structure measuring 30 nm. This is further coiled and condensed to compose a metaphase chromosome.

into a 30 nm thick chromatin fiber held together by another histone, H1, and other nonhistone proteins. Chromatin is further compacted into the highly condensed structures comprising each chromosome, with the maximum condensation occurring during the metaphase stage of mitosis (see Chapter 6).

Gene Function

The basic tenet of molecular genetics – often referred to as the central dogma – is that DNA encodes RNA, which in turn encodes the **amino acid** sequence of proteins. It is now clear that this is a simplified view of the function of the genome. As will be seen in Chapter 4, much of the DNA sequence does not encode protein. A large proportion of the genome consists of noncoding sequences, such as repeated DNA, or encodes RNA that is not translated into protein. Nevertheless, the

central dogma remains a critical principle of genome function. We will explore here the flow of information from DNA to RNA to protein.

Transcription

The process of copying the DNA sequence of a gene into **messenger RNA (mRNA)** is referred to as **transcription**. Some genes are expressed nearly ubiquitously. These are referred to as **housekeeping genes**. They include genes necessary for cell replication or metabolism. For other genes, expression is tightly controlled, with particular genes being turned on or off in particular cells at specific times in development or in response to physiological signals. Genomic studies are now being applied to analysis of gene regulation and are revealing remarkable details on the structure and function of regulatory elements in the human genome (Hot Topic 1.1).

ⓘ Hot Topic 1.1   Encode Project

The sequencing of the human genome (see Chapter 2) has made it possible to identify the full complement of genes, but does not in itself reveal how these genes are regulated. In 2003 a project was launched to characterize the entire set of coding elements in the genome, including identification of all genes and their corresponding regulatory sequences. The project is referred to as ENCODE, which is an acronym for *encyclopedia of DNA elements*. A pilot study was published in 2007 and more complete results were published in a series of papers in 2012.

The project has revealed a number of surprises. A total of 20 687 protein-encoding genes (not representing the full complement) were identified, each with, on average, 6.3 alternatively spliced transcripts. Among RNAs that do not encode protein, there were 8 801 small RNAs and 9 640 long non-coding transcripts. More than 80% of the genome was found to be transcribed into some kind of RNA in at least one cell type, a much higher level of transcriptional activity than expected. Ninety-five percent of the genome was found to be within 8 kb of a region involved in DNA/protein interaction. Nearly 400 000 regions were found to have features of enhancers and over 70 000 had features of promoter activity. Genetic variants associated with common disease (see Chapter 5) were found to be enriched in regions with functional elements that do not encode protein. It has become clear that much of the genome is dedicated to encoding elements responsible for fine control of gene expression in distinct cell types.

Gene expression is regulated by proteins that bind to DNA and either activate or repress transcription. The anatomy of elements that regulate gene transcription is shown in Figure 1.7. The **promoter region** is immediately adjacent to the transcription start site, usually within 100 base pairs. Most promoters include a base sequence of T and A bases called the TATA box. In some cases there may be multiple, alternative promoters at different sites in a gene that respond to regulatory factors in different tissues. Regulatory sequences may occur adjacent to the promoter or may be located thousands of base pairs away. These distantly located regulatory sequences are known as enhancers.

Enhancer sequences function regardless of their orientation with respect to the gene.

DNA-binding proteins may serve as repressors or activators of transcription, and may bind to the promoter, to upstream regulatory regions, or to more distant enhancers. Activator or repressor proteins are regulated by binding of specific ligands. Ligand binding changes the confirmation of the transcription factor and may activate it or inactivate it. The ligand is typically a small molecule, such as a hormone. Many transcription factors form dimers, either homodimers of two identical proteins or heterodimers of two different proteins. There may also be **corepressor** or **coactivator** proteins. Some transcription

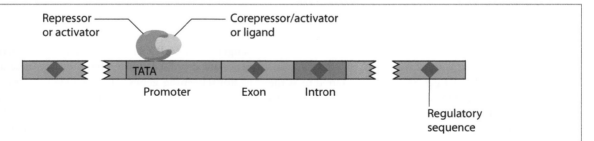

Figure 1.7 Cis-acting elements regulating gene expression. Transcription starts at the promoter by the binding of an RNA polymerase. Control of gene expression occurs via the binding of transcription factors upstream of the transcription start site at the TATA box. These factors can be either activators or repressors, and may bind coactivators or corepressors. Other DNA regulatory elements can occur within exons or introns or at some distance upstream or downstream of a gene.

factors stay in the cytosol until the ligand binds or some other activation process occurs, at which time they move to the nucleus to activate their target gene(s). In other situations, the transcription factors reside in the nucleus most of the time and may even be located at the response element sequences, but without the ligand they are inactive or even repress transcription.

Transcription begins with the attachment of the enzyme RNA polymerase to the promoter (Figure 1.8). There are three major types of RNA polymerase, designated types I, II, and

III. Most gene transcription is accomplished by RNA polymerase II. Type I is involved in the transcription of **ribosomal RNA (rRNA)**, and type III transcribes **transfer RNA (tRNA)** (see the "Translation" section of this chapter). The polymerase reads the sequence of the DNA template strand, copying a complementary RNA molecule, which grows from the 5′ to the 3′ direction. The resulting mRNA is an exact copy of the DNA sequence, except that uracil takes the place of thymine in RNA. Soon after transcription begins, a 7-methyl guanine residue is attached to the 5′-most base, forming the cap.

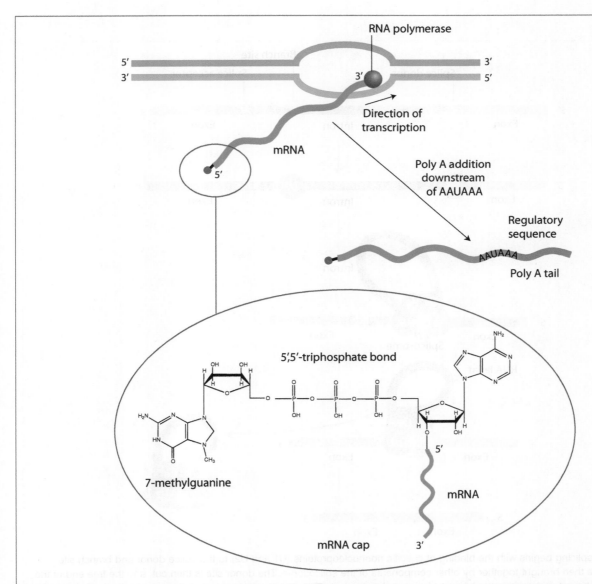

Figure 1.8 Transcription involves copying RNA from one strand of DNA. The reaction is catalyzed by RNA polymerase. A 7-methylguanosine cap is added to the 5′ end of most mRNA molecules before transcription is completed, and a poly-A tail is added enzymatically to the 3′ end downstream of an AAUAAA sequence.

Transcription proceeds through the entire coding sequence. Some genes include a sequence near the 3′ end that signals RNA cleavage at that site and enzymatic addition of 100 to 200 adenine bases, the poly-A tail. Polyadenylation is characteristic of housekeeping genes, which are expressed in most cell types. Both the 5′ cap and the poly-A tail stabilize the mRNA molecule and facilitate its export to the cytoplasm.

The DNA sequence of most genes far exceeds the length required to encode their corresponding proteins. This is accounted for by the fact that the coding sequence is broken into segments, called **exons**, which are interrupted by noncoding segments called **introns**. Some exons may be less than a hundred bases long, whereas introns can be several thousand bases in length; therefore, much of the length of a gene may be devoted to introns. The number of exons in a gene may be as few as one or two, or may number in the dozens. The processing of the transcript into mature mRNA requires the removal of the introns and splicing together of the exons (Figure 1.9), carried out by an enzymatic process that occurs in the nucleus. The 5′ end of an intron always consists of the two bases GU, followed by a consensus sequence that is similar, but not identical, in all introns. This is the **splice donor**. The 3′ end, the **splice acceptor**, ends in AG, preceded by a consensus sequence.

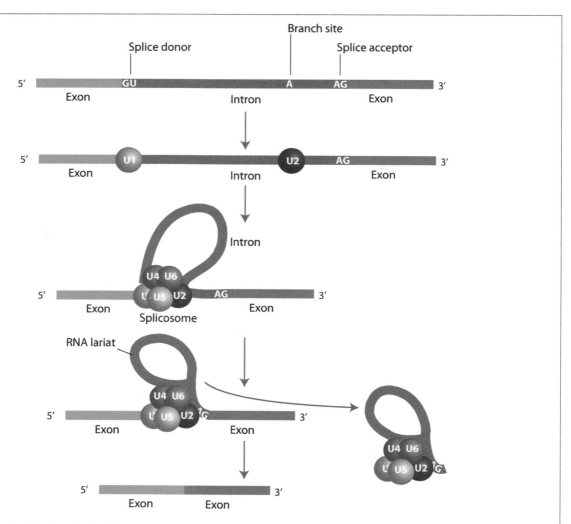

Figure 1.9 RNA splicing begins with the binding of specific ribonucleoproteins (U1 and U2) to the splice donor and branch site. These two sites are then brought together by other components of the splicosome. The donor site is then cut, and the free end of the intron binds to the branch point within the intron to form a lariat structure. Then the acceptor site is cleaved, releasing the lariat, and the exons at the two ends are ligated together.

The splicing process requires complex machinery composed of both proteins and small RNA molecules (**small nuclear RNA**, or **snRNA**), consisting of fewer than 200 bases. snRNA is also transcribed by RNA polymerase II. The splice is initiated by binding of a protein–RNA complex to the splice donor, at a point within the intron called the **branch point**, and the splice acceptor. First the RNA is cleaved at the donor site and this is attached in a 5′–2′ bond to the branch point. Then the acceptor site is cleaved, releasing a lariat structure that is degraded, and the 5′ and 3′ ends are ligated together. The splicing process also requires the function of proteins, **SR proteins**, which are involved in selecting sites for the initiation of splicing. These proteins interact with sequences known as **splice enhancers** or **silencers**. The splicing process is vulnerable to disruption by mutation, as might be predicted from its complexity (see Chapter 4).

The RNA-splicing process offers a point of control of gene expression. Under the influence of control molecules present in specific cells, particular exons may be included or not included in the mRNA due to differential splicing (Figure 1.10). This results in the potential to produce multiple distinct proteins from the same gene, adding greatly to the diversity of proteins encoded by the genome. Specific exons may correspond with particular functional domains of proteins, leading to the production of multiple proteins with diverse functions from the same gene. Some mRNAs are subject to RNA editing, wherein a specific base may be enzymatically modified. For example, the protein apolipoprotein B exists in two forms, a 48 kDa form made in the intestine and a 100 kDa form in the liver. Both forms are the product of the same gene. In the intestine the enzyme cytidine deaminase alters a C to a U at codon 2153, changing the codon from CAA (encoding glutamine) to UAA (a stop codon). This truncates the peptide, accounting for the 48 kDa form.

MicroRNA

Gene regulation is not limited to control at the level of gene transcription. There is another level of posttranscriptional control that involves RNA molecules that do not encode protein, referred to as **microRNAs (miRNAs)** (Figure 1.11). Several hundred distinct miRNAs are encoded in the human genome. These are transcribed by RNA polymerase II, are capped, and have poly-A tails added. miRNAs form hairpin structures through base pairing. The enzyme Drosha trims the hairpins, which are then exported to the cytoplasm, where the enzyme Dicer further cleaves them. After further processing, single-stranded miRNA molecules associate with a protein complex called the RNA-induced silencing complex (RISC). The RISC then binds to mRNA molecules by base sequence complementarity with the miRNA. This leads to either cleavage and degradation of the mRNA, or reduced rate of translation and eventual degradation of the mRNA. The overall effect is for miRNA to reduce the quantity of protein produced from a transcribed gene. Any specific miRNA might bind to many different mRNAs, leading to coordinated reduction in gene product from a large number of genes.

A similar process also occurs when double-stranded RNA is introduced into the cell by viral infection. The Dicer enzyme cuts the invading RNA into shorter fragments, called small interfering RNA (siRNA), which attach to the RISC. The RISC then binds to additional double-stranded RNA molecules and causes their degradation. This is referred to as RNA interference, and represents a kind of immune system

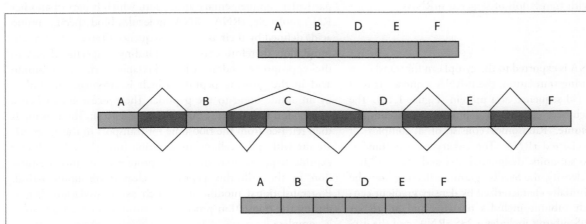

Figure 1.10 Alternative splicing. Splicing out each intron results in the inclusion of exons A–F in the mRNA. Alternatively, a splice can be made directly between exons B and D, skipping exon C. This results in the production of a distinct protein, missing the amino acids encoded by exon C.

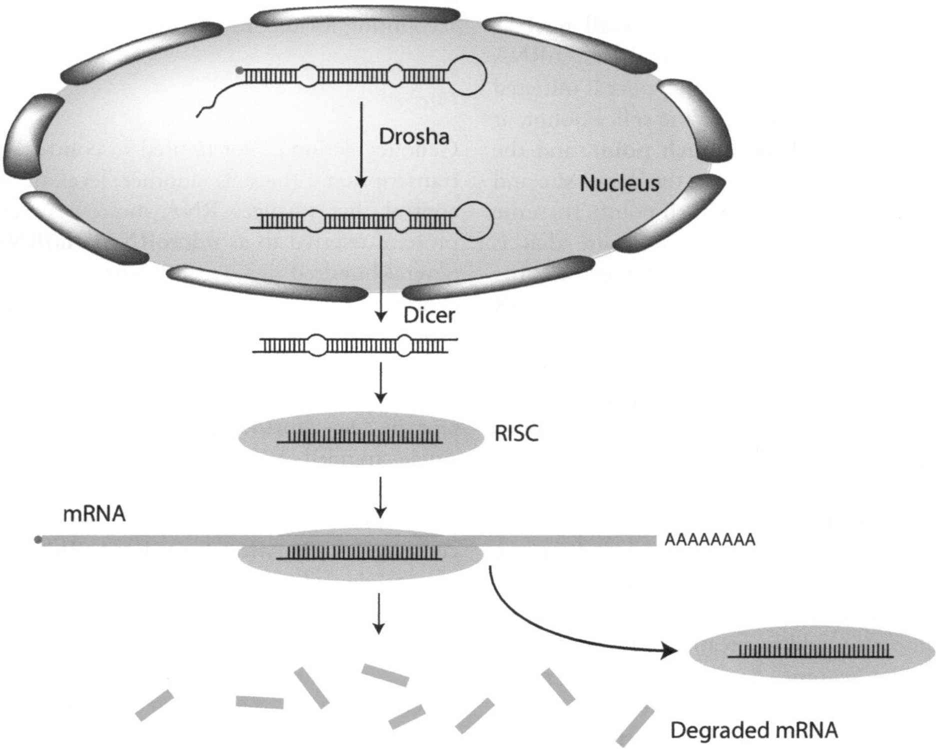

Figure 1.11 Mechanism of action of microRNA (miRNA). miRNA is transcribed and capped, and poly-A is added. The transcripts form hairpins due to internal base complementarity. The enzyme Drosha cleaves the miRNA in the nucleus, after which it is exported to the cytoplasm and further cleaved by Dicer. A single strand of the miRNA then associates with the RNA-induced silencing complex (RISC). Binding of the miRNA to a molecule of mRNA results in cleavage or, if the base pairing is not perfect, a reduced rate of translation.

within the cell. The process has also been used experimentally, wherein siRNA molecules are introduced into the cell to selectively interfere with translation of targeted mRNAs.

Translation

The mature mRNA is exported to the cytoplasm for translation into protein. During translation, the mRNA sequence is read into the amino acid sequence of a protein (Figure 1.12). The translational machinery consists of a protein–RNA complex called the **ribosome**. Ribosomes consist of a complex of proteins and specialized rRNA. The eukaryotic ribosome is composed of two subunits, designated 60S and 40S ("S" is a measurement of density, the Svedberg unit, reflecting how the complexes were initially characterized by density gradient centrifugation). Each subunit includes proteins and an rRNA molecule. The 60S subunit includes a 28S rRNA, and the 40S subunit an 18S rRNA. Ribosomes can be free or associated with the **endoplasmic reticulum (ER)**, also known as the rough ER.

The mRNA sequence is read in triplets, called codons, beginning at the 5′ end of the mRNA, which is always AUG,

encoding methionine (although this methionine residue is sometimes later cleaved off). Each codon corresponds with a particular complementary anticodon, which is part of another RNA molecule, tRNA. tRNA molecules bind specific amino acids defined by their anticodon sequence (Table 1.1). Protein translation therefore consists of binding a specific tRNA to the appropriate codon, which juxtaposes the next amino acid in the growing peptide, which is enzymatically linked by an amide bond to the peptide. The process ends when a stop codon is reached (UAA, UGA, or UAG). The peptide is then released from the ribosome for transport to the appropriate site within the cell, or for secretion from the cell. A leader peptide sequence may direct the protein to its final destination in the cell; this peptide is cleaved off upon arrival. Posttranslational modification, such as glycosylation, begins during the translation process and continues after translation is complete.

The process of translation consists of three phases, referred to as initiation, elongation, and termination. Initiation involves the binding of the first amino acyl tRNA, which always carries methionine, to the initiation codon, always AUG. A set of proteins, referred to as **elongation factors**, are involved in the

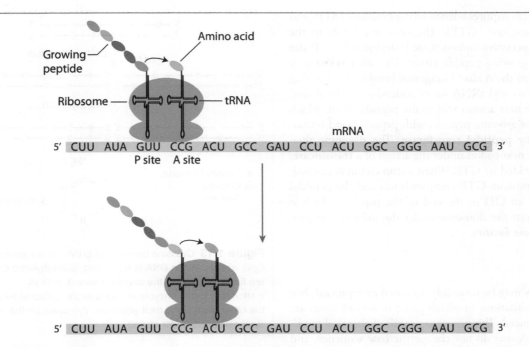

Figure 1.12 The process of protein translation. Translation takes place at the ribosome, which binds to the mRNA. Specific amino acyl tRNA molecules bind to the mRNA by base pair complementarity between a triplet codon on the mRNA and an anticodon on the tRNA. A peptide bond is formed between the growing peptide and the next amino acyl tRNA, transferring the growing peptide and elongating it by one amino acid. This continues until a stop codon is reached.

Table 1.1 The genetic code. A triplet codon is read from the left column, to the top row, to the full triplet in each box. Each codon corresponds with a specific amino acid, except for the three stop codons (labeled "Ter"). Most amino acids are encoded by more than one codon.

	T	C	A	G
T	TTT Phe (F)	TCT Ser (S)	TAT Tyr (Y)	TGT Cys (C)
	TTC "	TCC "	TAC "	TGC "
	TTA Leu (L)	TCA "	TAA Ter	TGA Ter
	TTG "	TCG "	TAG Ter	TGG Trp (W)
C	CTT Leu (L)	CCT Pro (P)	CAT His (H)	CGT Arg (R)
	CTC "	CCC "	CAC "	CGC "
	CTA "	CCA "	CAA Gln (Q)	CGA "
	CTG "	CCG "	CAG "	CGG "
A	ATT Ile (I)	ACT Thr (T)	AAT Asn (N)	AGT Ser (S)
	ATC "	ACC "	AAC "	AGC "
	ATA "	ACA "	AAA Lys (K)	AGA Arg (R)
	ATG Met (M)	ACG "	AAG "	AGG "
G	GTT Val (V)	GCT Ala (A)	GAT Asp (D)	GGT Gly (G)
	GTC "	GCC "	GAC "	GGC "
	GTA "	GCA "	GAA Glu (E)	GGA "
	GTG "	GCG "	GAG "	GGG "

process, which also requires adenosine triphosphate (ATP) and guanosine triphosphate (GTP). The ribosome binds to the mRNA at two successive codons. One is designated the **P site** and carries the growing peptide chain. The other is the next codon, designated the **A site**. Elongation involves the binding of the next amino acyl tRNA to its anticodon at the A site. This delivers the next amino acid in the peptide chain, which is attached to the growing peptide, with peptide bond formation catalyzed by **peptidyl transferase**. The ribosome then moves on to the next codon under the action of a **translocase**, with energy provided by GTP. When a stop codon is reached, a release factor protein–GTP complex binds and the peptidyl transferase adds an OH to the end of the peptide, which is then released from the ribosome under the influence of proteins called **release factors**.

Epigenetics

Individual genes may be reversibly activated or repressed, but there are some situations in which genes or sets of genes are permanently silenced. This occurs as a result of chemical modifications of DNA that do not change the base sequence, and also involves chemical changes in the associated histone proteins that result in compaction of the chromatin. Gene silencing is characteristic of one of the two copies of the X chromosome in females and on the maternal or paternal copy of imprinted genes. It also can occur on other genes in specific tissues and may be subject to environmental influences.

At the DNA level, gene silencing is accompanied by methylation of cytosine bases to 5-methylcytosine (Figure 1.13). This occurs in regions where cytosine is following by guanine (5'–CpG–3') near the promoter, sites referred to as **CpG islands**. Methylated sites bind protein complexes that remove acetyl groups from histones, leading to transcriptional repression. The silencing is continued from cell generation to generation because the enzymes responsible for methylation recognize the 5-methylcytosine on the parental strand of DNA and methylate the cytosine on the newly synthesized daughter strand.

X-chromosome inactivation provides a mechanism for equalization of gene dosage on the X chromosome in males, who have one X, and females, who have two. Most genes on one of the two X chromosomes in each cell of a female are permanently inactivated early in development (Figure 1.14). The particular X inactivated in any cell is determined at random, so in approximately 50% of cells one X is inactivated and in the other 50% the other X is inactivated. Regions of homology between the X and Y at the two ends of the X escape inactivation. These are referred to as **pseudoautosomal** regions. The inactive X remains condensed through most of the cell cycle, and can be visualized as a densely staining body during interphase, called the **Barr body**.

Initiation of inactivation is controlled from a region called the **X inactivation center (Xic)**. A gene within this region,

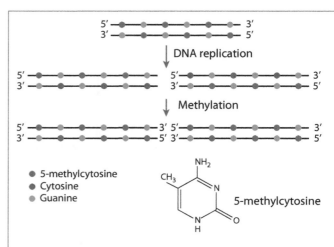

Figure 1.13 Cytosine bases 5' to guanines are methylated at CpG islands. When DNA is replicated, unmethylated cytosines are first inserted into the daughter strand. A DNA methyltransferase enzyme recognizes the 5-methylcytosine on the other strand and methylates the cytosines on the newly synthesized daughter strand.

known as Xist, is expressed on one of the two X chromosomes early in development. Xist encodes a 25 kb RNA that is not translated into protein, but binds to sites along the X to be inactivated. Subsequently, CpG islands on this chromosome are methylated and histones are deacetylated.

Genomic **imprinting** involves the silencing of either the maternal or paternal copy of a gene during early development (Figure 1.15). Like X chromosome inactivation, imprinting is probably accomplished through methylation of specific chromosome regions. The methylation "imprint" is erased in germ cells, so the specific gene copy to be inactivated is always determined by the parent of origin, regardless of whether that particular gene copy was active or inactive in the previous generation. Genomic imprinting applies to only a subset of genes, although the full extent of imprinting is not yet known.

Although methylation at a site tends to repress transcription, the effects of methylation can be complex (Figure 1.16). For example, there can be regulatory signals sent from one locus to another on a chromosome. If the signal is repression and the locus is methylated, this might disinhibit the target locus. Alternatively, a protein might bind to a site that blocks a signal transmitted from one locus to another. Methylation might prevent binding of the protein, permitting the interaction between the two loci. There are many clinical disorders that have been attributed to defects in imprinting. We will discuss these in Chapter 3.

Aside from having a role in X chromosome inactivation, epigenetic changes appear to be involved in silencing genes as a component of normal development or physiological responses

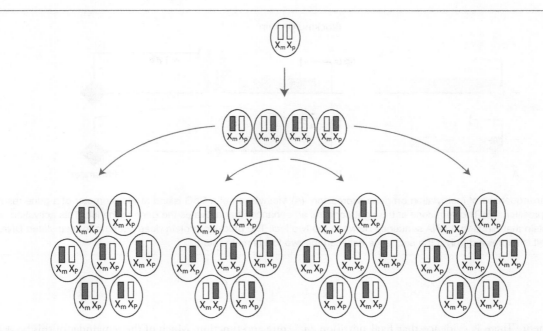

Figure 1.14 X chromosome inactivation. In the zygote, both the maternally and paternally derived X chromosomes (X_m and X_p) are active. Early in development, one of the two X chromosomes in each cell is inactivated (indicated as the red chromosome). This X chromosome remains inactive in all the descendants of that cell.

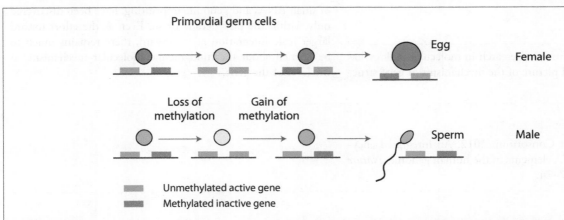

Unmethylated active gene

Methylated inactive gene

Figure 1.15 Concept of genomic imprinting. An imprinted gene will be methylated and inactive in somatic cells. In this example, a pair of adjacent genes is shown, one methylated if maternally inherited (left gene) and the other methylated if paternally inherited (right gene). In this illustration, both primordial germ cells (after meiosis) inherited the paternal allele; hence, the left-hand gene is unmethylated and the right-hand one is methylated. The methylation imprint is erased as the germ cell develops, and then reestablished according to whether the primordial germ cell is in a male (in which case the right-hand gene is methylated) or female (in which case the left-hand gene is methylated).

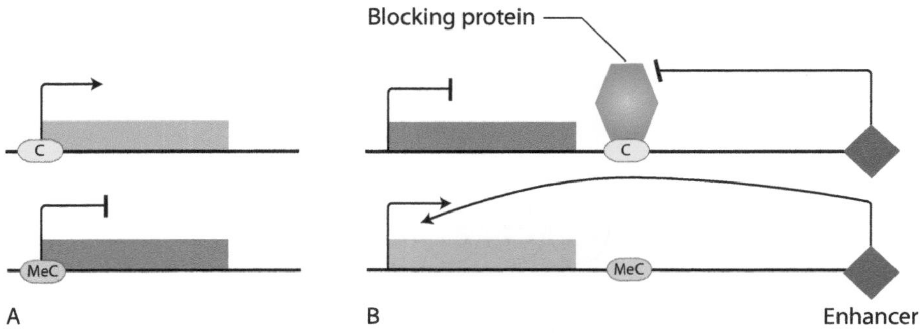

Figure 1.16 Consequences of methylation on gene expression. (A) Methylation of a CpG island at the promoter of a gene results in transcriptional repression. (B) The sequence at the right contains an enhancer that activates the gene at the left. This activation is blocked by a protein that binds to a DNA sequence between the two loci. The blocking protein does not bind to methylated DNA, so the gene at the left is expressed only if the sequence between the two loci is methylated.

to the environment. There is evidence that fetal nutrition *in utero* may influence the later risk of type 2 diabetes due to epigenetic marks laid down during fetal development, or that the response of an individual to stress may be mediated by epigenetic marks that occur during infancy in response to nurturing. The contribution of epigenetics to health and disease is an emerging important area of research on susceptibility to common disease.

Conclusion

More than half a century of research in molecular biology has resulted in a detailed picture of the mechanisms of gene struc-ture and function. Much of the remainder of this book will be devoted to exploration of the implications of dysfunction at the level of the gene or groups of genes and their interactions with the environment. We will see also that genetics research is moving to a new level of integration of basic molecular mechanisms, toward formation of a picture of how entire cells and organisms function. It is important to realize, however, that some fundamental molecular mechanisms, such as the role of small RNAs and genomic imprinting, have been discovered only within the past decade or so. Even as the effort toward larger scale integration goes forward, there remains much to be learned about the fundamental molecular mechanisms at the level of the gene.

REFERENCE

ENCODE Project Consortium 2012. An integrated ency-clopedia of DNA elements in the human genome. *Nature* vol. 489, pp. 57–74.

FURTHER READING

Alberts B, Johnson A, Lewis J, Raff M, Roberts K, Walter P 2007, *Molecular biology of the cell*, 5th edn, Garland Science, New York.

Krebs JE, Goldstein, ES, Kilpatrick ST 2009, *Lewin's genes X*, Jones & Bartlett, Sudbury, MA.

Lodish H, Berk A, Kaiser CA, Krieger M, Scott MP, Bretscher A *et al.* 2007, *Molecular cell biology*, 6th edn, Freeman, New York.

Find interactive self-test questions and additional resources for this chapter at **www.korfgenetics.com**.

Self-Assessment

Review Questions

1.1 The two strands of DNA separate when heated, and the temperature at which separation occurs is dependent on the base content. Specifically, DNA with a higher proportion of G–C base pairs tends to "melt" at a higher temperature than molecules with a higher A–T content. Why is this?

1.2 What is the role of transcription in DNA replication?

1.3 Consider this gene sequence. What is the base sequence of the mRNA that would be transcribed from this gene, and what is the amino acid sequence of the peptide that would be translated?

5'–promoter–ATG GTT GAT AGT CGT TGC CGC GGG CTG TGA–3'
3'–promoter–TAC CAA CTA TCA GCA ACG GCG CCC GAC ACT–5'

1.4 There are more proteins than there are genes. What are some of the mechanisms that account for this discrepancy?

1.5 A woman is heterozygous for an X-linked trait that leads to expression of two different forms of an enzyme. The two forms are separable as two distinct bands when the enzyme protein is run through an electric field by electrophoresis. If you were to test cultured skin fibroblasts and isolate enzyme, what would you expect to see? If you could isolate single fibroblasts and grow them into colonies before extracting the enzyme and subjecting it to electrophoresis, what would you expect to see?

CHAPTER 2
Genetic Variation

Introduction

The human genome contains variations in base sequence from one individual to another, on average every few hundred bases. Some sequence variants occur within areas that do not encode RNA or protein, and so have no visible effect. Others affect physical characteristics, or **phenotype**, by altering RNA or protein products. Genetic variants account for some physical differences between individuals, for example hair or eye color, body size, and facial appearance. Some underlie specific medical disorders. In this chapter, we will take a close-up look at DNA sequence variations and their effects on gene expression. Later in this book, we will see how these sequence variants exert their phenotypic effects.

Key Points

- DNA sequence variants are common in the population, and range from single base changes to large-scale DNA rearrangements.
- Sequence variants can be silent or may alter the quantity or quality of the gene product.
- Sequence variants can affect gene expression, the amino acid sequence of a protein, or splicing.
- Mutations may occur spontaneously or can be induced by chemical or radiation mutagens.
- Advanced paternal age is associated with increased rate of mutation.
- The fidelity of the DNA sequence is maintained by a DNA repair system.
- Genomic-level changes include copy number variants, inversions, and chromosomal changes.
- Polymorphisms are sequence variants that occur commonly in the population.

Human Genetics and Genomics, Fourth Edition. Bruce R. Korf and Mira B. Irons.
© 2013 John Wiley & Sons, Ltd. Published 2013 by John Wiley & Sons, Ltd.

DNA Sequence Variants

There is no canonical "human DNA sequence" (Ethical Implication 2.1). Genetic variation is being generated constantly, in both germ cells and somatic cells. Much of this variation either is repaired or is lethal to the cell. Sometimes, however, a variant will be neutral in its effect, or even convey a selective advantage. Selective advantage is the driving force of evolution at the population level, but in the individual selective advantage is the driving force of cancer.

Types of DNA Sequence Variants

DNA sequence variants can occur at many levels, ranging from a single nucleotide to an entire chromosome (Figure 2.1). The simplest change is a point mutation consisting of a single base substitution. This may occur as a consequence of misincorporation of a base into DNA during replication, or can be a result of changes due to chemical or physical mutagens (see "Causes of Nucleotide Mutation," this chapter). Deletions, duplications, insertions, and inversions are sequence rearrangements that may be as small as single base changes (for deletions, duplications, and insertions), can involve one or more exons within a gene, or can be as large as millions of base pairs. The latter may be visible through the microscope when chromosomal analysis is performed and are referred to as genomic changes. Deletions and insertions of bases in DNA are referred to as indels – sometimes there can be simultaneous deletion of some bases as well as insertion of others (Figure 2.2). A standardized nomenclature is used to describe mutations (Methods 2.1), and many databases are used to catalog mutations (Sources of Information 2.1).

Nucleotide-Level Changes

Nucleotide-level changes include alterations of single DNA bases or deletions, duplications, or insertions of a small number of bases. The effect of a genetic change on gene expression depends on whether the variant is located in a control region, exon, or intron, or whether it encompasses an entire gene or group of genes. Some very small changes can have profound phenotypic effects, whereas some large changes can be phenotypically silent.

A mutation within the promoter region or other control region, such as an enhancer element, can alter the level of expression of the gene (Figure 2.3). Expression levels may go up or down as a consequence of the mutation, depending on whether the change affects the binding of repressor or activator proteins or of the transcription initiation complex. Mutations in enhancer regions some distance from the gene can also have an effect on the level of expression. The various repressor and activator molecules are themselves gene products, so mutations

(?) Ethical Implications 2.1 Eugenics

What is the "normal" DNA sequence for any particular gene? Geneticists working with experimental systems, such as the fruit fly *Drosophila*, have coined the term "wild type" to indicate the most common version of a genetic trait in the population. Most fruit flies, for example, have red eyes, so the white-eyed phenotype is considered "mutant" and the red-eyed phenotype is the "wild-type" state. We will see that genetic variation is the rule, not the exception, so it is not possible to designate a "normal" or "wild-type" state for most genes at the level of DNA base sequence. Some genetic variants have a profound effect on gene function and may lead to clinically evident phenotypes that may be considered "abnormal." Other variations have no detectable phenotype, or are responsible for variations such as alteration of hair or eye color that are not important medically.

It has been known for a long time that selective breeding could increase or decrease the frequency of particular genetic traits in plants and animals, knowledge that has been used to great advantage in agriculture. As the science of human heredity began to emerge in the late 19th century, there were advocates of similar selective "breeding" in humans. Here, however, the notion of "desirable" or "undesirable" traits was in the eye of the beholder. The term "eugenics" was coined to describe the study of human traits and the application of selective breeding to increase the frequency of traits that were deemed desirable. The term has taken on sinister connotations, however, especially as eugenics became a tool of racist social policy. Eugenics has been invoked to deny the rights of individuals or groups, by means such as forced sterilization and genocide, to reproduce. The notion achieved its most grotesque form with the Nazi campaigns in the 1930s and 1940s to produce a "perfect" human race, largely through the mass murder of those deemed inferior.

Although modern medical genetics seeks to ameliorate or prevent the occurrence of disease due to genetic alterations, the goals are to alleviate individual suffering, not to "improve" the human race. We will see throughout this book that there are examples of genetic traits that are clearly and invariably deleterious, and others whose effects are more ambiguous, sometimes being advantageous in some circumstances and disadvantageous in others. At the least, it will become clear that there is no single "correct" DNA sequence, but genetic variation occurs, throughout the human genome, from individual to individual.

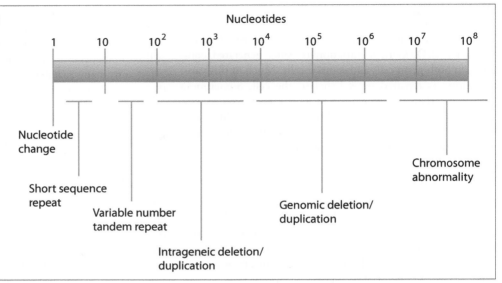

Figure 2.1 Scale of genetic and genomic variation, from the level of a single nucleotide (far left) to changes in entire chromosomes (right).

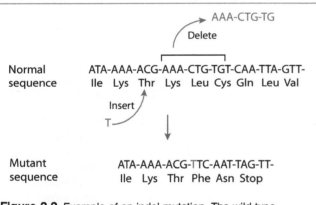

Figure 2.2 Example of an indel mutation. The wild-type (normal) sequence is shown at top, with the corresponding amino acid sequence. There is simultaneous deletion of eight bases and insertion of a single T. This leads to a frameshift in the mutant sequence, quickly resulting in a stop codon. (Courtesy of Dr. Ludwine Messiaen, University of Alabama at Birmingham.)

in these genes can alter the expression of the target gene for those regulators.

Mutations within an exon can alter the coding sequence of the gene (Figure 2.4). A single base substitution will change a codon. If the new codon encodes the same amino acid as the original, there will be no change in the protein, a silent mutation. If a different amino acid is encoded, the mutation is said

to be a **missense mutation**. The effect on protein function depends on whether the new amino acid changes the physical and chemical properties of the protein, and whether the change occurs at a critical site along the protein. Some changes substitute amino acids with similar chemical properties, for example two nonpolar amino acids such as isoleucine and valine. These may have little or no effect on the function of the protein, representing conservative mutations. Other times, the substitution may alter the protein, producing a detectable, but not necessarily deleterious, change in protein function. There are many sequence variants (**single-nucleotide polymorphisms**, or **SNPs**) between different individuals, and for that matter between proteins in humans and those in other species related through evolution (referred to as orthologous proteins), that represent such minor variants (Figure 2.5). Finally, in some cases, the amino acid change can have a profound effect on protein structure, perhaps obliterating function or leading to increased function, altered function, or aberrant response to control factors.

Some exon mutations lead to production of a truncated peptide by introducing a premature stop codon (Figure 2.6). There are three stop codons, and mutation of an amino acid–encoding codon to a stop will have this effect. Insertion or deletion of a nonintegral multiple of three bases will cause a **frameshift**, which results in misreading of the codons until a stop is reached. Mutations within exon splice enhancer sequences can alter splicing, and some mutations will create a new splice donor or acceptor sequence within the exon that also can disrupt splicing. In some cases, a single base change in an exon may affect splicing in addition to altering the amino acid sequence, causing a stop codon, or being a silent mutation.

✓ Methods 2.1   Mutation Nomenclature

A standardized nomenclature is used to describe mutations, which ensures that mutations are described in a consistent manner. These are codified on the website of the Human Genome Variation Society (www.hgvs.org). Genes are designated using official symbols designated by the Human Gene Nomenclature Committee (Wain *et al.* 2002). Mutations may be described at various levels, and the level used is identified by preceding the description with a letter: genomic = g.; coding sequence = c.; mitochondrial sequence = m.; RNA sequence = r.; and protein sequence = p. The reference sequence used should be specified; generally, genomic DNA should use the RefSeq database maintained by the National Center for Biotechnology Information (NCBI; see www.ncbi.nlm.nih.gov/RefSeq). For DNA-level changes, nucleotides are shown in capital letters; for RNA, small letters are used; and for proteins, three-letter abbreviations for amino acids are used. For coding DNA, the first nucleotide is the A of the ATG initiation codon; for genomic mutations at the 5′ end of an intron, the last nucleotide of the preceding exon is used with a "+" sign, and the number of nucleotides into the intron is shown; for mutations at the 3′ end of an intron, the first nucleotide of the next exon is shown with a "−" sign, and the number of nucleotides into the intron is shown. Specific symbols are used to designate changes:

>   Substitution in DNA
_   A range of affected bases
del Deletion
dup Duplication
ins Insertion
inv Inversion.

Some examples:

g.1346A>C: Change of A to C at position 1346 in the genomic DNA sequence

c.745delT: Deletion of T at position 745 in the coding sequence

g.1567_1568delAT: Deletion of AT at positions 1567–1568 in the genomic DNA sequence

c.145+1T: Change of splice donor (first position of intron after base 145 of preceding exon) to T

p.Arg54Gly: Change of arginine at codon 54 to glycine.

🔍 Sources of Information 2.1   Gene Mutation Databases

As efforts proceed to characterize mutations in various genes, there is a need to provide a central source of information regarding mutations and associated phenotypes. Some major mutations are annotated in the OMIM database (see Chapter 3), but the number of mutations identified in most genes exceeds what can be cataloged in OMIM. As a consequence, many locus-specific databases have been established. These databases are encouraged to utilize standardized nomenclature for their description of mutations (Methods 2.1) and a standardized reference DNA sequence, which is obtained from the NCBI's RefSeq database (www.ncbi.nlm.nih.gov/RefSeq). In addition, the Institute of Medical Genetics in Cardiff, Wales, maintains a Human Gene Mutation Database, which requires login to access (www.hgmd.cf.ac.uk/ac). Information about efforts to catalog human genome variants can also be found through the Human Variome Project (www.humanvariomeproject.org).

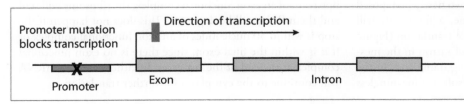

Figure 2.3 Mutation within a promoter sequence may lead to failure to initiate transcription.

TCC	CAA	ATC	GTC	CCT	CGA	GTT	Wild type
ser	gln	ile	val	pro	arg	val	sequence

TCC	(CAG)	ATC	GTC	CCT	CGA	GTT	Silent mutation
ser	gln	ile	val	pro	arg	val	

TCC	CAA	ATC	GTC	(GCT)	CGA	GTT	Amino acid
ser	gln	ile	val	ala	arg	val	substitution

Figure 2.4 Consequences of single base change mutations within an exon. If the amino acid is not altered, the mutation is silent. Missense mutations insert amino acids that may have an impact on protein function.

TCC	CAA	ATC	GTC	CCT	CGA	GTT	Wild type
ser	gln	ile	val	pro	arg	val	sequence

TCC	CAA	ATC	GTC	CCT	(TGA)	GTT	Stop mutation
ser	gln	ile	val	pro	stop		

TCC	CA(G)	AAT	CGT	CCC	TCG	AGT	T	Frameshift
ser	gln	asn	arg	pro	leu	ser		insertion

Figure 2.6 Mutations leading to premature termination of translation. A stop mutation changes an amino acid codon to a stop codon. A frameshift alters the amino acid sequence, and usually results in production of a stop codon.

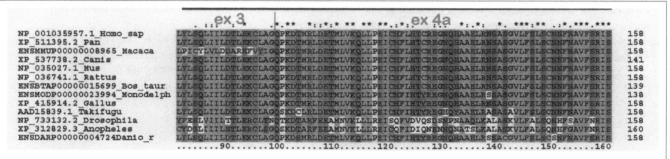

Figure 2.5 Conservation of amino acid sequence in orthologous proteins in various species. Amino acids are referred to by single-letter codes. Blocks of color indicate conserved amino acids. Amino acids that are not conserved are indicated by an absence of color.

Mutations within introns likewise lead to abnormal splicing (Figure 2.7). These include mutations that disrupt the splice donor, the acceptor, or the branch point sequences. The GT (in DNA) at the splice donor and the AG at the splice acceptor are highly conserved; mutation of any of these bases usually will disrupt normal splicing. Sometimes these mutations cause an exon to be skipped if the two flanking exons are spliced together. Other times, a sequence within either the exon or intron will substitute for the mutated donor or acceptor (the sequence, which is similar to a donor or acceptor sequence, is referred to as a "cryptic" donor or acceptor). Exon skipping can either result in a protein that is missing an essential domain (encoded by the skipped exon), or, if the two newly juxtaposed exons are not in the same reading frame, a frameshift will occur, leading to premature termination of translation (Figure 2.8). Loss of exon sequence or inclusion of intron in the messenger RNA (mRNA) can alter the reading frame and, in the case of inclusion of an intron sequence, result in a meaningless amino acid sequence. Any of these changes can result in premature termination of translation.

The presence of an abnormal stop codon, whether due to a nonsense mutation, a frameshift, or abnormal splicing, often leads to degradation of the mutant mRNA by a process referred to as nonsense-mediated decay (Figure 2.9). This occurs as the mRNA is being exported from the nucleus to the cytoplasm. At this point, the splicing ribonucleoproteins are still bound at the borders of newly spliced exons; these are referred to as exon junctional complexes. A ribosome binds to the mRNA and begins translation, displacing the exon junctional complexes as it passes. If a stop codon is reached more than 50 nucleotides upstream of an exon junctional complex, the ribosome will stall and the mRNA will be degraded. This does not happen if the stop is within 50 nucleotides of an exon junctional complex or if it is within the final exon, since there is no exon junctional complex at the end of the last exon. In either case, the mRNA will continue to the cytoplasm for further translation.

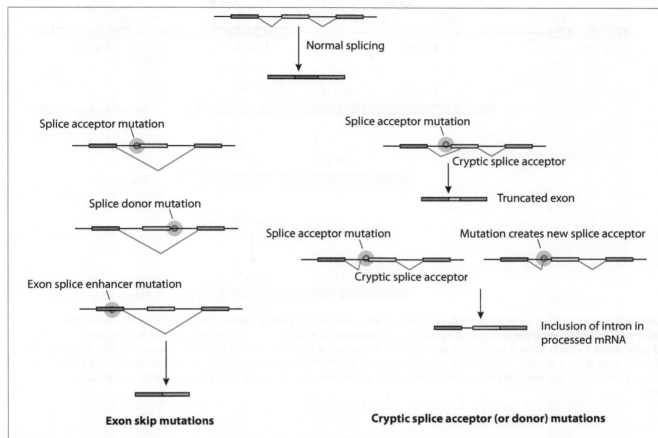

Figure 2.7 Various types of splicing mutations. Mutations of the splice donor or acceptor, or of an exon splice enhancer, all might lead to skipping of an exon in the mRNA due to splicing together of the flanking exons. In some cases, mutation of a splice donor or acceptor leads to an aberrant splice from a sequence within an intron or exon that can substitute for the splice donor or acceptor. This can result in the loss of some exon material or the inclusion of some intron material in the final processed mRNA.

Causes of Nucleotide Mutation

Mutations often occur spontaneously due to misincorporation of a base into DNA during replication. There are proofreading and repair mechanisms that identify base mismatches (see "DNA Repair," this chapter), but some errors nevertheless escape detection. Some mutations occur as a result of peculiarities of DNA structure, such as the presence of repeated sequences or intrastrand homologies that allow hairpin formation. The mutation rate is estimated to be about 10^{-8} per nucleotide per gamete, which equates to about 30 mutations per gamete. Most of these will reside in noncoding sequences and will not be associated with phenotypes, but if 1% of mutations are in coding regions, there will be millions of gametes in any individual with mutations with potential phenotypic significance (Hot Topic 2.1).

Although mutation is a natural process, and is the engine of evolutionary change, it is clear that there are chemical, physical, and biological circumstances that increase the likelihood of mutation. Study of these is important since mutations can lead to birth defects, genetic disorders, and cancer, and at least some of the agents that cause mutation consist of environmental exposures that might be controlled. Mutagens alter the chemical structure of a DNA base or induce breaks in the DNA strand. Some mutations cause deamination, for example conversion of cytosine to uracil, or alkylation, leading to cross-linking of the two DNA strands (Figure 2.10). Intercalating agents fit between bases in the double helix and cause a predisposition to insertion mutations. Another class of mutations results from the production of free radicals in the nucleus, which leads to DNA strand breakage. Ionizing radiation and ultraviolet light are two major physical

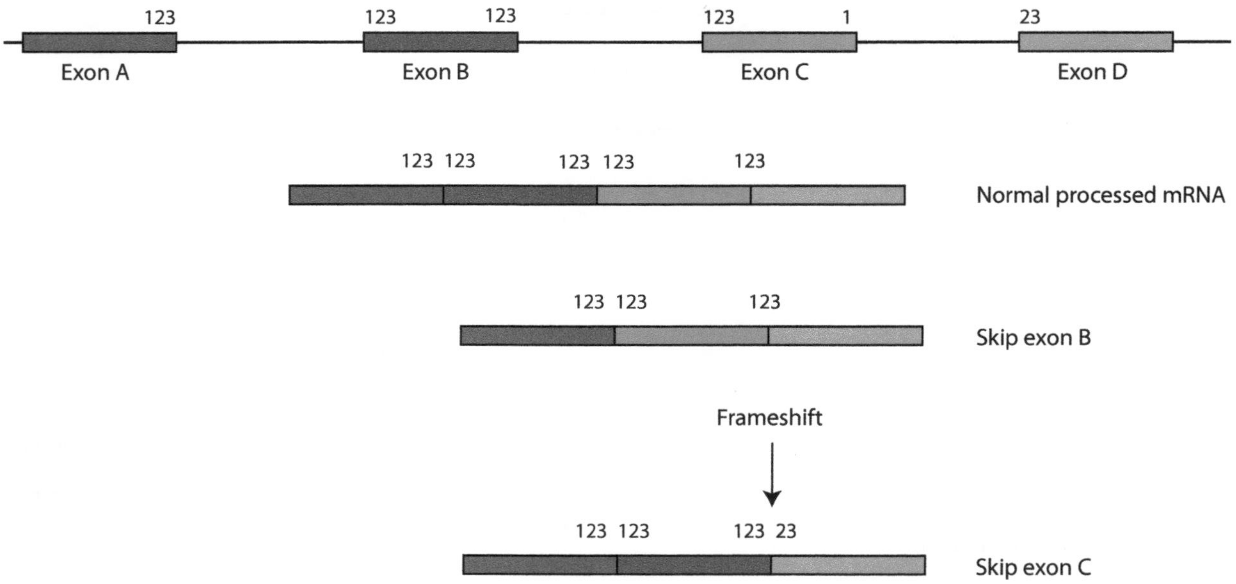

Figure 2.8 Exon skipping can result in the preservation or alternation of the reading frame in the final processed mRNA. The reading frame is indicated by the numbers above the end or beginning of each exon – 123 indicates the first, second, and third positions of a codon. Exon A ends at a 3 position, and B picks up at the next codon (1 position). The same is true for B and C. Exon C ends at the 1 position, and D picks up at the 2, preserving the reading frame. If exon B is skipped the reading frame is preserved, but if exon C is skipped there is a frameshift, as B, which ends at a 3 position, is juxtaposed with D, which begins at a 2.

mutagens. Ionizing radiation may act directly or indirectly by increasing free radicals in the cell. A wide variety of mutations can result, including point mutations and DNA strand breaks. The major effect of UV irradiation is the dimerization of adjacent thymine bases, which can result in a deletion mutation.

Biological factors may also increase the rate of mutation. Advanced paternal age is a risk factor for having a child with a genetic disorder due to a new mutation. Advanced maternal age does not convey similar risks, although there is an increased chance of chromosomal nondisjunction associated with advanced maternal age (see Chapter 6). The paternal age–related risk of mutation is thought to be due to the fact that male germ cells undergo mitotic divisions beginning in puberty and continuing throughout life (Figure 2.11). In contrast, oocytes complete all of their mitotic divisions during fetal life. Each round of DNA replication represents an opportunity for errors that result in mutation, so the older the father, the more mutations are likely to have accumulated in germ cells. The magnitude of the risk associated with advanced paternal age is small, however, and it is impossible to predict which genes might be affected, so it is difficult to provide specific counseling to a couple who may be concerned about risks.

DNA Repair

As noted, there are built-in mechanisms to repair DNA damage. Much of what is known about DNA repair was originally learned from the study of microorganisms, such as bacteria. Similar repair pathways exist in eukaryotic cells, including those in humans. Aberrations in DNA repair pathways underlie a set of inherited disorders (Table 2.1; Clinical Snapshot 2.1), as well as contribute to the pathogenesis of cancer.

Three major systems exist for repair of three types of damage (Figure 2.13). The nucleotide excision repair system removes DNA bases that have been damaged by chemicals or radiation. An endonuclease nicks the DNA several bases to each side of the damaged base, and the bases are excised by DNA helicase. The strand is then filled in by a DNA polymerase using the intact strand as a template, and the newly synthesized segment is then ligated to the DNA strand. Base excision repair removes chemically modified bases through a glycosylase enzyme. The sugar–phosphate to which the base was attached is then removed by an endonuclease, and finally the correct base is inserted and ligated to the strand. Mismatch repair removes bases that are erroneously introduced during DNA replication and do not pair correctly. The system recognizes the short

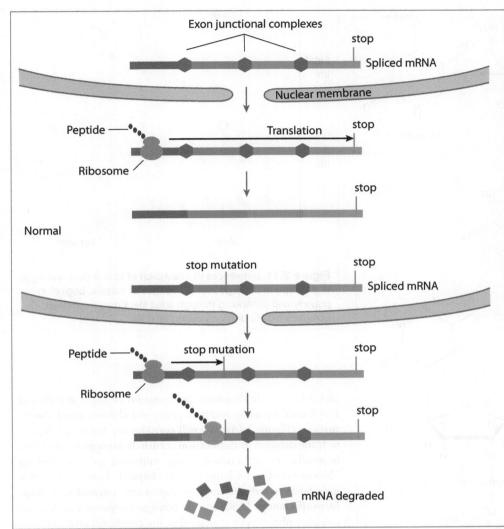

Figure 2.9 Nonsense-mediated decay. Normally (top), the spliced mRNA is exported from the nucleus into the cytoplasm with exon junctional complexes still attached at the exon borders. A ribosome binds and begins translation, displacing exon junctional complexes as translation proceeds until the stop codon is reached. If there is a premature stop codon 50 nucleotides or more in front of an exon junctional complex, the ribosome stalls and the mRNA is then targeted for degradation. This will not occur if the stop mutation is in the last exon (as would be the case for the normal stop), since there is no downstream exon junctional complex.

ⓘ Hot Topic 2.1   1000 Genomes Project

With the complete human genome sequence in hand, there is now an effort underway to more fully characterize the degree of genetic variation. The 1000 Genomes Project is intended to characterize 95% of human genome variants having a minor allele frequency of at least 1% (hence defined as polymorphism). Results of a pilot project have been published (1000 Genomes Project Consortium 2010). Three pilot studies were done: "low coverage" sequencing (i.e., a limited number of sequence "reads" for each base) on 179 individuals, deep resequencing (i.e., a large number of sequence "reads" for each base) on two trios (child and both parents), and sequencing of 8140 exons in 697 individuals from seven populations. Based on these studies, it was estimated that an individual has 10 000–11 000 variants that would change the amino acid sequence of a protein and an additional 10 000–12 000 that would not affect protein sequence. They estimate 190–210 in-frame indels, 80–100 premature stop mutations, 40–50 variants that would affect splicing, and 220–250 deletions that would lead to frameshift. They also found approximately 50–100 variants per genome that have been associated with inherited disorders (though not usually homozygous). The study of trios allowed an estimation of the mutation rate at approximately 10^{-8} per base pair. The full 1000 Genomes Project will sequence genomes of 2500 individuals from five regions of the world.

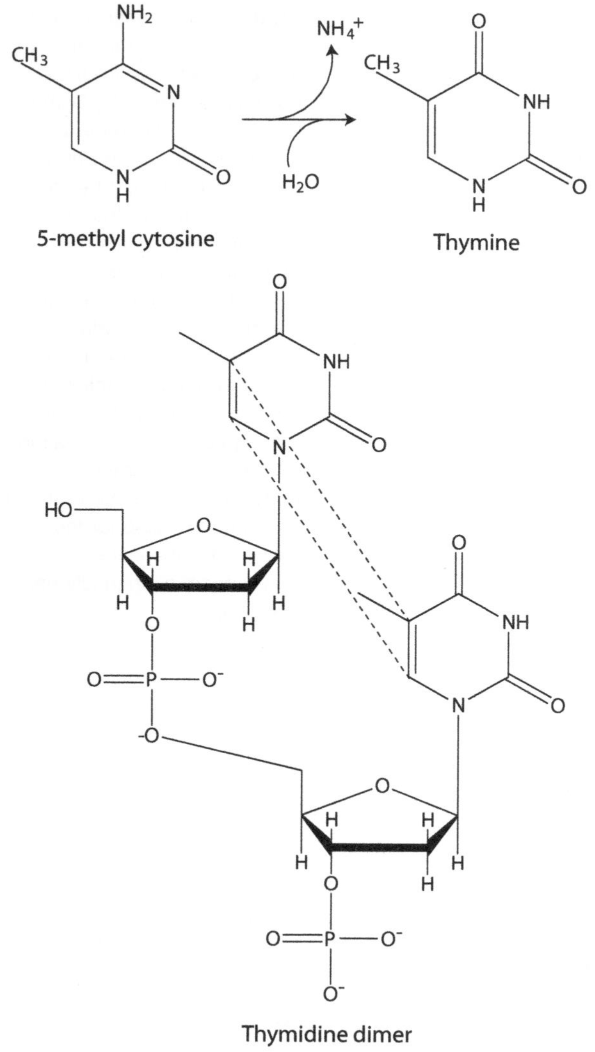

Figure 2.10 Deamination of 5-methyl cytosine to thymine (top), and thymidine dimer resulting from UV irradiation (bottom).

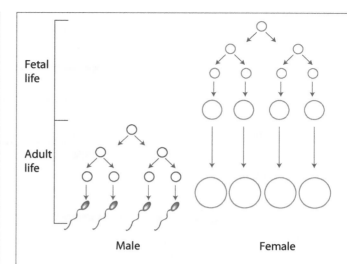

Figure 2.11 Differences in maturation of sperm (left) and eggs (right). Sperm undergo multiple rounds of mitosis, beginning at puberty and continuing through adult life. Eggs, in contrast, complete mitotic divisions during fetal life.

mismatched segment, excises the stretch of bases from the region of the newly replicated strand, and then recopies the excised segment from the other strand. Single- and double-strand DNA breaks may occur as a result of a chemical mutagen or radiation exposure. Single-strand breaks are filled in by copying from the intact strand. Double-strand breaks are repaired by enzyme systems that juxtapose the two ends and ligate them together, referred to as nonhomologous end joining.

Genomic Changes

Longer range genomic mutations include deletions, duplications, and inversions involving multiple exons within a gene, and deletions, duplications, or inversions of larger stretches of DNA encompassing multiple genes and chromosomal abnormalities (Figure 2.14). We will consider the latter in Chapter 6. If the deletion or duplication is entirely intragenic, the effect is similar to an exon-skipping mutation as described in "Nucleotide-Level Changes" (this chapter). Loss of the entire gene leads to reduced levels of expression, referred to as **haploinsufficiency**. Deletions of contiguous genes can lead to complex phenotypes representing the combined effect of haploinsufficiency at many loci. Duplications may lead to increased levels of gene expression.

Genomic mutations can be classified into two groups: recurrent mutations in which the size of the deletion or duplication is similar from individual to individual, and changes that are unique to an individual. The former are typical of a group of microdeletions or duplications that produce defined syndromes, such as Charcot–Marie–Tooth disease (Clinical Snapshot 2.2) and a wide variety of others that will be discussed in detail in Chapter 6. The basis for the size consistency of the deleted or duplicated segment is that these changes are bounded by repeated DNA sequences known as low-copy repeats (LCRs) or segmental duplications. An LCR is defined as a set of DNA segments ranging in size from 1 kb to hundreds of kb, with at least 95% sequence homology repeated several times in the genome. In some cases there are just two copies per genome, but in others there can be many more. LCRs are often clustered on the chromosome, and given their sequence similarity are prone to mispairing during meiosis or even in somatic cells. Recombination between mispaired LCRs (referred to as nonallelic homolo-

Table 2.1 Major medical disorders resulting from mutation in the DNA repair system.

Syndrome	Features	Genetic cause
Ataxia-telangiectasia MIM 208900	Ataxia, telangiectasia, immune deficiency, and lymphoma	Mutations in ataxia telangiectasia mutated (ATM) gene; cell cycle checkpoint for repair of DNA damage
Bloom syndrome MIM 210900	Short stature, photosensitive skin, risk of malignancy, and increased frequency of sister chromatid exchange	Mutations in helicase gene involved in DNA replication and recombination
Werner syndrome MIM 277700	Short stature, premature aging, and malignancy	Helicase gene mutations (distinct from Bloom syndrome gene)
Fanconi anemia MIM 227650	Congenital anomalies, aplastic anemia, and chromosome breakage increased with alkylating agents or mitomycin C	Genetically heterogeneous; various genes involved in DNA repair.
Xeroderma pigmentosum MIM 278700	Photosensitive skin, freckling, and skin cancer	Defective excision repair of ultraviolet-induced DNA damage
Trichothiodystrophy MIM 234050	Abnormal skin and hair, short stature, and developmental impairment	Defective excision repair of ultraviolet-induced DNA damage; possible effect on transcription
Cockayne syndrome MIM 216400	Photosensitive skin, white matter degeneration, cerebral calcification, and dwarfism	Defective excision repair of ultraviolet-induced DNA damage; possible effect on transcription
Nijmegen breakage syndrome MIM 251260	Progressive microcephaly, growth retardation, immunodeficiency, and cancer predisposition	Defective response to DNA double-strand breaks

gous recombination, or NAHR) will result in deletion and duplication products (Figure 2.16); the reason that the size of deletion or duplication is consistent for a given chromosomal region is that the size is dependent on spacing between LCRs, which will be similar in different individuals. However, there can be some differences in size attributable to recombination happening between different pairs of LCRs if there are several clustered in a region. Inversions can result from recombination events between an LCR located within a gene and an LCR outside the gene (Figure 2.17). This is the predominant mutational mechanism in the Factor VIII gene underlying hemophilia A.

The second group of rearrangements arises through more complex mechanisms. High-resolution analysis has revealed that some of these are not "simple" deletions or duplications, but in fact are highly complex rearrangements, for example consisting of multiple deletions of noncontiguous sequences. The precise mechanism of origin of these rearrangements is not known, but they are thought to arise as a consequence of aberrant events during DNA synthesis, where a replication fork can be disrupted by a break in DNA, leaving one of the strands undergoing synthesis to "invade" an adjacent replication fork, leading to deletion. This can occur multiple times, leading to complex noncontiguous deleted segments.

Gene Duplication and Evolution

Gene duplication events have played an important role in the evolution of the genome. Over the course of many generations after the duplication event, the gene copies may undergo subsequent mutation, altering function of the respective gene products. This can result in gene families, with different members having similar, but not identical, functions. Examples include the various globin genes (alpha, beta, gamma, etc.), genes that encode opsin proteins involved in color vision, genes involved in olfaction, and many, many others. Genes that are derived by evolution from a common ancestor are referred to as orthologous genes; genes derived from duplication events are referred to as paralogous genes (Figure 2.18).

Genetic Polymorphism

Many genetic loci exhibit a high frequency of variation from individual to individual. These are referred to as polymorphisms. A polymorphism is formally defined as a locus with two or more alleles in which at least one minor allele has a frequency of at least 1%.

◉ Clinical Snapshot 2.1   DNA Repair Disorders

Timothy is a 2-year-old referred because of unusual skin findings. He was born after a full-term pregnancy and was healthy as a newborn. By the end of the first year of life, however, his parents noted that his face was becoming covered with freckles. This seemed odd for a baby, and especially odd since no one else in the family has freckles. Recently, his family spent some time at the beach and Timothy developed severe sunburn. His parents were surprised, since they had tried to keep him out of the sun and had applied sunscreen. Now, one month later, his skin appears dry and scaly, and there are innumerable freckles on the face, arms, and trunk – all areas where he had been exposed to the sun. Timothy is in the 50th centile for height and weight, but his head is in the 20th centile. No one else in the family has had similar problems.

Timothy has signs typical for xeroderma pigmentosum (XP) (MIM 278700). The disorder usually presents in the early years of life with freckling and extreme sun sensitivity of the skin (Figure 2.12). Affected children may develop severe sunburn even with minimal ultraviolet exposure. There is a very high risk of skin cancer, with onset usually in the childhood years. There may be ocular problems due to ultraviolet (UV) light–induced damage and some children develop neurological problems, including small head size, developmental delay, deafness, ataxia, and seizures. Xeroderma pigmentosum is due to defective excision repair. Cultured cells obtained from affected individuals display increased cell death on exposure to UV. At least eight distinct genes are known to be associated with XP. These genes encode proteins involved in the excision repair process. Care of persons with XP involves

protection from UV exposure and careful monitoring for the development of skin cancer. The disorder is inherited as an autosomal recessive trait.

Xeroderma pigmentosum is one of a number of disorders of DNA repair or DNA replication. Some are described in Table 2.1. Most are associated with an increased risk of malignancy due to the accumulation of mutations in cells that cannot repair DNA damage. Short stature is another common feature. Management is focused on symptomatic treatment and surveillance for cancer. No primary therapy exists for any of these disorders. Each is inherited as an autosomal recessive trait.

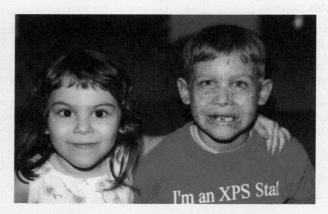

Figure 2.12 Two children affected with xeroderma pigmentosum. Some children, such as the boy at the right, are more fair-skinned and sun-sensitive than others and develop freckling at a younger age. (Courtesy of Xeroderma Pigmentosum Society.)

Types of Polymorphisms

There are four major types of DNA polymorphisms. SNPs consist of a single base change, and may occur anywhere in a gene, including an exon, as well as between genes (Figure 2.19). SNPs are usually detected by a variety of DNA sequencing–based techniques.

Simple sequence repeats comprise a second type of polymorphism. These are stretches of DNA in which a di-, tri-, or tetranucleotide sequence is repeated multiple times. The exact number of repeats can vary from individual to individual, and can be measured by **polymerase chain reaction (PCR)** amplification (Methods 2.2) of the segment containing the repeat and measurement of the size of the resulting fragment by electrophoresis in a polyacrylamide gel, which has sufficient

resolution to detect a difference of as few as two bases (Figure 2.21). **Simple sequence repeats** tend to have multiple alleles, making it likely that an individual will be found to be heterozygous.

A third type of polymorphism involves short tandem repeats. These are repeats of tens to hundreds of bases, with the exact number of repeats being polymorphic (Figure 2.22). Short tandem repeats can be detected with PCR-based approaches.

The fourth type is the copy number variation, which consists of different numbers of copies of a specific genetic sequence. This often occurs due to NAHR between LCRs. It has been estimated that as much as 12% of the genome consists of repeated sequences where differences in numbers of repeats exist between individuals. We will explore possible clinical implications of some of these differences in Chapter 6.

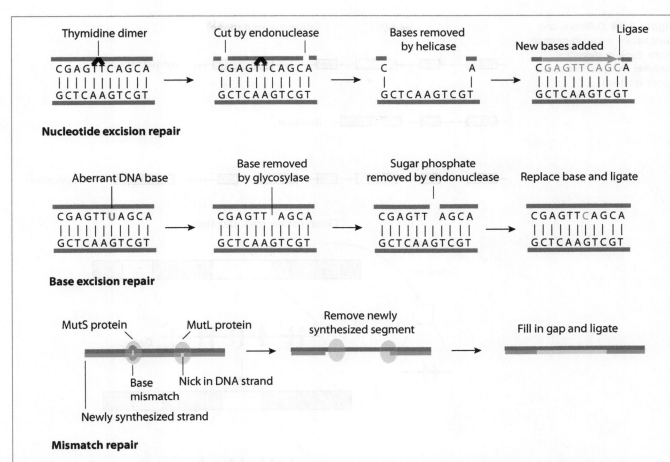

Figure 2.13 Three major systems of DNA repair. Nucleotide excision repair removes a segment of DNA around a damaged base, and the gap is then filled in using the intact strand as a template. Base excision repair first removes the damaged base, then the sugar–phosphate, and then fills in the correct base. Mismatch repair repairs instances of misincorporation of a base on the newly synthesized strand. The protein MutM binds to the mismatch, and MutL scans the DNA for a nearby nick. Bases between the nick and just upstream of the mismatch are then removed from the newly synthesized strand and filled in using the parental strand as a template.

Significance of Genetic Polymorphisms

The term "polymorphism" does not imply whether a DNA variant will have phenotypic effect. Many polymorphisms are silent, occurring in regions that do not encode RNA or protein, but some occur within or nearby coding or regulatory sequences. These may produce medically insignificant phenotypes or, in some cases, phenotypes that contribute to disease. We will explore this further in Chapters 3 and 7. Study of genetic polymorphisms has been of critical importance in gene mapping and in searching for genes that are involved in common disorders. We will return to this in Chapters 4 and 5.

Conclusion

Although we speak of a "human genome sequence," in fact the genome is fluid, with constant changes occurring as cells divide. Although many of these changes are repaired, some escape repair and may persist at the level of the cell or, if they occur in the germ line, at the level of the organism. Some do not change gene function, whereas others have profound effects. The discipline of medical genetics is based on the effects of genetic variation on health and the development of diagnostic tests and interventions to deal with these changes when they impair health.

Figure 2.14 Deletions and duplications involving multiple exons (top), or deletions involving multiple contiguous genes (bottom).

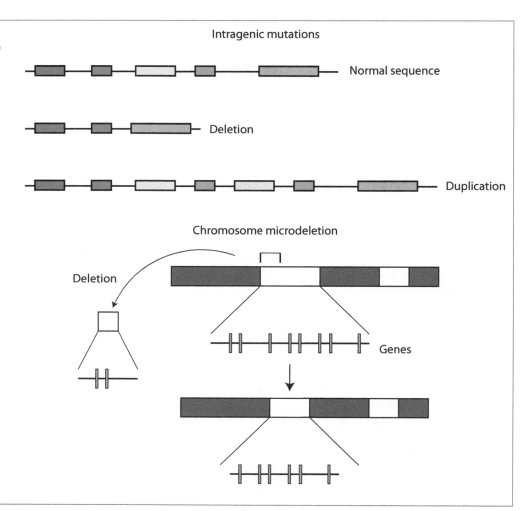

👁 Clinical Snapshot 2.2 Charcot–Marie–Tooth Disease

George is 22 years old and is undergoing his second orthopedic procedure for high arches. He has known that he has Charcot–Marie–Tooth disease since he was a teenager. At that time he began to notice weakness in his feet, which progressed to difficulty walking due to a foot drop (his toes tend to scrape the ground when he walks). The weakness has gradually spread to include his lower legs, and he has some weakness in his hands as well. He occasionally has pain in his feet, but he is not aware of any sensory loss. He has very high arches (Figure 2.15), which has required wearing special shoes. He has depressed knee and ankle jerk reflexes. Otherwise, though, George is in good health, and he has no cognitive problems. His initial diagnosis was made on the basis of these clinical findings and also the fact that his father is similarly affected. His father has had genetic testing, showing duplication of the *PMP22* gene on chromosome 17. His paternal grandmother and a paternal uncle are also affected.

Charcot–Marie–Tooth disease is a form of hereditary motor and sensory neuropathy. The disorder affects the myelin sheath of sensory and motor nerves, causing slow nerve conduction and both motor and sensory deficits. Long nerves, such as nerves to the feet, are affected earliest and most severely. The most prominent clinical sign is weakness of distal muscles, especially of the feet, lower legs, and hands. Sensory deficits may also be present, but may be less prominent than the motor deficits clinically. Deep tendon reflexes will be depressed or absent.

Charcot–Marie–Tooth disease is genetically heterogeneous, with various modes of inheritance in different families, including autosomal recessive, autosomal dominant, and X-linked. The most common form, CMT1A (MIM 118220), is autosomal dominant and is associated with duplication of the *PMP22* gene on chromosome 17. *PMP22* encodes a myelin protein gene and is flanked by a set of LCRs that can lead to unequal crossover events. In addition to Charcot–Marie–Tooth disease resulting from duplication, a separate disorder, hereditary neuropathy with liability to pressure palsies (HNPP), results from deletion of *PMP22*. Deletion is the reciprocal product of an aberrant crossover that leads to duplication. The phenotype of HNPP is also a peripheral neuropathy, with a tendency for neuropathy to occur as a consequence of chronic physical pressure on nerves.

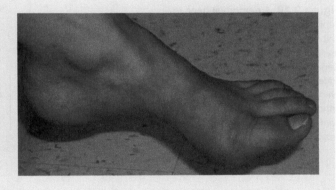

Figure 2.15 Pes cavus (high arches) in a person with Charcot–Marie–Tooth disease.

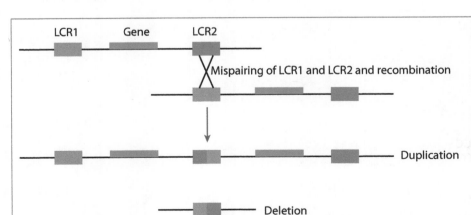

Figure 2.16 Nonallelic homologous recombination between two low-copy repeats (LCRs) that bound a region that includes one of more genes (green box). The two LCRs are homologous, though not necessarily identical in sequence. A crossover between them generates a duplication allele and a deletion allele.

Figure 2.17 Nonallelic homologous recombination between an LCR within an exon in a gene and an LCR outside the gene results in an inversion and splitting of the gene, rendering it inactive.

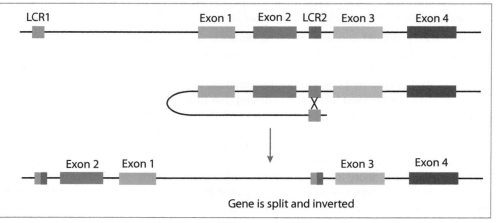

Gene is split and inverted

Figure 2.18 A primordial gene is duplicated, generating two copies that subsequently acquire mutations leading to divergent functions. Genes derived from a common ancestral gene through speciation events are designated as orthologous genes; genes derived from a gene duplication event are designated as paralogous genes.

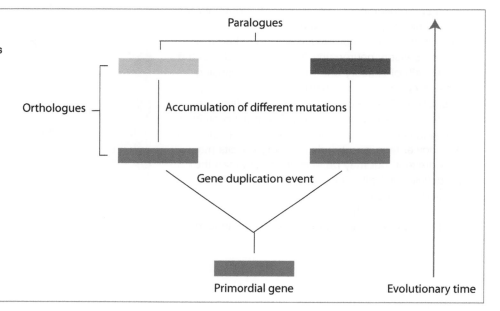

```
ACTTGGATTCATACAGGC
TGAACCTAAGTATGTCCG
        ↕
ACTTGGATCCATACAGGC
TGAACCTAGGTATGTCCG
```

Figure 2.19 Single-nucleotide polymorphism, in which two sequences differ at a single base pair.

Methods 2.2   Polymerase Chain Reaction (PCR)

The PCR provides a means of amplifying a specific DNA sequence against a background of an entire genome (Figure 2.20). It begins with the synthesis of a pair of primers – oligonucleotides of 20–25 bases – that are homologous to a pair sequence that flanks a region of interest. The distance between the primer binding sites is limited, usually to around 1000 bases or fewer. The primers are designed to bind to opposite strands of the target DNA, which is separated into single strands by heat. The primers serve as a starting point for a DNA synthesis reaction, using DNA polymerase and a supply of the four nucleotides, as the temperature of the solution is cooled. This produces a pair of hybrid molecules, which are once again separated into single strands by heating. Again the primers bind and a DNA synthesis reaction is allowed to begin. The DNA polymerase is derived from a bacterium that thrives at high temperatures, allowing the same polymerase to be used in spite of multiple cycles of heating and cooling of the reaction mixture. The process is iterated multiple times, 20 or more, using an automated system, which leads to an exponential increase in the target DNA sequence. This results in over a million copies of the target sequence, sufficient to be visualized by staining the DNA following electrophoresis in an agarose gel.

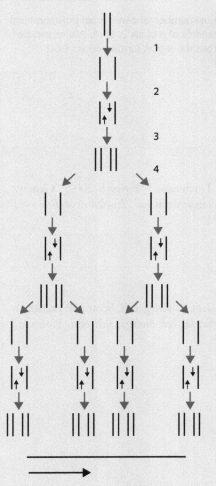

Figure 2.20 Diagram of polymerase chain reaction (PCR). Strands of target DNA are separated (1), and primers are allowed to bind to opposite strands (2). A DNA synthesis reaction then is allowed to proceed, copying the target DNA (3). This process is repeated cyclically (4), resulting in exponential amplification of the target sequence.

Arrows indicate oligonucleotide primers bound to single-stranded DNA molecules.

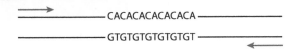

CA repeat, consisting of 7 copies of CA sequence

Figure 2.21 Simple sequence repeat. In this case, the dinucleotide CA is repeated several times. The allele shown has seven repeats, but other alleles might have five, six, seven, eight, nine, or even more copies of the CA sequence. The copy number is determined by PCR amplification of the region (arrows denote PCR primers in flanking DNA) and determination of the product's size by polyacrylamide gel electrophoresis.

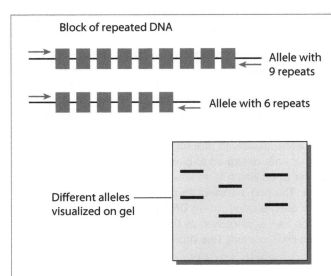

Figure 2.22 A variable-number tandem repeat polymorphism consists of multiple repeats of a block of DNA. Alleles can be detected by PCR across the region (arrows depict PCR primers).

REFERENCES

1000 Genomes Project Consortium 2010, "A map of human genome variation from population-scale sequencing", *Nature*, vol. 467, pp. 1061–73.

Wain HM, Lush M, Ducluzeau F, Povey S 2002, "Genew: the human nomenclature database", *Nucleic Acids Research*, vol. 30, pp. 169–71.

FURTHER READING

Alberts B, Johnson A, Lewis J, Raff M, Roberts K, Walter P 2007, *Molecular biology of the cell*, 5th edn, Garland Science, New York.

Krebs JE, Goldstein, ES, Kilpatrick ST 2009, *Lewin's genes X*, Jones & Bartlett, Sudbury, MA.

Lodish H, Berk A, Kaiser CA, Krieger M, Scott MP, Bretscher A *et al.* 2007, *Molecular cell biology*, 6th edn, Freeman, New York.

Find interactive self-test questions and additional resources for this chapter at **www.korfgenetics.com**.

Self-Assessment

Review Questions

2.1   Some silent mutations have been found to be associated with disease. Suggest a possible mechanism for this. How would you test this hypothesis?

2.2   What types of mutations are most likely to be associated with haploinsufficiency?

2.3   You are trying to find mutations in a gene and choose to look at RNA rather than DNA. The rationale is that by sequencing RNA, you will see not only base substitutions but also the effects of mutations that alter splicing. A colleague points out, however, that this strategy might miss some stop mutations. Why might this be so?

2.4   Given the frequency of spontaneous mutation, and assuming that mutation occurs at random in the genome, approximately how many mutations might be expected in a germ cell compared with the individual from whom that germ cell was derived?

2.5   Under what circumstances might a polymorphism be associated with a pathological phenotype?

CHAPTER 3
Patterns of Inheritance

Introduction

It is likely that people have recognized that some traits – and some diseases – cluster in families long before there was any semblance of a modern concept of disease or even of medical practice. It was not until the beginning of the 20th century, however, that specific patterns of inheritance were recognized in humans. The groundwork for understanding single-gene inheritance was laid by Gregor Mendel, a monk who in the 1860s experimented with pea plants at a monastery in Moravia, now in the Czech Republic. Mendel's work lay unrecognized for decades, until it was discovered at the turn of the 20th century by three botanists who performed similar experiments. Within a few years, the British physician Archibald Garrod recognized the existence of families in which traits segregated in accordance with Mendel's laws, launching the discipline of medical genetics.

Human Genetics and Genomics, Fourth Edition. Bruce R. Korf and Mira B. Irons.
© 2013 John Wiley & Sons, Ltd. Published 2013 by John Wiley & Sons, Ltd.

Key Points

- An autosomal recessive trait is expressed only in individuals who are homozygous.
- An autosomal dominant trait will be expressed in homozygotes or heterozygotes. Many human autosomal dominant disorders are lethal in the homozygous state, however.
- Sex-linked traits are transmitted with the X or Y chromosome. An X-linked trait never displays male-to-male transmission.
- Pseudodominant inheritance occurs when a homozygous individual and a heterozygous individual mate. A recessive trait will thereby exhibit vertical transmission. It occurs mostly with traits that are relatively common.
- Digenic inheritance involves the occurrence of a trait in an individual who is heterozygous at two loci simultaneously.
- Penetrance is defined as the existence of a phenotype in an individual with the at-risk genotype. Nonpenetrant individuals do not express the phenotype. There may be a range of expressivity among individuals who are phenotypically affected.
- New mutations may account for sporadically affected individuals. Some individuals are mosaics for a mutation if the mutation arose postzygotically. In some cases, the mutation is confined to the germline.
- Genomic imprinting effects may lead to a disorder being manifest only if the gene was inherited from the parent whose gene copy is expressed.
- Disorders associated with the mutational mechanism of triplet repeat expansion display the phenomenon of anticipation, where a disorder becomes more severe with each passing generation.
- Each mitochondrion contains multiple copies of a circular, double-stranded DNA molecule that encodes some of the proteins involved in oxidative phosphorylation, as well as a set of transfer RNAs (tRNAs) and ribosomal RNAs (rRNAs).
- Mitochondrial DNA is maternally inherited, so mitochondrial traits are always passed from a female to all of her children.
- Mitochondria are passively segregated in cell division. There may be a mixture of mutant and wild-type mitochondria in the same cell, which is referred to as heteroplasmy.

The study of traits determined by single genes remains the mainstay of human genetics. More than 10 000 such traits have been catalogued. From a medical point of view, many are rare, affecting fewer than one in 100 000 individuals. Some are more common, though the most common conditions tend to be determined by combinations of genes interacting with one another and with the environment. In this chapter, we will focus on patterns of genetic transmission, including Mendelian inheritance, multifactorial inheritance, and some recently identified special cases and exceptions to the Mendelian paradigm. We will also see how modern tools of molecular genetics are beginning to reveal the mechanisms that underlie these patterns. As detailed clinical information on rare genetic disorders can be difficult to find, online sources such as GeneReviews have been developed to provide assistance to physicians caring for patients with these conditions (Sources of Information 3.1).

Sources of Information 3.1
GeneReviews

Access to comprehensive clinical information regarding rare genetic syndromes is often difficult to obtain easily. GeneReviews are comprehensive, peer-reviewed sources of clinical and diagnostic information on many genetic conditions written by clinical experts. The reviews contain clinical, diagnostic, management, molecular, and genetic counseling information, as well as information on resources available to patients and families and additional references on the condition. The reviews are updated periodically in order to reflect new diagnostic and therapeutic information. GeneReviews can be accessed at its website, www.genereviews.org.

Mendelian Inheritance

The foundation for our modern understanding of genetic segregation is that a diploid organism contains two copies of every gene (excepting those carried on the sex chromosomes). One copy of each gene is inherited from each parent. These gene copies separate during the formation of haploid germ cells and are reunited at fertilization. The individual copies of a particular gene are called **alleles**. The genetic constitution of an individual with respect to a particular trait is referred to as the genotype, whereas the corresponding physical manifestation of the trait is the phenotype. In human genetics, traits can be transmitted as autosomal or sex linked, and as **dominant** or **recessive**. Sex is determined by the X and Y chromosomes: A male has an X and a Y chromosome, and a female has two X chromosomes. Genes located on a sex chromosome are said to be **sex-linked gene**s, whereas the non-sex-linked genes are referred to as autosomal. Geneticists use standard symbols to depict the inheritance of traits within a family tree, or pedigree (Methods 3.1). These symbols are illustrated in Figure 3.1.

Autosomal Recessive Inheritance

The traits described by Garrod displayed the properties of recessive inheritance elucidated by Mendel. These traits are expressed only in individuals who possess two mutant gene copies (alleles) inherited from each parent (Figure 3.2). Such individuals are said to be **homozygous**, since both gene copies are mutated. We will see later that the specific mutation in each allele may be different, but both nevertheless are mutated. The parents are both carriers (i.e., they are **heterozygous**), having one mutated copy and one nonmutated (**wild-type**) copy (Figure 3.3). The parents, as a couple, face a one-in-four chance of each passing mutated copies to any offspring. Probably the trait has been in the family for generations, with many individuals being heterozygous carriers, but only in instances where the trait comes together in a homozygous state does the disorder surface. The likelihood of this occurring is increased if the parents are related to one another (consanguineous), in which case they both inherit what may be a rare recessive allele from a common ancestor (Figure 3.4). Rare recessive disorders are therefore more common in the offspring of consanguineous parents, but not all consanguineous matings result in recessive disorders and not all recessive disorders require consanguinity to be uncovered.

Garrod coined the term "inborn errors of metabolism" to describe the human genetic traits he characterized. Two of them, albinism (MIM 203100) and alkaptonuria (MIM 203500), are disorders of tyrosine metabolism (Figure 3.5). The conditions result from a deficiency of specific enzymes due to a mutation in the genes that encode the enzymes. Lack of enzyme activity results in buildup of a substrate, which may be toxic, and/or deficiency of a product (Figure 3.6). In albinism, there is a deficiency of the pigment melanin due to lack

> ### ✓ Methods 3.1 Taking a Family History
>
> Obtaining an accurate family history is a fundamental skill that will be increasingly crucial in the practice of medicine. It is of obvious importance if a person seeks care because of a family history of a genetic disorder. Often, however, a person will not realize the importance of a medical condition in a relative and will not volunteer the information unless it is explicitly sought. A three-generation family history, including information about siblings, parents, and grandparents, should be obtained as a standard component of medical practice. A "pedigree" should be constructed, using the symbols in Figure 3.1. Some tips for taking a complete and accurate family history are as follows:
>
> - If a person is seeking medical advice about a specific problem, ask specifically whether relatives have a similar problem.
> - When asking about brothers and sisters, inquire whether there was ever a sibling who had died; some people will only remember to mention their living sibs.
> - Inquire about neonatal deaths, miscarriages, and infertility.
> - Be alert to sibships in which not all sibs share the same two parents.
> - Ask about consanguinity.
> - Ask about the ethnic origins of different branches of the family.
> - Where possible, try to obtain documentation (i.e., medical records) for important points of family history; often family members will conclude that a relative has a disorder believed to "run in the family" based on superficial information that may be inaccurate.

of activity of the enzyme tyrosinase (MIM 606933). The problem in alkaptonuria is the buildup of a toxic substance due to an enzyme deficiency. Another defect of phenylalanine metabolism, phenylketonuria (PKU) (MIM 261600), is due to deficiency of the enzyme phenylalanine hydroxylase. Phenylalanine and its metabolites accumulate to toxic levels. There is also a deficiency of downstream products of phenylalanine, including the neurotransmitter DOPA and the pigment melanin. We will revisit PKU in other chapters of this book when we consider newborn screening.

The biochemical basis for the dominance of wild-type alleles over mutant alleles in inborn errors of metabolism can be understood by considering how enzymes function (Figure 3.7). Enzymes are proteins that catalyze chemical reactions. An

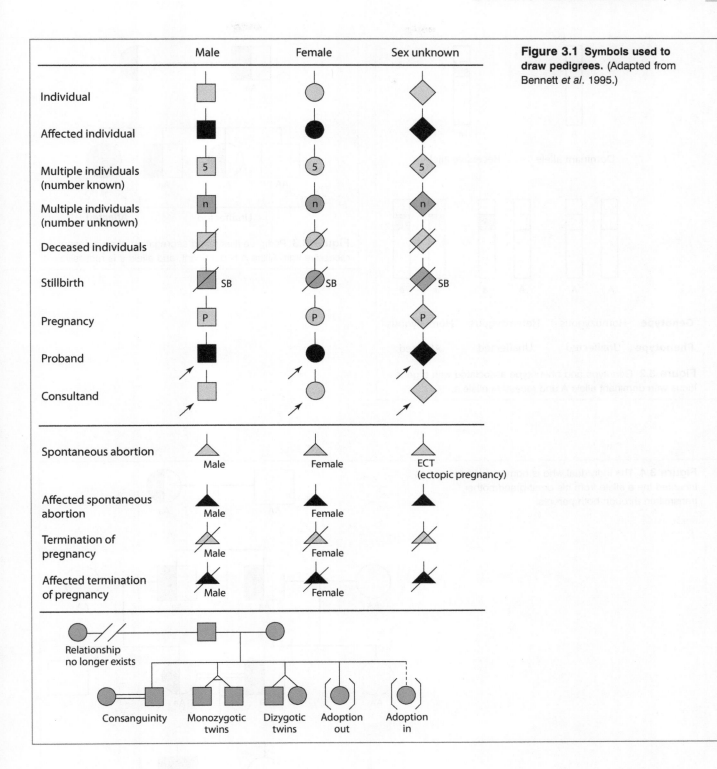

Figure 3.1 Symbols used to draw pedigrees. (Adapted from Bennett *et al*. 1995.)

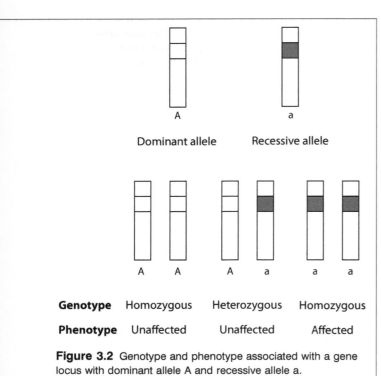

Figure 3.2 Genotype and phenotype associated with a gene locus with dominant allele A and recessive allele a.

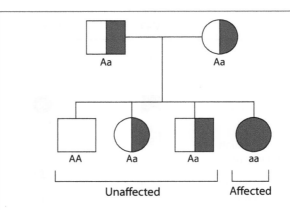

Figure 3.3 Pedigree illustrating segregation of an autosomal recessive trait. Allele A is dominant, and allele a is recessive.

Figure 3.4 The individual who is homozygous for aa has inherited the a allele from his great-grandmother, transmitted through both parents.

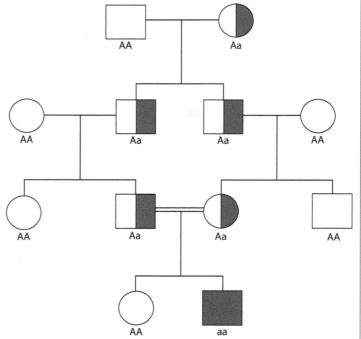

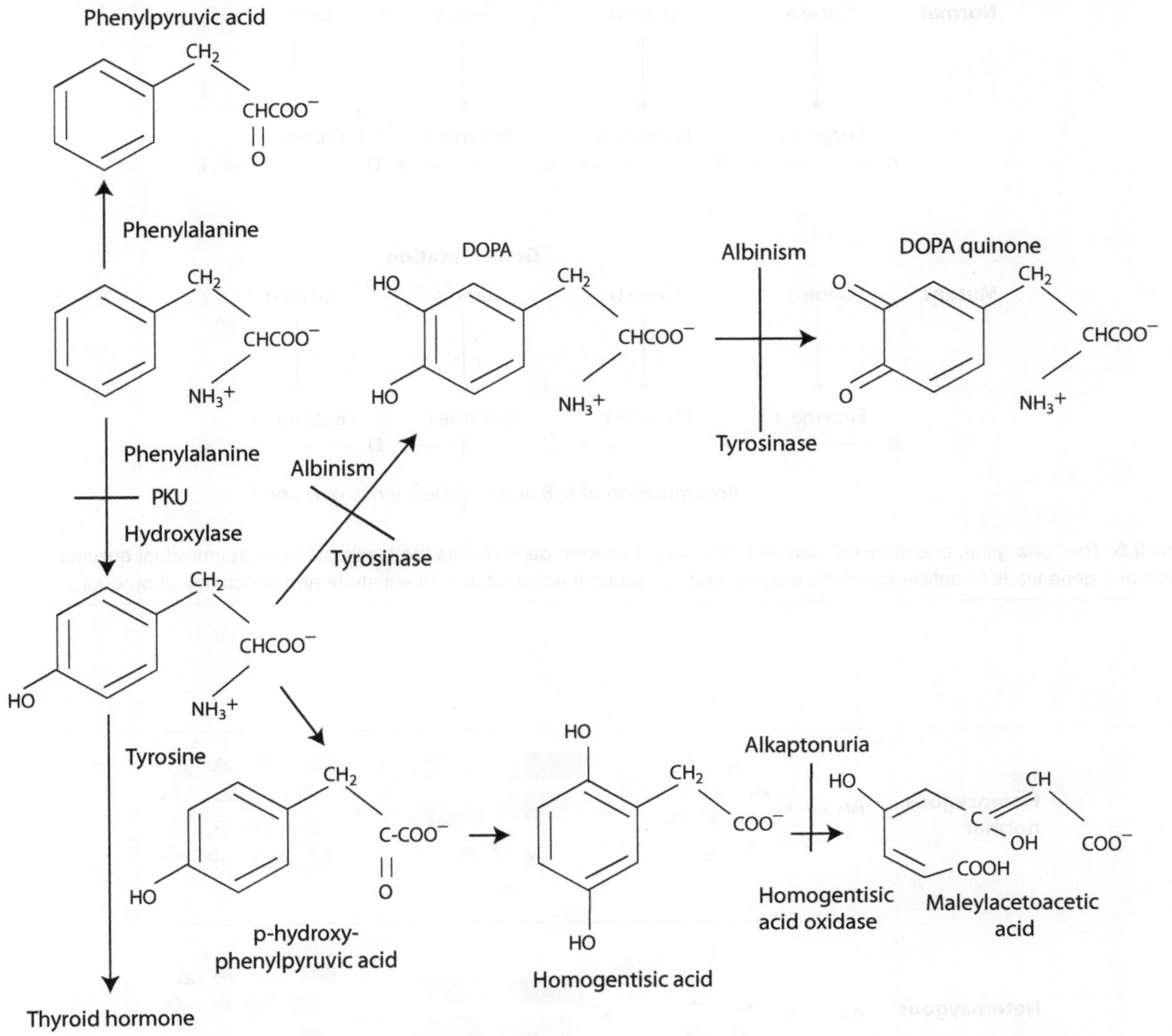

Figure 3.5 Metabolic pathways involving tyrosine. Phenylalanine is converted to tyrosine by phenylalanine hydroxylase, the enzyme blocked in phenylketonuria. Lack of homogentisic acid oxidase leads to alkaptonuria and deficiency of tyrosinase to albinism.

enzyme is not consumed during the reaction, so only small quantities are required for a reaction to be carried out. In a person homozygous for a mutation in the gene encoding an enzyme, little or no enzyme activity is present, so he or she will manifest the abnormal phenotype. A heterozygous individual expresses 50% of the normal level of enzyme activity due to expression of the wild-type allele. This is usually sufficient to prevent phenotypic expression.

Not all recessive traits are due to enzyme deficiency. Cystic fibrosis (MIM 219700) is a recessive disorder in which there is marked thickening of secretions, especially in the lung and in ducted glands such as the pancreas. The disorder is due to mutations in a gene that encodes a chloride channel. Deficient chloride transport across the cell membrane leads to a reduction in the water content of extracellular fluid. Apparently, a 50% reduction in chloride transport in heterozygous carriers is still compatible with adequate hydration of extracellular fluid.

In general, recessive traits are associated with a reduced level of activity of a gene product in systems that have sufficient reserve function so that loss of half the activity in the heterozygous state does not perturb the system. The mutations responsible for recessive traits tend to lead to lack of gene expression, as with promoter mutations; lack of protein production, for example due to mutations that lead to premature termination of translation; or production of a protein with

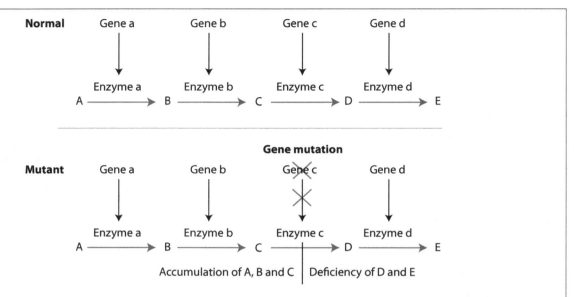

Figure 3.6 The "one gene, one enzyme" concept. Normally a specific gene directs the synthesis of each individual enzyme. Mutation of a gene leads to deficiency of the enzyme and consequent accumulation of substrate and deficiency of product.

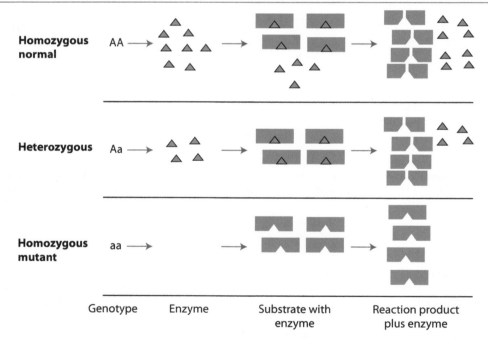

Figure 3.7 Model explaining recessive transmission of most enzyme deficiencies. Normally, more than sufficient enzyme is synthesized to carry out a reaction. A heterozygote still has sufficient enzyme, but a homozygote for a mutation does not make enough enzyme to complete the reaction.

Clinical Snapshot 3.1   Autosomal Recessive Congenital Deafness

Seth is a 4-week-old boy who is referred to a genetics clinic for evaluation for congenital deafness. His deafness was first detected by newborn screening, and subsequently found by further testing to represent a profound sensorineural deafness. His health has been excellent, and there is no known family history of deafness. A careful physical examination is performed, and no congenital anomalies are noted. Genetic testing is performed looking for mutation in the GJB2 gene, and he is found to have a mutation in both alleles.

Deafness is subdivided into sensorineural and conductive causes. The former involves dysfunction in the cochlea, the auditory nerve, or in connections of the nerve to the brain. Conductive deafness is due to problems from the external ear up to the cochlea. Approximately one-half of cases of congenital sensorineural deafness are due to genetic causes, with 30% of these classified as syndromic (deafness associated with other abnormalities) and 70% as nonsyndromic. Of the nonsyndromic forms,

approximately three-quarters are inherited in an autosomal recessive manner. In accordance with this mode of transmission, one expects to see that both parents are unaffected with the disorder, yet they face a one-in-four recurrence risk with each pregnancy. The most common cause of autosomal recessive congenital deafness (MIM 220290) is due to mutation in the gene GJB2 (MIM 121011), which encodes the protein Connexin 26. Hexamers of Connexin 26 aggregate in the cell membrane to form gap junctions and are critical for the flux of potassium ions in the inner ear necessary for normal hearing (Figure 3.8). The most common mutation is a deletion of one G from a run of six in the gene, which leads to a frameshift and lack of expression of the gene product. The carrier frequency of this mutation is as high as 3% in some populations. A wide variety of additional mutations may occur. Many affected individuals are compound heterozygotes, having two different mutant alleles.

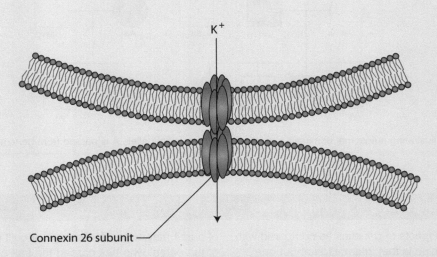

Figure 3.8 Connexin 26 subunits aggregate into hexameric gap junctions to connect adjacent cells. In the inner ear, the gap junctions serve to transfer potassium ions between cells.

reduced or absent function, such as due to amino acid substitution (Clinical Snapshot 3.1).

Autosomal Dominant Inheritance

Autosomal dominant traits are expressed in both the heterozygous and the homozygous states (Figure 3.9). Actually, many human dominant disorders are not "pure" dominants; the

homozygote may actually be more severely affected, and even may not survive, so clinically affected individuals will be heterozygotes. For rare traits this distinction is largely academic, since usually only one of the parents carries the mutant allele (Figure 3.10). In such families, the affected individual faces a 50% risk of any offspring being affected (Ethical Implications 3.1).

Individuals with the connective tissue dysplasia Marfan syndrome (MIM 154700) have lax joints and floppy heart

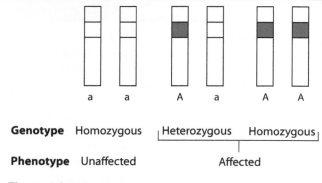

Genotype	Homozygous	Heterozygous	Homozygous
Phenotype	Unaffected	Affected	

Figure 3.9 The phenotype of a dominant allele is expressed in individuals who are either homozygous or heterozygous for the allele.

valves and are prone to aortic dissection, among other problems. The disorder is due to deficient production of the protein fibrillin–1 (MIM 134797), which is a component of connective tissue. Mutations that lead to reduction of fibrillin–1 by 50% lead to weakening of connective tissue and signs of mild Marfan syndrome (Figure 3.11). This is referred to as haploinsufficiency. Some fibrillin–1 mutations result in production of normal quantities of fibrillin–1, but the fibrillin–1 interacts abnormally with other proteins in connective tissue. This mechanism is referred to as a dominant negative effect. The abnormal protein, in effect, "poisons" the system, leading to a more severe form of Marfan syndrome than occurs with haploinsufficiency.

Osteogenesis imperfecta (MIM 166200) is a disorder in which there is abnormal bone matrix, leading to brittle bones

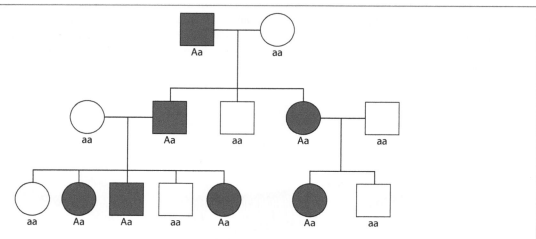

Figure 3.10 Pedigree illustrating autosomal dominant transmission. The dominant allele A is passed from generation to generation.

ⓘ Ethical Implications 3.1   Family Ties

One of the unique aspects of genetics as compared with other areas of medicine is that information about one family member may have an impact on other relatives. This has many implications that are important to consider when discussing family history with patients. Firstly, relevant information may not be widely known within the family. It may be necessary to ask specific questions of relatives in order to learn of family traits that have not been openly discussed. In some cases, this may unlock family secrets that can cause discomfort or even disrupt relationships. For example, it may reveal instances where an individual stated to be the parent of a child is not the biological parent, or instances of miscarriage, termination of pregnancy, or death that have not been revealed. Secondly, genetic transmission of a trait may engender feelings of guilt on the part of the parent who has passed the trait on to a child. It is important to realize that taking a family history may raise such feelings, and addressing them can be helpful. Thirdly, information learned about one member of a family may indirectly provide information about another. For example, a dominant trait known to be present in a grandparent and diagnosed by genetic testing in a child can also be assumed to be present in the parent. The parent may not wish to know of his or her diagnosis, but will probably learn of it from the child's test result. This is a risk of genetic testing that may not be obvious to the family, but should be pointed out as the possibility of testing is discussed.

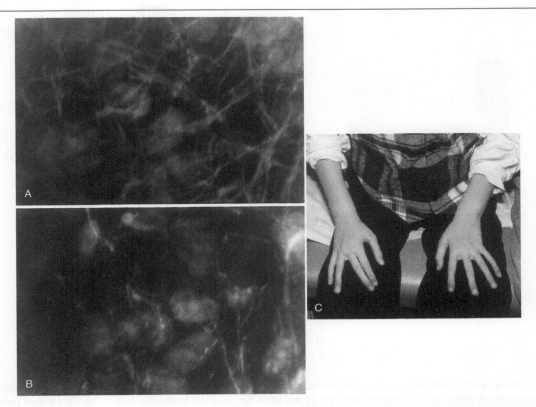

Figure 3.11 Immunofluorescence photomicrograph of normal (A) and Marfan syndrome (B) fibroblast sample stained for fibrillin, showing deficient fibrillin – 1 in the Marfan sample. (Courtesy of Dr. Heinz Furthmayr, Department of Pathology, Stanford University.) (C) Arachnodactyly seen in a child with Marfan syndrome. (Courtesy of Dr. Ronald Lacro, Department of Cardiology, Children's Hospital, Boston.)

and frequent fractures. The condition is due to mutations in the gene that encodes components of type I collagen. Collagen is a triple helical molecule consisting of two chains of alpha$_1$(I) collagen (MIM 120150) and one of alpha$_2$(I) collagen (MIM 120160). Mutation in one allele that encodes alpha$_1$(I) can lead to disruption of 75% of collagen triple helices due to the polymeric nature of the mature molecule (Figure 3.12) – another example of a dominant negative effect.

An example of a dominant disorder due to a gain-of-function mutation is achondroplasia (MIM 100800). Achondroplasia is a form of dwarfism due to mutation in the fibroblast growth factor type 3 receptor (MIM 134934) (Figure 3.13). This is a transmembrane receptor that, when activated by ligand binding at the cell surface, promotes the differentiation of cartilage into bone. A specific mutation in the gene for the receptor constitutively activates the system, causing premature conversion of the growth plate into bone, severely stunting growth. Gain-of-function mutations tend to be highly selective in that they require amino acid substitution at strategic sites in a protein.

The molecular basis of dominant traits tends to be diverse. One additional important mechanism of dominant inheritance

is associated with a unique set of genes involved in predisposition to malignancy, referred to as tumor suppressor genes. We will defer discussion of these genes, however, until Chapter 8, where the genetics of cancer is discussed.

X-Linked Inheritance

The third major pattern of genetic transmission is referred to as sex linked, and it involves genes on the X and Y chromosomes (Figure 3.14). A mutation on the X chromosome will more likely be expressed in males, who receive a single X from their mothers and a Y from their fathers. Males are said to be hemizygous for genes on the X chromosome. Females will express the trait only if they inherit it from both parents, which will occur much more rarely. A female carrier for an X-linked recessive trait faces a 50% risk of transmission of the trait to any offspring. Females who inherit the trait will be carriers, whereas males who inherit the trait will be affected (Figure 3.15). Males never transmit an X-linked trait to their sons. An X-linked trait can also be transmitted as a dominant. In this case, an affected female has a 50% chance of passing the trait to any offspring, whereas males transmit the trait to all of their

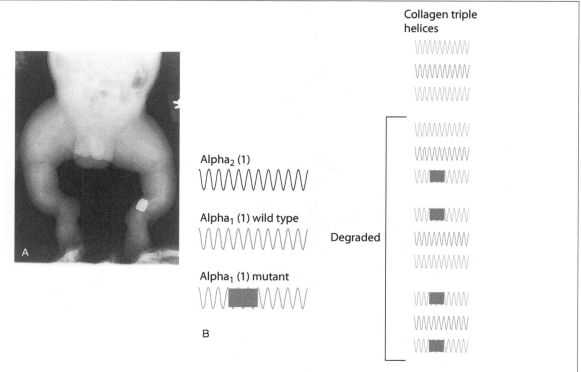

Figure 3.12 (A) X-ray of infant with osteogenesis imperfecta, showing multiple fractures. (B) Dominant negative model. Although only one allele for alpha$_1$(I) procollagen is mutant (depicted by the black box over the molecule), 75% of the triple-helical molecules incorporate at least one mutant protein and are degraded in the cell.

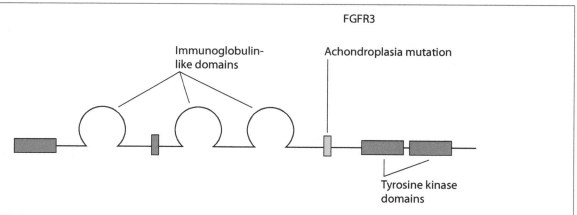

Figure 3.13 Diagram of an FGFR3 molecule, showing the site of gain-of-function mutation responsible for achondroplasia.

daughters but none of their sons. Some X-linked dominant traits are lethal in males, and therefore are expressed only in females (Figure 3.16; Clinical Snapshot 3.2).

The distinction between dominant and recessive X-linked traits is complicated by the phenomenon of X-chromosome inactivation introduced in Chapter 1. Most X-linked alleles are expressed on one of the two X chromosomes in any specific cell in a female. A female who is heterozygous for an X-linked trait will therefore express the mutant allele in approximately half her cells and the nonmutant allele in the other half. There may be some phenotypic expression of the trait based on the mutant allele being expressed in 50% of cells. Sometimes there is nonrandom X inactivation, that is, one X chromosome is active in more than 50% of cells. This can occur by chance, or may occur if there is a structural abnormality on one X chromosome that causes a cell that expresses this X to die due to severe genetic imbalance. If nonrandom X inactivation leads to a preponderance of cells expressing an X-linked mutant gene, then the individual will express the phenotype. Another way that a female can express the phenotype of an X-linked recessive condition is if she has only one X chromosome. This is the case for phenotypic females with Turner syndrome, who have only 45 chromosomes and only a single sex chromosome. We will revisit Turner syndrome elsewhere in this book.

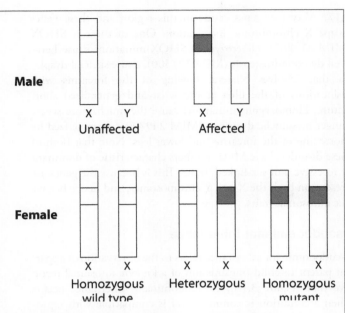

Figure 3.14 Males who carry a mutation on the X chromosome will express the phenotype associated with that mutation. Females can be homozygous for either the wild type or the mutant allele or can be heterozygous. Whether they express the mutant allele depends on whether it behaves as a recessive or a dominant trait.

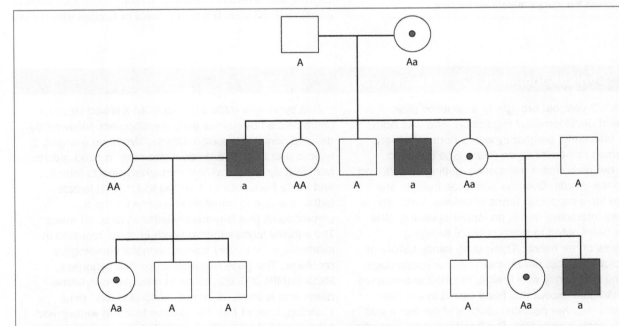

Figure 3.15 Pedigree illustrating X-linked recessive transmission. Note the absence of male-to-male transmission.

Y-Linked Inheritance

Pedigrees exhibiting Y-linked inheritance will show only male-to-male transmission, with only males being affected. Only a few such conditions exist. Mutations of Y-linked genes manifest primarily as male infertility and are therefore usually not passed on to future generations. This is changing, however, with the advent of assisted reproduction techniques that allow those with Y-linked genetic infertility to pass their genetic differences to future generations.

Of special note is the pseudoautosomal region, the small region of homology shared by the tips of the short and long arms of the X and Y chromosomes (Xp/Yp and Xq/Yq) (Figure 3.17). Very few genes reside in this region and these genes escape X chromosome inactivation. One of these is SHOX (MIM 312865). Heterozygous SHOX mutations cause Leri–Weil dyschondrosteosis (MIM 127300), a rare skeletal dysplasia that involves bilateral bowing of the forearms with dislocations of the ulna at the wrist and generalized short stature. Homozygous mutations cause the much more severe Langer mesomelic dwarfism (MIM 249700), characterized by shortening of the forearms and lower legs. Note that both of these disorders have MIM numbers characteristic of dominant or recessive, not sex-linked, traits. This is because the genes are present on both the X and Y chromosomes, and hence behave like autosomal traits.

Pseudodominant Inheritance

Pseudodominant inheritance refers to the observation of apparent parent-to-child transmission of a known autosomal recessive trait (Figure 3.18). Pseudodominant inheritance occurs when a condition is common and is compatible with reproduction. Vertical transmission occurs when one parent is homozygous and the other is heterozygous. An example is hemochromatosis (MIM 235200), a disorder in which there is excessive absorption of iron. Iron deposits in tissues such as the heart, liver, and pancreas, where it is toxic. Hemochromatosis is an autosomal recessive trait with a carrier frequency as high as one in 10 in individuals of Celtic ancestry. In this population, it would not be rare for a homozygous individual to have a heterozygous partner.

Digenic Inheritance

Digenic inheritance is a relatively recently recognized form of genetic transmission. It was first noted in families with the eye

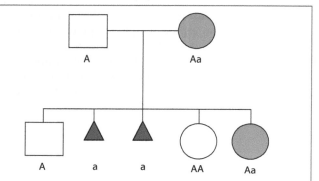

Figure 3.16 Pedigree illustrating X-linked dominant transmission with male lethality. Only females are affected. Males who inherit the mutant allele a die in utero.

 Clinical Snapshot 3.2   Rett Syndrome

Emma is a 3 year old brought to a genetics clinic because of developmental regression. She was born after an uneventful pregnancy with a normal delivery, and seemed to be well as an infant. She began to achieve her early motor milestones, getting to walk and saying a few words. Over the past year, though, she seems to have slipped in terms of development. She is much less interactive and is no longer speaking. She also has been noted to make unusual wringing movements of her hands. There is no family history of similar problems, but her mother had one miscarriage before the pregnancy with Emma. Physical examination is unremarkable except that head size is in the 10th centile, whereas her pediatric records show that it was in the 50th centile a year ago. The hand wringing is readily evident. A clinical diagnosis of Rett syndrome is made.

Rett syndrome (MIM 312750) is an X-linked disorder characterized by normal early development, followed by developmental regression. Compulsive hand wringing is typical, and there is a gradual decrease in head growth rate. Rett syndrome almost exclusively affects females, and has a frequency of 1:10000 to 1:15000 female births. It is due to mutation in a gene on the X chromosome that is generally lethal in affected males. The lethality leads either to death in utero, resulting in miscarriage, or to very severe neonatal neurological problems. The gene responsible for Rett syndrome, MECP2 (MIM 300005), binds to methylated cytosine bases and is involved in methylation-induced gene silencing. Loss of MECP2 function leads to widespread gene dysregulation, which underlies the neurological phenotype.

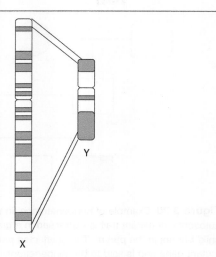

Figure 3.17 Regions of homology on the short and long arms of the X and Y chromosomes are referred to as pseudoautosomal regions. The X and Y pair in this region at their short arms and long arms. Genes in the pseudoautosomal region of the X are not subject to X-chromosome inactivation.

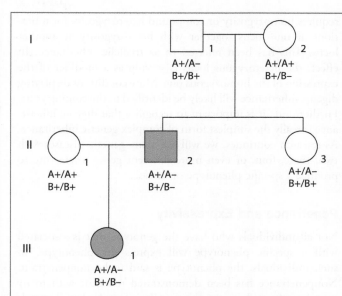

Figure 3.19 Digenic inheritance. Individual I-1 is heterozygous for a mutation in gene A (A–), and I-2 is heterozygous for a mutation in gene B (B–). One of their children, II-2, inherits A– from father and B– from mother, and, being doubly heterozygous, is affected. Sibling II-3 is heterozygous only for A– and is not affected. A child of II-2, III-1, inherits both A– and B– from her father and is also affected.

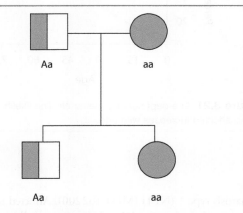

Figure 3.18 Pseudodominant inheritance. A heterozygous male and homozygous female transmit a recessive disorder to their daughter, giving the appearance of dominant transmission. This is most likely to occur when the mutant allele is common in the population.

disorder retinitis pigmentosa (RP) (MIM 268000), in children of parents who each carried a mutation in different RP-associated genes, ROM1 (MIM 180721) and peripherin (MIM 170710) (Figure 3.19). Both parents had normal vision, as one would expect, since ROM1 and peripherin typically cause RP only when an individual is homozygous for mutated alleles. Offspring who were double heterozygotes, however, developed RP.

With digenic inheritance, normal parents, one of whom carries a "gene A" mutation and the other a "gene B" mutation, will have a one-in-four risk of having a child who inherits both gene A and gene B mutations and will express the mutant phenotype. For the affected generation, inheritance may appear like an autosomal recessive trait (affected sibs, unaffected parents, and one-in-four recurrence risk). An affected child will have a one-in-four chance of passing on both alleles (gene A and B mutations), but transmission will appear as vertical (dominant).

Known examples of digenic inheritance include RP, holoprosencephaly (MIM 236100), hereditary hearing impairment (MIM 220290), one form of Antley–Bixler syndrome (abnormal formation of the skull and facial features, and developmental delay) (MIM 207410), and autosomal dominant familial exudative vitreoretinopathy (MIM 133780). A variation on this theme has been discovered in some individuals with Bardet–Biedl syndrome (MIM 209900). This disorder is characterized by obesity, retinitis pigmentosum, and renal anomalies, among other features, and is inherited as an autosomal recessive trait. There are several distinct genes that can cause Bardet–Biedl syndrome. In some cases, the disorder requires homozygosity or compound heterozygosity for mutations at one locus together with heterozygosity at another locus. This has been referred to as triallelic inheritance. In effect, the heterozygous locus is serving as a modifier of the expression of the homozygous one. More conditions displaying digenic inheritance will likely be identified in the coming years. Furthermore, it is important to recognize that digenic inheritance is really the simplest form of complex genetic inheritance. As research continues, we will see many genetic diseases with two, three, four, or even more different genes interacting to produce a specific phenotype or disease.

Penetrance and Expressivity

Not all individuals who have the genotype that is associated with a specific phenotype will express the phenotype. In such individuals, the phenotype is said to be nonpenetrant. Nonpenetrance has been demonstrated to occur with many genetic traits and can be most easily inferred when a grandparent and child have a disorder that does not appear to be expressed in the parent (Figure 3.20). In deciding whether a person is nonpenetrant for a genetic trait, it is important to define the phenotype carefully and examine the individual for all clinical manifestations of the condition. Some individuals will be very mildly affected, so the phenotype might escape detection unless a careful examination is performed.

Sometimes a rate of penetrance will be specified for a disorder. This rate applies to a population, not to an individual. For example, if 60% of individuals who carry a mutant gene express the phenotype, the rate of penetrance is 60%. A particular individual, however, either expresses the phenotype or does not. The individual is either penetrant or nonpenetrant; it does not make sense to speak in terms of partial penetrance, although the person may have mild expression of the trait.

Some disorders display age-dependent penetrance. These are typically adult-onset disorders, where the likelihood of a phenotype in a person with the mutation increases with age. An example is Huntington disease (MIM 143100), a dominantly inherited neurodegenerative disorder in which there is a progressive dementia and movement disorder. Virtually all mutation carriers will express the disorder if they live long enough, but children are very rarely affected (Figure 3.21). It is important to realize that clinical evaluation of young children at risk for disorders that display age-dependent penetrance does not provide a reliable indication of whether they have inherited the disorder.

Penetrance sometimes is confused with another genetic term, expressivity. Expressivity refers to the degree of phenotypic expression of a genetic trait. Many genetic traits exhibit a wide range of expressivity, which means that the characteristics of affected individuals differ from person to person. This is illustrated by the autosomal dominant disorder neurofi-

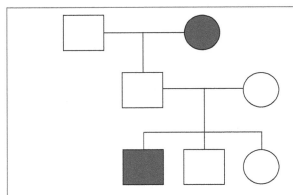

Figure 3.20 Example of nonpenetrance, in which an autosomal dominant trait is expressed in a grandparent and child but not in the parent. The unaffected parent must carry the mutant gene and is said to be nonpenetrant.

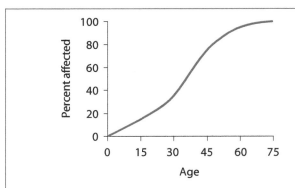

Figure 3.21 Age-dependent penetrance. The likelihood of being affected increases with age.

bromatosis type 1 (NF1) (MIM 162200). Affected individuals develop tumors along peripheral nerves, as well as patches of brown pigmentation on the skin (café-au-lait spots). Other features include bone deformities, learning disabilities, and brain tumors, but manifestations vary widely from person to person, even within the same family. Some people have innumerable skin tumors and life-threatening malignant growths, whereas others have only a few skin spots. NF1 exhibits a wide range of expressivity, yet the penetrance is high: Virtually all persons who carry the NF1 gene mutation express at least some signs of the disorder.

Genetic Heterogeneity

We have already encountered situations in which a single phenotype is caused by mutation in multiple distinct genes (e.g., retinitis pigmentosum and deafness). This is an example of locus heterogeneity. It reflects the fact that genes whose products participate in specific biological pathways or functions can result in similar phenotypes when mutated. Often, it is not possible to determine which gene is responsible for a phenotype solely by analyzing the phenotype. This is the case, for example, with deafness. There are dozens of genes that can cause deafness, and the phenotype for most of these is the same – lack of hearing. In some cases there may be distinct but overlapping phenotypes such as can be seen in Pendred syndrome (MIM 274600), which causes deafness and goiter, or Waardenburg syndrome (MIM 193500), which causes deafness and characteristic facial features. Another example of locus heterogeneity occurs with café-au-lait macules. For example, multiple café-au-lait macules can be seen in NF1, which causes multiple café-au-lait macules, skinfold freckling, and neurofibromas; Legius syndrome (MIM 611431), which causes multiple café-au-lait macules and skinfold freckling; and McCune–Albright syndrome (MIM 174800), which causes large café-au-lait macules, precocious puberty, and bone abnormalities.

There is a second form of genetic heterogeneity, referred to as allelic heterogeneity. A specific phenotype may result from mutation in a specific gene, but the exact mutation may differ from one affected individual to another. Sometimes the phenotypes due to specific mutations can be distinguished from one another; sometimes not. Indeed, in some cases, different mutations in the same gene can give totally different conditions. For example, specific mutations in the RET (MIM 164761) gene give rise to Hirschsprung disease (MIM 142623), a disorder in which there is aberrant migration of ganglion cells in the intestine that leads to intestinal obstruction. Other mutations in this same gene cause multiple endocrine neoplasia type 2 (MEN2, also known as phenochromocytoma and amyloid-producing medullary thyroid carcinoma, or PTC syndrome) (MIM 171400). Allelic heterogeneity is very common in genetic disorders. In autosomal recessive disorders, the two mutant alleles may differ from one another; this is referred to as compound heterozygosity. To some extent, allelic heterogeneity contributes to variable expression of a specific phenotype. Another major contributor is the occurrence of genetic modifiers, that is, alleles at other loci that contribute to expression of the phenotype.

Mutation and Mosaicism

Some mutations have existed in the population a long time, and they segregate through families for multiple generations. There are instances, however, where an individual represents the first occurrence of a new mutation in the family. This is especially apparent in completely penetrant dominant traits, where a child may be affected but neither parent displays the phenotype. It is presumed that the mutation has occurred in the sperm or egg cell that formed the child. We

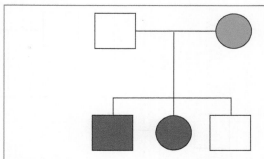

Figure 3.22 The mother of the two affected children is a mosaic for the mutation. She does not show signs of the disorder, or signs may be exceptionally mild or limited to a restricted region of the body. If she is a germline mosaic, only egg cells would carry the mutation.

considered the phenomenon of new mutation in Chapter 2, where we noted that there is a slightly increased risk of new mutation as a function of advanced paternal, but not maternal, age.

There are two special instances of new mutation that deserve mention (Figure 3.22). One is germline mosaicism, in which the mutation occurs during germ cell development and may involve multiple sperm or egg cells. This is of importance because an individual with germline mosaicism is at risk of having more than one affected child in spite of not being affected with the trait him or herself. The other phenomenon is somatic mosaicism. Here, the mutation occurs during early embryonic development, so the individual has multiple cells with or without the mutation. Such individuals may express mild manifestations of the phenotype, or may express the phenotype in a restricted region of the body. If the mutation is present in the germline, there is a risk of having affected children.

Genomic Imprinting

We have encountered the phenomenon of genomic imprinting in Chapter 1, wherein some genes are expressed only from the maternal or paternal copy. If a mutant gene is imprinted, the phenotype will be expressed only in offspring who inherit the gene from the parent whose copy is expressed. That parent, however, may not be affected if he or she inherited the mutation from the parent whose copy is not expressed. For example, familial paragangliomas (MIM 168000) are inherited as an autosomal dominant trait with an imprinting effect. The tumors arise from autonomic ganglia located at various sites in the body. The trait tends to be expressed only when inherited from the father. The responsible gene, succinate dehydrogenase complex subunit D (SDHD) (MIM 602690), is inactivated in the female germline and therefore expressed only from the paternal copy. Looking at a pedigree (Figure

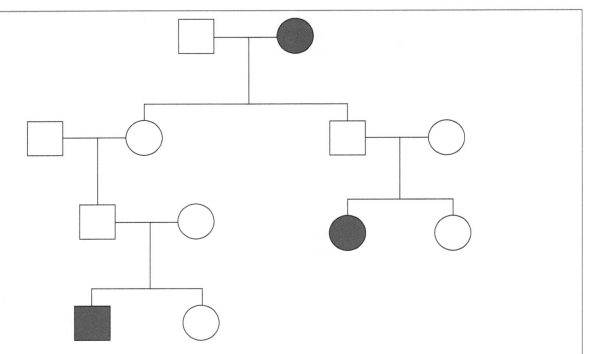

Figure 3.23 Pedigree of family with hereditary paragangliomas, in which the mutant gene is expressed only if inherited from the father. Examples of apparent nonpenetrance are due to inheritance of the mutation from a female.

3.23), the trait appears to skip generations if it is transmitted from a female.

Another example of a condition that is caused by an imprinted gene is Angelman syndrome (MIM 105830), which results from deficient expression of the maternally inherited UBE3A (MIM 601623) allele on chromosome 15. Affected individuals typically have intellectual disability, absent or limited speech, abnormal gait, and seizures. There are several mechanisms that can lead to disruption of the maternal UBE3A allele (see also Chapter 6), including deletion of maternal chromosome 15, paternal uniparental disomy of chromosome 15, mutation of the UBE3A gene, or an abnormality of the imprinting center (which is important in resetting the parental imprint during gametogenesis). Either deletion or abnormal methylation (epigenetic modification) of the imprinting center can lead to an inherited form of Angelman syndrome. The pedigree of a family with Angelman syndrome secondary to an abnormality of the imprinting center may resemble that of an autosomal dominant condition with nonpenetrance because the condition will be expressed only if inherited from the mother (Fig. 3.24).

Triplet Repeat Disorders and Anticipation

It has long been recognized that there is a set of genetic disorders in which signs and symptoms tend to be more severe and have earlier age of onset from generation to generation. This phenomenon is referred to as anticipation. An example is the muscle disorder myotonic dystrophy (MIM 160900). Affected individuals have muscle weakness and difficulty with muscle relaxation after a sustained period of contraction. The condition is transmitted as an autosomal dominant trait and tends to become more severe as the gene mutation is passed from generation to generation.

The basis for anticipation was unknown for a long time, and some doubted that the phenomenon was real, attributing it to bias of ascertainment – the disorder in a family would go unnoticed until it was brought to attention by a severely affected, young family member. The true explanation came to light with the discovery of a group of disorders associated with triplet repeat expansions in a variety of genes.

Many genes include regions of simple sequence repeats – dinucleotides, trinucleotides, and so on. The exact number of repeats in a specific gene may differ from one individual to another, usually with no impact on gene function. There is a subset of these genes, however, with trinucleotide repeats in which expansion of the number of repeats beyond a threshold leads to abnormal gene function (Figure 3.25). In myotonic dystrophy, the repeat expansion occurs near the 3' end of the gene. The region with the triplet repeat encodes a segment of messenger RNA (mRNA) that binds a nuclear protein. Expansion of the CTG (represented as CUG in the RNA)

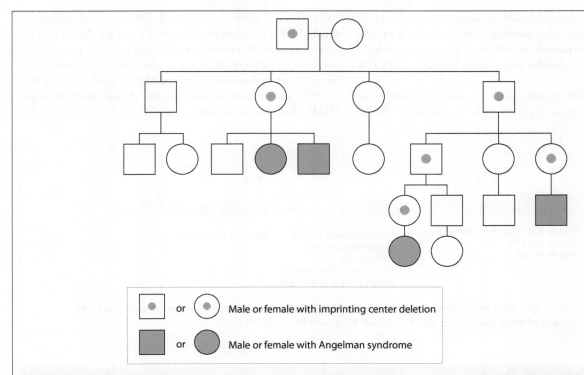

Figure 3.24 Pedigree of a family with Angelman syndrome in which the imprinting center deletion is expressed only if inherited from the mother. This is an example of apparent nonpenetrance due to inheritance of the imprinting center deletion from a male.

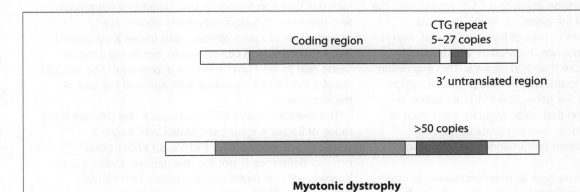

Figure 3.25 There is a CTG repeat expansion in the 3′ untranslated region of the gene that encodes the protein involved in myotonic dystrophy. The repeat may be 5–27 copies in the general population, but having an expansion in excess of 50 copies is associated with myotonic dystrophy.

repeat in this region causes binding of excessive protein, leading to dysfunction of this gene product, which encodes a muscle cell membrane ion channel, as well as of other gene products encoded by RNA molecules that would normally bind this nuclear protein.

All known triplet repeat expansion disorders affect the nervous system (Figure 3.26). Fragile X syndrome (MIM 300624) is a form of X-linked intellectual disability in which there is deficient production of a protein due to a CGG expansion near the promoter region that causes hypermethylation and consequent silencing of the gene (Hot Topic 3.1). There is a set of disorders, including Huntington disease (MIM 143100) and various forms of spinocerebellar ataxia (multiple MIM), that are due to CAG expansion in an exon within dif-

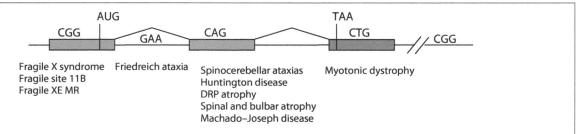

Figure 3.26 Generic gene with three exons and two introns showing the location of triplet repeats in genes associated with neurological disorders. Each of these disorders is due to a repeat expansion in a different gene.

ⓘ Hot Topic 3.1 Fragile X–Associated Tremor Ataxia Syndrome

Fragile X syndrome (MIM 300624) is a form of X-linked intellectual disability. It is called fragile X because of a tendency for the tip of the long arm of the X chromosome to be broken off from the chromosome when chromosomes are analyzed cytologically. It is due to a triplet repeat expansion in the gene FMR1 (MIM 309550). The expansion involves a CGG repeat near the promoter region of the gene. Normally, there are approximately 15–45 copies of the CGG repeat, with no phenotypic consequence. Individuals with fragile X syndrome have more than 200 repeats. This expansion is associated with methylation of the promoter region and inactivation of the gene. The FMR1 protein is an RNA-binding protein that helps regulate translation of transcripts for dendritic-forming proteins, thereby preventing unregulated and uncontrolled dendritic formation.

Fragile X syndrome is most often expressed in males, but some females express the phenotype if a high proportion of activated X chromosomes contain the expanded allele. Expansion to full mutation occurs from preexisting premutation alleles. These alleles contain 55–200 repeats. The expanded size tends to be unstable during meiosis, leading to expansion to full mutation. Expansion occurs only in female meiosis, so premutation males do not transmit full-mutation alleles to their daughters.

Premutation female carriers do not have features of fragile X syndrome, but those with larger expansions (typically >80) can have abnormal phenotypes. These include psychiatric disturbances and premature ovarian failure. The mechanisms that underlie these changes are not known. Premutation males are at risk for fragile X–associated tremor and ataxia syndrome (FXTAS), which also affects some females. The syndrome includes intention tremor, ataxia, peripheral neuropathy, and dementia. Affected individuals usually are grandfathers of males affected with fragile X syndrome. Because of this, the condition was not recognized as being due to the FMR1 gene for a long time. The risk of developing FXTAS increases with age and the size of the expansion.

The mechanisms of FXTAS appear to be different from those of fragile X syndrome. Males with fragile X syndrome do not develop FXTAS, so FMR1 gene product deficiency is not the mechanism. Unlike fragile X males with full mutations, the males with FXTAS express their FMR1 gene at aberrantly high levels, not low levels. It has been proposed that the excessive number of CGG repeats in FMR1 premutation transcripts binds to RNA-binding proteins, depleting the pool of these proteins and preventing their interaction with other transcripts (Figure 3.27). The protein–RNA complexes are then degraded in the proteosome, leading to intranuclear inclusion bodies that are seen in the brain cells of males with FXTAS.

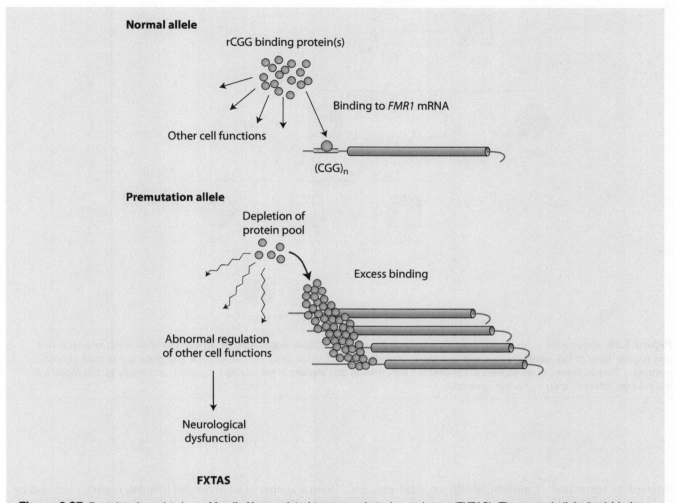

Normal allele

rCGG binding protein(s)

Binding to *FMR1* mRNA

Other cell functions

(CGG)n

Premutation allele

Depletion of
protein pool

Excess binding

Abnormal regulation
of other cell functions

Neurological
dysfunction

FXTAS

Figure 3.27 Postulated mechanism of fragile X–associated tremor and ataxia syndrome (FXTAS). The normal allele (top) binds an RNA-binding protein at the CGG repeat site, and normal FMRP is produced. The binding protein also interacts with other mRNA species. In individuals with a premutation allele, increased numbers of transcripts with long CCG tracts bind excessive amounts of protein, depleting the pools required for other cellular functions. The protein–FMR1 complex is complexed with ubiquitin and is degraded in the proteosome. (Redrawn from Hagerman and Hagerman 2004.)

ferent genes that leads to a polyglutamine repeat expansion in the encoded proteins. Friedreich ataxia (MIM 229300) is due to a GAA repeat expansion within an intron, which causes abnormal mRNA processing. It is the only one of the triplet repeat expansion disorders that is inherited as an autosomal recessive trait.

How does triplet repeat expansion lead to anticipation? Understanding this requires knowledge of two points. Firstly, the larger the repeat is, the more severe the disorder, and the earlier the age of onset. Secondly, the larger the repeat, the more unstable it is, and hence the greater the chance that it will expand further as it is passed from generation to generation. This is illustrated for myotonic dystrophy in Figure 3.28.

Mitochondrial Inheritance

It used to be assumed that the entire DNA complement of a cell was contained within the nucleus, but it has become clear that this is not the case. DNA is also found within another cellular organelle, the mitochondrion. Mitochondria are responsible for the generation of adenosine triphosphate (ATP) via aerobic metabolism, and each mitochondrion contains multiple copies of a double-stranded, circular DNA molecule of 16 569 base pairs (Figure 3.29). This DNA encodes 13 peptides that are subunits of proteins required for oxidative phosphorylation. In addition, there is a complete set of 22 transfer RNAs and two ribosomal RNAs. These RNAs are

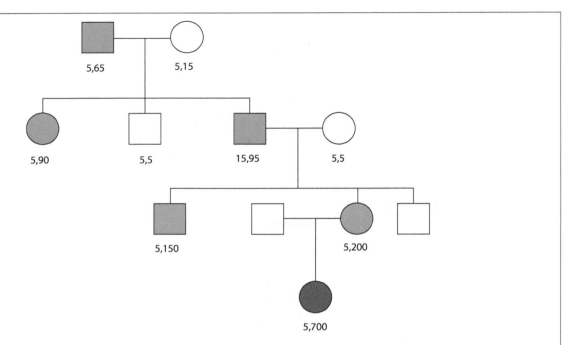

Figure 3.28 Anticipation in myotonic dystrophy. The number of CTG repeats is indicated below each symbol. Each individual has one normal allele of five repeats. In the first generation, the affected individual has a 65-repeat allele that gives rise to mild myotonic dystrophy. This increases to 95 repeats in his affected son, then to 200 repeats in his affected daughter, and finally to 700 repeats in the severely affected child in the last generation.

involved in translation of mitochondrially encoded proteins within the mitochondrion.

The process of oxidative phosphorylation requires more than 60 proteins. Most are encoded in the nucleus and are transported into the mitochondrion from the cytoplasm. Only a minority of the mitochondrial proteins is encoded in the mitochondrial genome and synthesized within the mitochondrion. The structure of the mitochondrial genome bears more resemblance to prokaryotic than to eukaryotic genomes. The genes lack introns and are transcribed as polycistronic messages from two promoters. The spaces between genes consist of tRNAs, whose excision from the polycistronic message releases the individual gene transcripts. There are also two sites for initiation of DNA synthesis, one on each strand of the double helix.

A number of clinical disorders have been identified that are due to mutations within mitochondrial genes (Clinical Snapshot 3.3; Table 3.1). As might be expected, these traits are associated with failure of mitochondrial energy production. Mitochondrial DNA exhibits two critical differences from the nuclear genome that account for unusual patterns of inheritance of mitochondrial genetic traits. These are maternal transmission and heteroplasmy. A pedigree displaying maternal transmission is shown in Figure 3.30. The trait is transmitted from a mother to all of her children, but is not transmitted by males. This is due to the fact that essentially all of the mitochondria are maternally inherited. At the time of fertilization only, the sperm nucleus enters the egg. Mitochondria in the sperm are shed prior to fertilization. There may be minor exceptions to this rule but, for the most part, mitochondrial traits are maternally inherited.

Although all of the children of a woman with a mitochondrial mutation might be expected to inherit the mutation, there is usually a wide range of variation in expression. This is due to the phenomenon of heteroplasmy. Unlike the nuclear genome, which is represented by one complete copy per cell, there are hundreds of mitochondrial DNA molecules in each cell. These mitochondria separate passively when a cell divides, in contrast to the orderly separation of chromosomes in the nuclear genome during cell division. If some of the mitochondria contain a mutation and others do not, the result can be unequal distribution of mutant and nonmutant mitochondria to daughter cells (Figure 3.31). During egg cell production, this can result in different oocytes receiving widely differing numbers of mutant or nonmutant mitochondrial DNA molecules, which translates into offspring who inherit the mutation to different degrees. In somatic cells it results in some

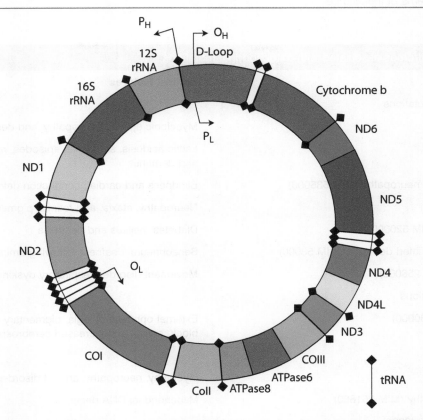

Figure 3.29 Map of the mitochondrial genome. ND6, ND5, ND4, ND4L, ND3, ND2, and ND1 are components of complex I. COIII, COII, and COI are components of complex IV. Adenosine triphosphatase (ATPase) 6 and ATPase 8 are components of complex V. Cytochrome b is part of complex III. O$_H$ and O$_L$ are the origins of replication of the heavy and light strands, respectively; P$_H$ and P$_L$ are promoters for these strands.

⊙ Clinical Snapshot 3.3 MELAS

Evan is a 12 year old with severe developmental delay and seizures. His seizures began around 2 years of age and have been difficult to control with medication. Although his early developmental milestones were normal, he has gradually lost developmental skills and has had a number of sudden episodes of neurological deficits that have been diagnosed as strokes. He has mild, diffuse muscle weakness, as well as partial loss of use of his right arm and leg since one of the strokes. A recent blood test during a stroke-like episode revealed a high lactic acid level. No one else in the family is similarly affected, though his sister has had several seizures, and his mother has a history of severe migraine headaches. A diagnosis of MELAS is made.

MELAS (MIM 540000) is an acronym for mitochondrial encephalomyopathy, lactic acidosis, and stroke-like episodes. The disorder may present at any time in life with progressive neurological deterioration and seizures. There are events in which there is sudden onset of neurological deficit that have the time course of strokes.

The mechanism is not the typical vascular occlusion of strokes, though the exact pathophysiology is not known. Lactic acid tends to accumulate in the blood, especially during stroke-like episodes. Lactic acid is a byproduct of the failure of aerobic metabolism in the mitochondria. Various mitochondrial mutations can be responsible for MELAS. The most common is a mutation in the mitochondrial gene for leucine tRNA (MIM 590050). MELAS follows maternal transmission, as expected for a mitochondrial trait, but there can be a wide range of variable expression within a family. This is accounted for by heteroplasmy for the mitochondrial mutation. Some individuals inherit only a small proportion of mutant mitochondria and are mildly affected or entirely escape clinical signs. Others inherit a larger proportion and are more severely affected. Furthermore, the specific signs and symptoms may depend on the proportion of mutant and nonmutant mitochondria in specific tissues, such as brain or muscle.

Table 3.1 Major syndromes associated with mitochondrial mutations.

Syndrome	Clinical features
Mitochondrial point mutations	
MERRF (MIM 545000)	Myoclonic epilepsy, myopathy, and dementia
MELAS (MIM 540000)	Lactic acidosis, stroke-like episodes, myopathy, seizures, and dementia
Leber hereditary optic neuropathy (MIM 535000)	Blindness and cardiac conduction defects
NARP (MIM 551500)	Neuropathy, ataxia, and retinitis pigmentosa
Diabetes/deafness (MIM 520000)	Diabetes mellitus and deafness
Aminoglycoside-associated deafness (MIM 58000)	Sensorineural deafness following aminoglycoside exposure
Leigh syndrome (MIM 256000)	Movement disorder, respiratory dyskinesia, and regression
Deletions and duplications	
Kearns–Sayre (MIM 530000)	External ophthalmoplegia, pigmentary retinopathy, heart block, ataxia, and increased cerebrospinal fluid protein
Nuclear mutations	
MNGIE (MIM 603041)	Myopathy, neuropathy, and GI disorder
Fatal infantile neuropathy (MIM 251880)	Mitochondrial DNA depletion

Source: Shanske *et al.* (2001).

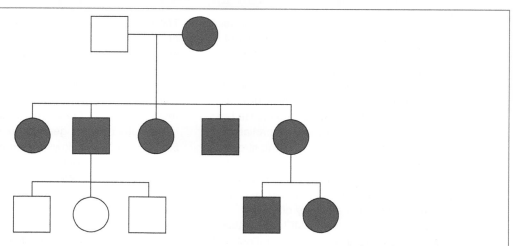

Figure 3.30 Maternal genetic transmission. An affected woman transmits the trait to all of her children. Affected men do not pass the trait to any of their offspring.

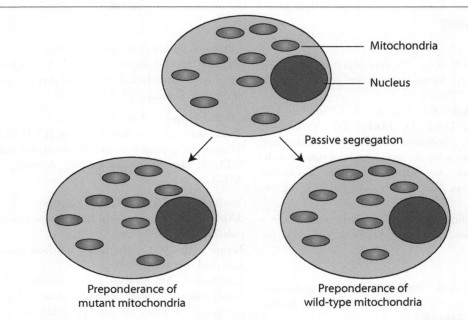

Figure 3.31 Concept of heteroplasmy. Both wild-type (copper) and mutant (blue) mitochondria are included in the hundreds of mitochondria in a cell. These mitochondria segregate passively when the cell divides. The proportions of mutant and wild-type mitochondria can change dramatically due to chance segregation. This can lead to variation in the proportion of affected mitochondria in different tissues or different individuals in a family.

tissues having a preponderance of mutant or nonmutant mitochondrial DNA molecules, and consequent tissue-specific effects of the mitochondrial mutation.

Conclusion

We have come a long way since the days of Mendel and Garrod, and now have an understanding of single-gene inheritance at the molecular level. With this increased understanding, however, we also have a new appreciation for the complexity of genetic systems. There are no true single-gene disorders – no gene acts in isolation to determine a phenotype without interacting with other genes and with the environment. We will consider multifactorial traits elsewhere in this book, and traditionally these have been considered separately from monogenic traits. This distinction is beginning to blur, however. All traits are complex traits; some involve the action of one or a few genes of major effect, and some a larger number of genes. Understanding how these networks function remains one of the challenges in research in genetics and is likely to be translated into further advances in diagnosis and treatment.

REFERENCES

Bennett RL, Steinhaus KA, Uhrich SB, O'Sullivan CK, Resta RG, Lochner-Doyle D, Markel DS, Vincent V, Hamanishi J 1995, "Recommendations for standardized human pedigree nomenclature: update and assessment of the recommendations of the National Society of Genetic Counselors", *American Journal of Human Genetics*, vol. 56, pp. 745–52.

Hagerman PJ, Hagerman RJ 2004, "The fragile X permutation: a maturing perspective", *American Journal of Human Genetics*, vol. 74, pp. 805–16.

Shanske AL, Shanske S, DiMauro S 2001, "The other human genome", *Archives of Pediatrics and Adolescent Medicine*, vol. 155, pp. 1210–16.

FURTHER READING

General References

Badano JL, Katsanis N 2002, "Beyond Mendel: an evolving view of human genetic disease transmission", *Nature Reviews Genetics*, vol. 3, pp. 779–89.

Bennett RL, Steinhaus KA, Uhrich SB, O'Sullivan CK, Resta RG, Lochner-Doyle D, Markel DS, Vincent V, Hamanishi J 1995, "Recommendations for standardized human pedigree nomenclature: update and assessment of the recommendations of the National Society of Genetic Counselors", *American Journal of Human Genetics*, vol. 56, pp. 745–52.

Guttmacher A, Collins FS 2002, "Genomic medicine – a primer", *New England Journal of Medicine*, vol. 347, pp. 1512–20.

Mosaicism

Youssoufian H, Pyeritz RE 2002, "Mechanisms and consequences of somatic mosaicism in humans", *Nature Reviews Genetics*, vol. 3, pp. 748–58.

Zlotogora J 1998, "Germ line mosaicism", *Human Genetics*, vol. 102, pp. 381–6.

Digenic Inheritance

Kajiwara K, Berson EL, Dryja TP 1994, "Digenic retinitis pigmentosa due to mutations at the unlinked peripherin/RDS and ROM1 loci", *Science*, vol. 164, pp. 1604–8.

Triplet Repeat Disorders

Everett CM, Wood NW 2004, "Trinucleotide repeats and neurodegenerative disease", *Brain*, vol. 127, pp. 2385–405.

Mitochondrial Genetics

Taylor RW, Turnbull DM 2005, "Mitochondrial DNA mutations in human disease", *Nature Reviews Genetics*, vol. 6, pp. 389–402.

Clinical Snapshot 3.1: Congenital Deafness

Nance WE 2003, "The genetics of deafness", *Mental Retardation and Developmental Disabilities Research Reviews*, vol. 9, pp. 109–19.

Clinical Snapshot 3.2: NF1

Ward BA, Gutmann DH 2005, "Neurofibromatosis 1: from lab bench to clinic", *Pediatric Neurology*, vol. 32, pp. 221–8.

Clinical Snapshot 3.3: Rett Syndrome

Weaving LS, Ellaway CJ, Gecz J, Chritodoulou J 2005, "Rett syndrome: clinical review and genetic update", *Journal of Medical Genetics*, vol. 42, pp. 1–7.

Clinical Snapshot 3.4: MELAS

Thambisetty M, Newman NJ, Glass JD, Frankel MR 2002, "A practical approach to the diagnosis and management of MELAS: case report and review", *Neurologist*, vol. 8, pp. 302–12.

Methods 3.1: Taking a Family History

AMA Family History Tools, http://www.ama-assn.org/ama/pub/category/2380.html

Bennett RL 2004, "The family medical history", *Primary Care*, vol. 31, pp. 479–95.

Guttmacher AE, Collins FS, Carmona RH 2004, "The family history – more important than ever", *New England Journal of Medicine*, vol. 351, pp. 2333–6.

Ethical Implications 3.1: Family Ties

Taub S, Morin K, Spillman MA, Sade RM, Riddick FA, Council on Ethical and Judicial Affairs of the American Medical Association 2004, "Managing familial risk in genetic testing", *Genetic Testing*, vol. 8, pp. 356–9.

Hot Topic 3.1: FXTAS

Hagerman PJ, Hagerman RJ 2004, "The fragile X permutation: a maturing perspective", *American Journal of Human Genetics*, vol. 74, pp. 805–16.

Genomic Imprinting

Buiting K 2010, "Prader-Willi syndrome and Angelman syndrome", *American Journal of Medical Genetics, Part C*, vol. 154C, pp. 365–76.

Genetic Heterogeneity

Shah KN 2010, "The diagnostic and clinical significance of café-au-lait macules", *Pediatric Clinics of North America*, vol. 57, pp. 1131–53.

Find interactive self-test questions and additional resources for this chapter at **www.korfgenetics.com**.

Self-Assessment

Review Questions

3.1   You take a family history and obtain the pedigree shown in Figure 3.1Q. How would you counsel the family given this information?

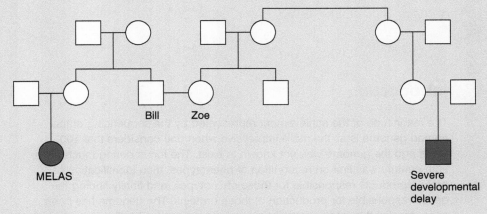

3.2   What is the most likely mode of inheritance represented in the pedigree in Figure 3.2Q?

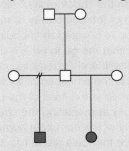

3.3   Individuals II-3 and II-4 wish to know the risk of having a child with an autosomal dominant disorder that affects I-2, II-1, and II-3 (see Figure 3.3Q). The penetrance of the disorder is 75%.

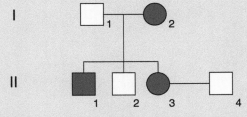

3.4   How could the pedigrees shown in Figure 3.4Q be explained by genetic imprinting?

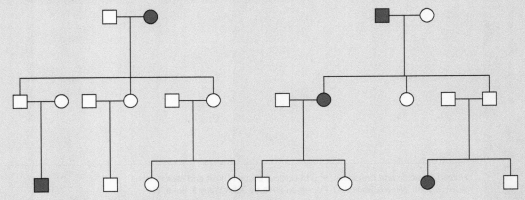

3.5   What is the genetic basis for the phenomenon of anticipation?

CHAPTER 4
The Human Genome

Introduction

The magnitude of the achievement represented by the sequencing of the human genome is all the more impressive when one considers that 100 years ago the genome was not known to exist. The focus during much of the 20th century was first on recognition of phenotypes, then identification of protein products responsible for those phenotypes, and finally finding the genes responsible for production of those proteins. The genome has been conceptualized by many metaphors, such as a parts list for the organism, a computer program, or even the "book of life." None of these quite capture the emerging appreciation of the complexity of the genome. We now know that only a small proportion is devoted to encoding the amino acid sequence of proteins. We also know that the genome is a dynamic system, constantly monitoring and repairing itself, and undergoing changes at multiple time scales – minutes to hours in the timespan of a cell cycle, years in the lifespan of an individual, and millennia at the level of the population and the species. We are a long way from fully appreciating the structure and function of the genome, but the availability of the complete human genome sequence has brought us to a point where the tools are at hand to explore the complexity of human biology with the promises of new appreciation for the physiology of health and disease and new approaches to diagnosis and treatment.

Human Genetics and Genomics, Fourth Edition. Bruce R. Korf and Mira B. Irons.
© 2013 John Wiley & Sons, Ltd. Published 2013 by John Wiley & Sons, Ltd.

Key Points

- Genes can be isolated by cloning in organisms such as bacteria and yeast. This provides purified DNA corresponding to a gene of interest that can be studied in detail.
- Genetic linkage analysis provides a means for mapping the genome using the frequency of recombination between loci as a measure of genetic distance.
- Linkage analysis in humans is accomplished by the calculation of lod scores.
- A variety of DNA sequence polymorphisms can be used as markers for linkage analysis.
- Positional cloning allows genes to be identified by first mapping the genes and then cloning the DNA within the mapped region until the gene of interest has been found.
- The Human Genome Project is an international effort that has succeeded in sequencing the human genome.
- The human genome includes around 23000 genes, but genes comprise less than 5% of the genome. There are many RNA transcripts that are not translated into protein.
- Multiple forms of repeated sequence are scattered throughout the genome.
- The ability to study the human genome has spawned new disciplines, including genomics, proteomics, and systems biology.

Gene Cloning

The possibility of determining the sequence of the human genome began with the ability to isolate specific genes. This technology, referred to as gene **cloning**, began to be developed in the 1970s. The basic goal is to isolate a specific segment of DNA so that it can be studied in great detail, including determination of its base sequence. DNA cloning is based on the construction of recombinant DNA molecules, inserting a fragment of interest, such as human DNA, into a vector that is capable of replication within a bacterial or yeast cell. Creation of recombinant molecules relies on the use of **restriction endonuclease**s that cut DNA at specific sequences of 3–8 bases. Some of these enzymes leave unpaired overhangs (Figure 4.1), so mixing human DNA cut by a restriction enzyme with vector DNA cut with the same enzyme allows hybrid molecules to form that can be "stitched" together with DNA ligase. A vector must be capable of being introduced into a host cell, such as a bacterium, and must be able to replicate itself within the host. The first vectors for such recombinant DNA experiments were plasmids, which consist of an origin of replication, one or more antibiotic resistance genes, and several unique cutting sites for various restriction enzymes that serve as points of insertion of foreign DNA. The antibiotic resistance genes allow selection of bacteria that have successfully taken up the vector. The plasmid vector accommodates only a small quantity of DNA (about 10000 base pairs, or 10kb). Very large fragments can be cloned in **yeast** or **bacterial artificial chromosomes** (YACs or BACs).

Initial cloning efforts focused on genes that encode proteins of known function. For example, the gene that encodes the enzyme tyrosinase (MIM 606933), involved in the synthesis

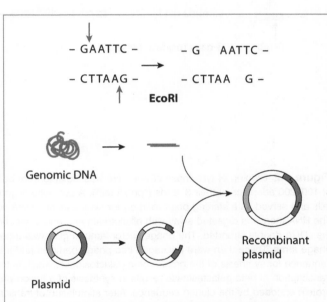

Figure 4.1 The restriction enzyme EcoRI recognizes the palindromic hexamer GAATTC and cleaves asymmetrically to result in non-base-paired ends. To create a recombinant plasmid, genomic DNA is cut into fragments with non-base-paired ends. A plasmid cloning vector is cut with the same enzyme, also producing non-base-paired ends. Mixing the two together permits hybrid molecules to be formed, which result in a double-stranded, closed circular molecule when the ends are joined with a DNA ligase. The two genes on the plasmid are antibiotic resistance genes, one of which is interrupted by the inserted DNA.

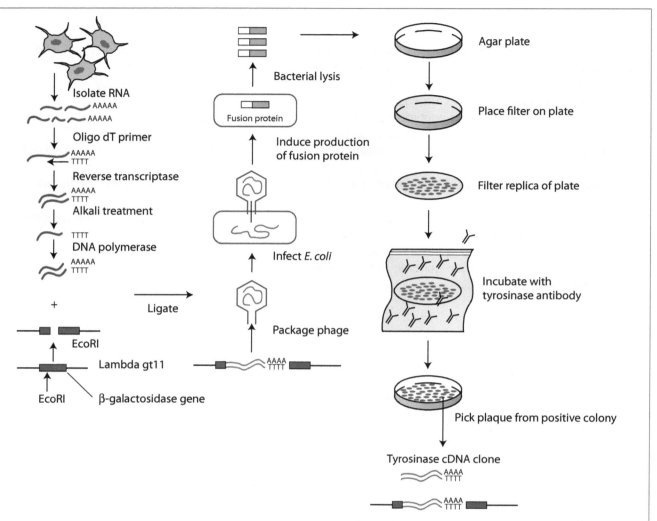

Figure 4.2 Cloning of tyrosinase cDNA. RNA was isolated from cells that express tyrosinase. Most mRNA molecules contain a "tail" of 100–200 adenines at their 3′ ends ("polyA tail"). A synthetic oligo dT sequence (a string of thymidines) was bound to these polyA tails and served as a starting point (primer) for synthesis of a DNA copy of the RNA (cDNA) using the enzyme reverse transcriptase. The RNA then was digested away with alkali treatment, and a second DNA copy made with the enzyme DNA polymerase, rendering the cDNA double stranded. The phage vector lambda gt11 was digested with EcoRI, and cDNA molecules were ligated with the phage arms. These then were packaged into phage particles and infected into *Escherichia coli* cells. Lambda gt11 contains a sequence for synthesis of the protein beta-galactosidase, which is located at the site into which foreign DNA is cloned. Stimulation of transcription of beta-galactosidase results in synthesis of a fusion protein consisting of part of beta-galactosidase and part of the protein encoded by the cloned sequence. After stimulation of transcription, bacteria were plated on agar and plaques of lysed bacteria were absorbed onto filters. The filters were incubated in a bag with tyrosinase antibody. The antibody became bound to tyrosinase on the filter, and the binding was detected with an immunologic staining reaction. This identified the clones containing tyrosinase cDNA, which then were isolated and used as a source of tyrosinase cDNA. (Source: Kwon *et al.* 1987.)

of the skin pigment melanin, was cloned in a bacteriophage vector (Figure 4.2). First, the entire coding sequence for the gene was cloned. This was accomplished using a **complementary DNA (cDNA) library** obtained from cells known to synthesize large quantities of melanin. Messenger RNA (mRNA) was isolated from these cells, and a DNA copy was made from the mRNA using the enzyme **reverse transcriptase**, which copies RNA into DNA. The resulting DNA sequences are referred to as cDNA. The cDNA segments were then randomly cloned into bacteriophages, which then were used to infect bacteria. The vectors were designed so that the inserted cDNA would be transcribed and translated into protein within the bacteria. Those that, by chance, had incorporated the tyrosinase cDNA could be identified using a tagged antibody to tyrosinase. The tyrosinase gene itself could then be cloned by using the cDNA to detect other bacteriophages that had incorporated genomic DNA sequences rather than cDNA. The tyrosinase cDNA was radioactively labeled, separated into single strands, and used to identify homologous genomic DNA sequences in the bacteriophage-infected bacterial colonies. The cloned DNA could then be sequenced (Methods 4.1), from which the amino acid sequence of the tyrosinase protein could be inferred from the genetic code.

A variety of similar approaches have been used with great success in cloning dozens of genes, but these approaches are limited to genes of known function. Most genes of medical interest are known through their associated phenotypes, and the gene products have been unknown, so different approaches are necessary to identify genes involved in these disorders. Beginning in the 1980s, an approach was introduced that is referred to as **positional cloning**, which has proved to be enormously successful. The approach is based on identification of a gene by cloning DNA at the site in the genome to which the gene has been mapped. To understand the approach, though, we first have to look at how gene mapping is done.

Gene Mapping

Approaches to gene mapping began to be developed during the early decades of the 20th century, initially through work with plants and other experimental organisms such as the fruit fly *Drosophila* and the mouse. The basic principle is that genes are linearly arrayed on the chromosome and that the order of genes is the same from one individual to another in a species. During meiosis, homologous chromosomes pair and may exchange segments. Although this does not alter the order of loci on the chromosome, it does result in changes in the specific alleles that are present on a particular copy of a chromosome (Figure 4.4). The set of specific alleles on the same DNA strand on a particular chromosome is referred to as a **haplotype**.

Linkage Analysis

The frequency of recombination between a pair of genes is a function of distance; the farther apart they are, the more often a crossover event will occur between them. If two genes are very close together, recombination between them will be rare. For extremely closely linked genes, alleles that are part of a haplotype tend to remain so from generation to generation (Figure 4.5). Only rarely will new combinations be created by crossing over.

The opposite situation is illustrated by genes that are located on different chromosomes. In this case, alleles segregate randomly to gametes. For an unlinked pair of loci, there is a 50% chance that the parental combination of alleles will be found in an offspring and a 50% chance that a nonparental combination will occur. Fifty percent **recombinant** and nonrecombinant genotypes is the outcome of random segregation (Figure 4.6).

Suppose that two genes are separated by a distance such that recombination occurs between them 10% of the time. On average, then, 10% of germ cells will be recombinant and 90% nonrecombinant. This expectation would be realized if a very large number of offspring were sampled. The ideal mating experiment matches a doubly heterozygous individual with a homozygous partner and samples an extremely large number of offspring. Such experiments are commonly done with fruit flies or mice but are not useful for mapping the human genome.

To circumvent this difficulty, a statistical approach has been developed to extract linkage information from smaller families. What is calculated is the relative likelihood (the odds) that a particular set of family information would be obtained if a pair of genes is linked rather than if they segregate randomly. For a family with four children, the chance of any combination of recombinant and nonrecombinant genotypes given nonlinkage (i.e., the result of random segregation) is $(1/2)(1/2)(1/2)(1/2) = 1/16$. (Note that birth order is ignored, since this factor will be the same in the numerator and denominator of the odds ratio.) The chance of seeing any combination of recombinant and nonrecombinant genotypes if the genes are linked depends on how closely they are located. For example, if the rate of recombination between a set of genes is 10%, then the probability of a recombinant individual is 0.1 and of a nonrecombinant individual is 0.9. In a family of four (Figure 4.7), the probability of seeing one recombinant and three nonrecombinant offspring if the rate of recombination is 10% is $(0.1)(0.9)(0.9)(0.9) = 0.0729$.

In this family of four with one recombinant and three nonrecombinant combinations of alleles, which is more likely: linkage with a recombination frequency of 10%, or nonlinkage? We can compare the relative likelihood of these two possibilities by creating an odds ratio. In this case, $0.0729/0.0625 = 1.167$; linkage is slightly favored over nonlinkage. The same can be done for other values of the frequency of recombination between the two genes. The frequency of recombination usually is expressed as a variable θ, the recombination fraction. At $\theta = 0$, the probability of linkage will be 0 if any recombinants occur at all, because at this value of θ, no recombination is possible. At a value of $\theta = 0.5$, the odds ratio will be 1, because 50% recombination is equivalent to nonlinkage. Between $\theta = 0$ and $\theta = 0.5$, the probability of linkage depends on family size and the number of recombinant and nonrecombinant individuals. A family with some recombinant individuals, but fewer than expected by random segregation, will be better explained by an intermediate value of θ: If θ is too low, few or no recombinants are expected, and if θ is too high, more are expected.

Although this approach can help extract data from small families, there is a limit to what can be learned. In a family of

Methods 4.1   DNA Sequencing

Determination of DNA sequence has been a critical component of the study of the structure and function of individual genes, and was of key importance in the Human Genome Project. The most commonly used approach is illustrated in Figure 4.3. A DNA synthesis reaction is carried out in a reaction mixture that contains a primer sequence, DNA polymerase, the four nucleotides, and a set of four dideoxynucleotides, each labeled with a different fluorescent color. As new DNA is synthesized from the template, on some strands a dideoxynucleotide will be incorporated in the place of a deoxynucleotide. This will cause synthesis of that strand to cease. The reaction mixture is then subjected to electrophoresis in a polyacrylamide gel, separating the partially synthesized strands by size. The gel is scanned with a laser and the color of emitted light is analyzed, indicating the size of each strand that ends in a particular dideoxynucleotide.

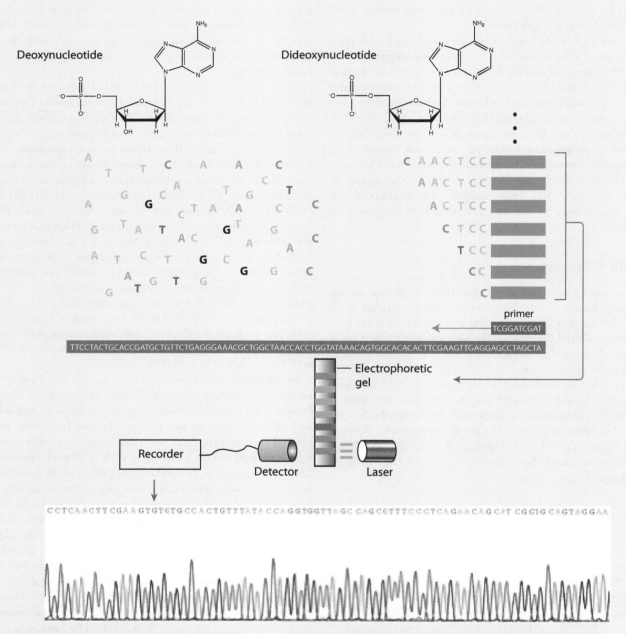

Figure 4.3 DNA sequencing. A DNA synthesis reaction is carried out using a DNA primer that binds to the segment to be sequenced. DNA polymerase is added along with the four nucleotides, including some dideoxynucleotides, each labeled with a specific fluorescent dye. This is indicated by the colored nucleotides in the figure. As DNA synthesis proceeds, sometimes a dideoxynucleotide will be incorporated, causing synthesis of that strand to cease, as there is no 3′ hydroxyl group to bind the next nucleotide. The collection of fragments is then separated according to size by electrophoresis, and the gel is scanned with a laser to detect the color of the fragment, determined by the terminal fluorescently labeled dideoxynucleotide. A readout consists of the different colors of each fragment, which indicates the base sequence.

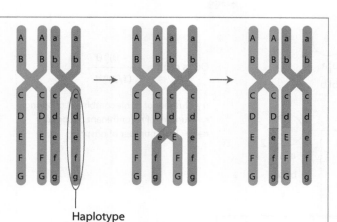

Figure 4.4 Crossing over during meiotic pairing of homologous chromosomes. Although the relative locations of genes A, B, C, D, E, F, and G are not changed, the particular sets of alleles on the two chromosomes change. Initially, alleles E, F, and G were on one member of the pair, and e, f, and g on the other. After the crossover, A, B, C, and D are together on one chromosome arm along with e, f, and g, and a, b, c, and d are on the other arm with E, F, and G. A set of alleles together on the same chromosome arm is referred to as a haplotype.

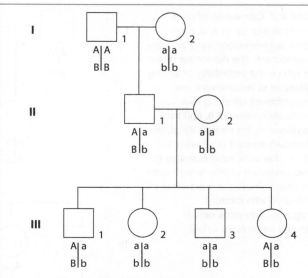

Figure 4.5 Tight linkage between a pair of loci, with no recombination between them. Individual II-1 is heterozygous at the two loci; his partner is doubly homozygous. Each offspring in generation III gets a and b from the mother and either AB or ab from the father. None gets the recombinant Ab or aB from the father.

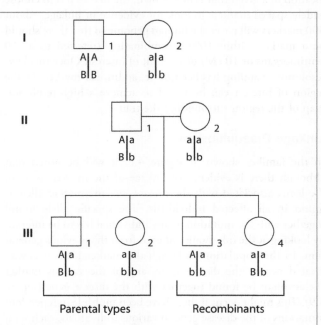

Figure 4.6 Random segregation of alleles at two unlinked loci. Individual II-1 is doubly heterozygous and produces four types of sperm: AB, Ab, aB, and ab. Each of these four combinations is represented in one of the offspring, resulting in equal numbers of parental (nonrecombinant) and recombinant offspring.

four, chance segregation of alleles can lead to no recombinant offspring even if genes are unlinked. There is no substitute for the statistical power of large numbers. How can this be achieved?

One way is to pool data from many families – in effect, to consider many different sibships as if they were all one large sibship. In figuring the probability of linkage or nonlinkage for a family, each child is viewed as an independent statistical event, and the total probability of the recombinants and non-recombinants in the sibship is the product of the individual probabilities for each offspring. If data from multiple sibships are obtained, the probability for each offspring can be multiplied together. This becomes unwieldy if many individuals are studied, but recall that adding logarithms is the equivalent of multiplying the numbers to which they correspond. Therefore, the odds ratio can be calculated for each sibship, the fraction converted to a logarithm, and then the log of the odds ratio added from family to family to obtain a final log of the odds ratio for the entire dataset. "Log of the odds" is abbreviated with the acronym lod. **Lod scores** are calculated family by family for multiple values of θ and then are summed for each value of θ. How high does a lod score need to be to indicate probable linkage or nonlinkage of a pair of genes? Evidence for linkage generally is accepted when a lod score is 3 or greater, indicating at least a 1000:1 odds ratio favoring linkage. Lod scores of −2 or less are accepted as evidence against linkage, indicating at least a 100:1 ratio favoring nonlinkage. The value

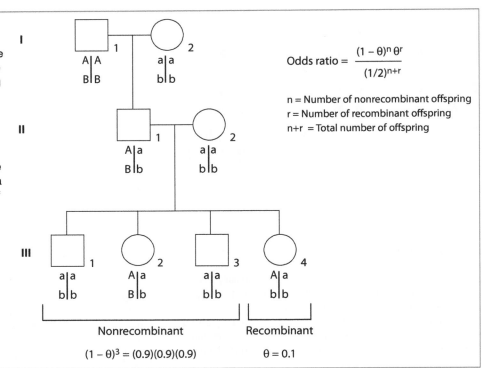

Figure 4.7 Calculation of odds ratio. In this sibship of four, three children are nonrecombinant and one is recombinant. The numerator of the odds ratio is the probability of seeing this number of recombinant and nonrecombinant offspring at a recombination value of θ, and the denominator is the probability given random segregation (equivalent to θ = 0.5). This odds ratio indicates the relative likelihood of this family's data given recombination at a set value of θ compared with random segregation. The odds ratio is computed for multiple values of θ.

$$\text{Odds ratio} = \frac{(1-\theta)^n \, \theta^r}{(1/2)^{n+r}}$$

n = Number of nonrecombinant offspring
r = Number of recombinant offspring
n+r = Total number of offspring

Nonrecombinant
$(1-\theta)^3 = (0.9)(0.9)(0.9)$

Recombinant
$\theta = 0.1$

of θ at which the peak lod score is obtained is taken as the maximum likelihood value of θ (Figure 4.8).

There is one important caution that must be applied to the study of linkage by pooling data from many families. This is the possibility of genetic heterogeneity. If different genes at different locations are responsible for a trait in different families, no one marker will be linked to them all. Data favoring linkage in one family will be canceled out by data favoring nonlinkage in another, with the net result that random segregation will be favored. It is always safer to analyze linkage data from individual large families to avoid the pitfall of genetic heterogeneity.

Genetic Polymorphism and Linkage

The search for linkage requires that individuals be heterozygous for the two loci that are being mapped. If one locus is associated with a phenotype such as a genetic disorder, the heterozygous individual is either affected with a dominant trait or a carrier for a recessive one. It is unlikely, however, that there will be another gene locus nearby that can also be assessed phenotypically. The advent of DNA markers, however, has provided the ability to map almost any genetic trait anywhere in the genome. The fundamental property of a useful genetic marker is that there must be at least two alleles, and these alleles must be common enough so that heterozygosity is common. As we saw in Chapter 2, the techniques of molecular genetics have revealed many different types of polymorphisms. If the

location of a given trait is not known, the first step is to choose widely spaced markers to look for evidence of linkage. About 300 markers will cover the human genome so that there should be a marker within 10% recombination (referred to as 10 centimorgans or 10 cM) of the trait of interest. Once this low-resolution mapping has been done, additional markers in the region of interest can be tested to achieve a high-resolution map of the region surrounding the trait.

Linkage Disequilibrium

In the families shown in Figure 4.8, it will be noted that although there is evidence of linkage of the marker locus to the locus associated with the disease, no one marker allele is found in all affected individuals. The specific allele found together with the mutation in any individual has to be inferred by looking at the inheritance of each from the previous generation. In the population, although the marker locus is always located nearby the disease gene, any of the various marker alleles might be found together with the disease gene (Figure 4.9). This might occur if there have been multiple independent mutations of the disease gene in various individuals, each with a different allele at the nearby marker. Alternatively, it is possible that the mutation arose once in a common ancestor of those with the disease gene, and over a long period of time sufficient genetic recombination has occurred so that any marker allele might be found together with the disease locus. This is referred to as linkage equilibrium; it means that the

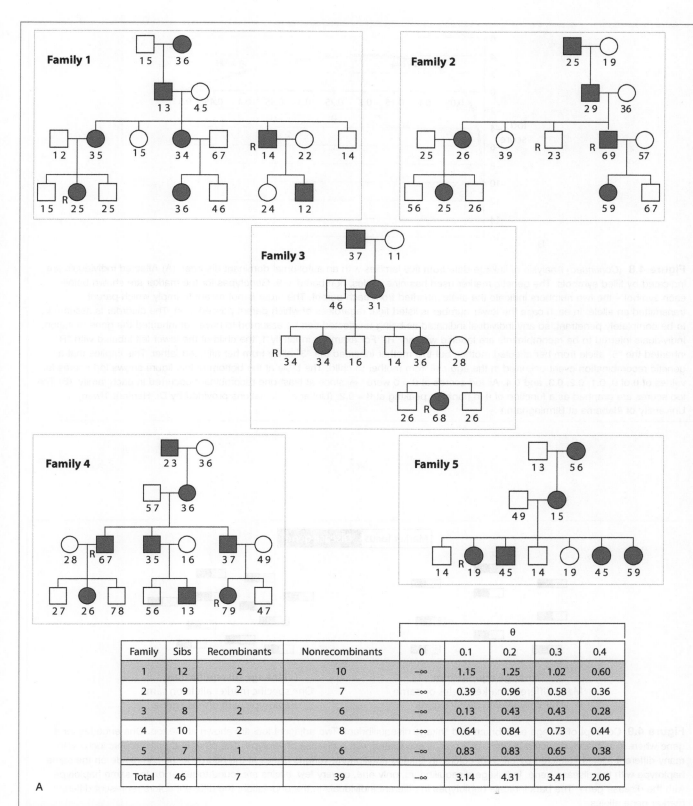

				θ				
Family	Sibs	Recombinants	Nonrecombinants	0	0.1	0.2	0.3	0.4
1	12	2	10	−∞	1.15	1.25	1.02	0.60
2	9	2	7	−∞	0.39	0.96	0.58	0.36
3	8	2	6	−∞	0.13	0.43	0.43	0.28
4	10	2	8	−∞	0.64	0.84	0.73	0.44
5	7	1	6	−∞	0.83	0.83	0.65	0.38
Total	46	7	39	−∞	3.14	4.31	3.41	2.06

A

Figure 4.8 (Continued overleaf)

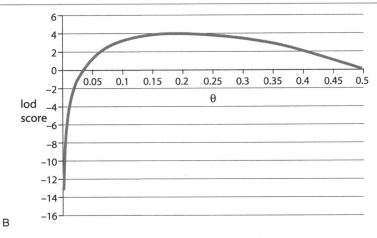

B

Figure 4.8 (*Continued*) Analysis of linkage data from five families with an autosomal dominant disorder. (A) Affected individuals are indicated by filled symbols. The genetic marker used has nine alleles, numbered 1–9. Genotypes for the marker are shown below each symbol – the two numbers indicate the allele inherited from each parent. The order is not meant to imply which parent transmitted an allele; in each case the lower number is listed first, regardless of which parent passed it on. The disorder is assumed to be completely penetrant, so any individual indicated as being unaffected can be assumed to have not inherited the gene mutation. Individuals inferred to be recombinants are labeled with an "R." For example, in family 1, the child at the lower left labeled with "R" inherited the "5" allele from her affected mother, but this mother inherited the "3" allele from her affected father. This implies that a genetic recombination event occurred in the egg cell from mother to child. The table at the bottom of this figure shows lod scores for values of θ of 0, 0.1, 0.2, 0.3, and 0.4. All lod scores at θ = 0 were −∞, since at least one recombinant occurred in each family. (B) The lod scores are graphed as a function of θ in panel B, peaking at θ = 0.2. (Linkage calculations provided by Dr. Hemant Tiwari, University of Alabama at Birmingham.)

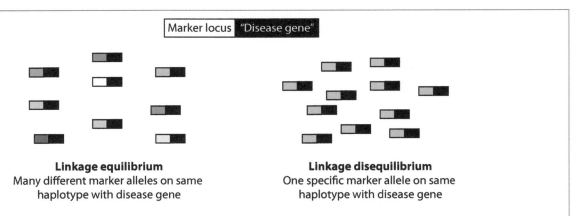

Figure 4.9 Concept of linkage equilibrium and linkage disequilibrium. Two adjacent loci are shown at the top. One encodes for a gene where a mutation, depicted by the black box, is associated with a disease phenotype. The other is a polymorphic locus with many different alleles, depicted by different colors. In linkage equilibrium, various alleles at the nearby locus can reside on the same haplotype with the disease gene. In linkage disequilibrium, only one, or very few, alleles are found together on the same haplotype with the disease gene. The bars indicate haplotypes in different individuals in the population; the different colors represent different marker gene alleles.

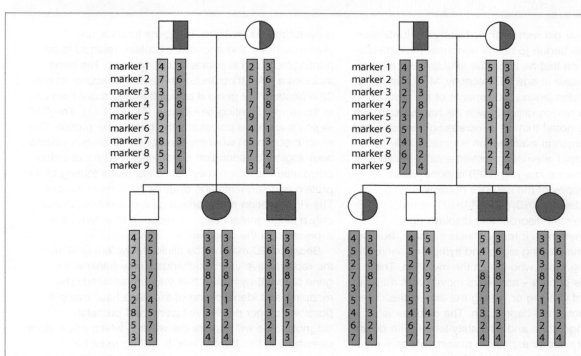

Figure 4.10 Haplotype analysis of nine marker loci in two families with an autosomal recessive disorder. The haplotype that includes the disease mutation is outlined in purple. Note that the two carrier parents share the same haplotype for the chromosome with the mutation in two unrelated families. Affected individuals are homozygous for the entire haplotype, indicating a large block of linkage disequilibrium. Also note two crossover events, one in each family. This localizes the disease gene between markers 3 and 7.

frequency of any particular haplotype of the disease gene and the marker is the product of the frequency of the two individual alleles.

In contrast, in some situations there is a preferential association of any set of alleles in a haplotype together, including potentially a mutation associated with disease and nearby markers. This is referred to as linkage disequilibrium. It usually reflects a mutation having occurred only once or very few times in history, so that recombination with nearby loci has not occurred sufficiently to achieve linkage equilibrium. When a segment of DNA with loci in linkage disequilibrium is found, this provides strong evidence that there is very tight linkage with the target (disease) gene (Figure 4.10).

Positional Cloning

As DNA polymorphisms began to become available in the early 1980s, efforts were initiated to map the genes responsible for various human genetic disorders. One of the first major successes was localization of the gene for Huntington disease to the short arm of chromosome 4 (Clinical Snapshot 4.1). Gradually, the location of many other disorders came into focus. Gene mapping began to provide tools for molecular diagnosis, since the same linkage approach that resulted in

mapping a gene could also be used to track the gene mutation in a specific family. We will explore this approach later in this book. Another benefit, however, was the ability to clone the DNA for the disease gene by positional cloning.

The basic principle of positional cloning is to first determine the location of a gene by gene mapping and then to isolate DNA in the region and identify a segment that corresponds to the gene of interest. If one begins from a polymorphic locus that is found to be linked to the disease, one can use that locus to identify segments of DNA cloned in a vector that accommodates large inserts, such as a cosmid (a plasmid that is injected into bacterial cells like a phage) or a yeast artificial chromosome, that accommodates very large segments of inserted DNA. Eventually the sequence of interest will be cloned (Figure 4.12). This is determined by the fact that the gene is expressed in tissues affected by the disorder and that mutations are found in affected individuals. Ultimate proof that the correct gene has been found may involve reproducing the disorder in model systems, such as a mouse model, by introduction of the mutant gene (Methods 4.2).

Beginning in the mid-1980s, a major series of successes led to an increasing number of genes identified by positional cloning. These include chronic granulomatous disease (MIM 3064.00), Duchenne muscular dystrophy (MIM 310200),

Clinical Snapshot 4.1 Huntington Disease

Mark is a 35-year-old with a family history of Huntington disease. He has begun to notice abnormal movements and is concerned that he might be affected. His mother died of the disease at age 55. Recently, Mark has noted occasional sudden jerking movements of his arms or legs, and he is having difficulty with his handwriting. His family has also noted that he is increasingly irritable and forgetful. His physical examination is notable only for difficulty with rapid alternating movements of his fingers. Magnetic resonance imaging (MRI) is done, which shows mild atrophy of the caudate nucleus.

Huntington disease (HD) (MIM 143100) is an autosomal dominant disorder that displays age-dependent penetrance. It rarely affects children, but the probability of manifesting signs and symptoms increases with age among those who inherit the mutation. The hallmark sign is chorea – abnormal movements that can take the form of writhing or jerking the extremities. There is also a dementia and depression. The disorder is relentlessly progressive and ultimately lethal, with death most commonly due to aspiration pneumonia as a result of abnormal control of swallowing. Suicide is also common. Abnormal movements may be treated with medications, but there is no treatment that slows the progression.

Huntington disease was one of the first disorders to be mapped using restriction fragment length polymorphisms, in 1984. The gene locus is on chromosome 4 and encodes a protein, referred to as huntingtin, which is expressed in neurons. The gene includes a CAG trinucleotide repeat, with approximately 22 repeats in the general population and more than 36 in those with Huntington disease (Figure 4.11). The CAG region encodes a polyglutamine tract in the protein. The exact mechanism whereby the abnormal protein causes neurological deterioration is not known. The expanded polyglutamine region may cause abnormal folding of the protein and sequestration of other proteins in the cell. The HD mutation represents a gain of function, in that only a single mutant allele is required to achieve full expression of the disorder.

Because HD may not be clinically evident until after the reproductive years, individuals may transmit the gene before they realize that they are affected. The mapping and identification of the gene have made it possible to offer predictive testing and prenatal diagnosis. We will explore the ways in which this is done elsewhere in this book. Genetic testing must be provided with great care and sensitivity, though, since presymptomatic diagnosis of an unpreventable neurological disorder can impose a major psychological burden on the affected individual and members of the family.

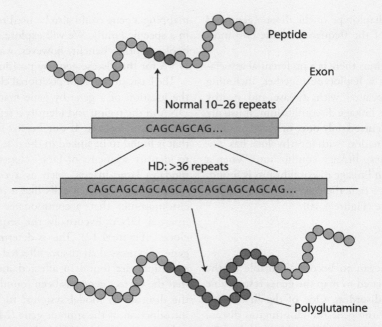

Figure 4.11 Huntington disease results from expansion of a CAG triplet repeat from a normal number of 10–26 repeats to greater than 36 repeats. This results in expansion of a polyglutamine sequence in the corresponding protein.

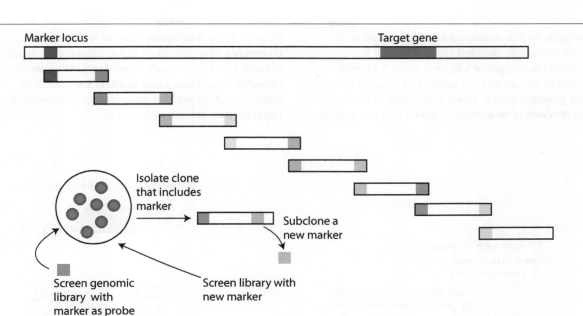

Figure 4.12 Schematic of gene walking, in which a linked marker is used to identify a clone that includes the marker, along with additional DNA. This process is iterated until a large region of overlapping clones has been obtained. Eventually, the gene of interest will have been cloned (although it remains to be identified). A unidirectional walk is illustrated here.

Methods 4.2   Animal Models of Human Disease

Animal models offer major advantages for study of disease and test of new treatments. There are many natural animal models of human genetic disorders, but the repertoire is limited. Technologies now permit creation of a wide variety of models in many different types of organisms.

Among the most powerful are mouse models. Specific genes can be inserted into the mouse by the injection of DNA from a gene of interest into the nucleus of a fertilized oocyte. The inserted gene will integrate at random into the DNA and produce transgenic mice that express the inserted gene. It is also possible to target specific mouse genes with mutations (Figure 4.13). Embryonic stem (ES) cells are isolated from blastocysts and can be maintained in culture. A mutant version of the gene of interest is transfected into the ES cells. The gene is part of a vector that includes a selectable marker. In a small proportion of cells, the inserted gene will undergo homologous recombination with the normal mouse gene and replace the normal gene with the mutant form. The selectable marker permits these cells to be isolated, and they are then injected into mouse blastocysts to produce chimeric animals. The chimeric mice are mated to produce "gene knockout" animals. In some cases, the knockout proves to be lethal. To avoid this problem, conditional knockout mice can be created (Figure 4.14). In this case, the inserted gene is normal but is flanked by a pair of DNA sequences (loxP sites) that undergo homologous recombination if another gene called cre recombinase is activated. The cre recombinase is transfected into the ES cells next to a promoter that is active only in specific cell types. Activation of cre in these cells leads to homologous recombination between the loxP sites and excision of the inserted gene in those cells. Other cells that do not express cre remain unaffected. This approach permits the function of a disrupted gene to be studied in specific tissues or at specific times in development.

There are many other model organisms that are amenable to genetic manipulation. The worm *Caenorhabditis elegans* offers the advantage that development has been precisely cataloged from fertilization through the fully developed organism, with each cell identified. Many of the developmental

(Continued)

pathways in higher eukaryotes are functional in *C. elegans*, permitting detailed study. The fruit fly *Drosophila melanogaster* has long been a favorite organism of geneticists because of its ease of manipulation for genetic studies. Gene knockouts in *Drosophila* permit analysis of mutations in genes that are homolo-

gous to those that cause disease in humans. Another commonly used organism is the zebrafish, a small tropical fish that is nearly transparent. Mutagenized zebrafish have been used to study the effects of disruption of genes that replicate developmental and physiological defects in humans.

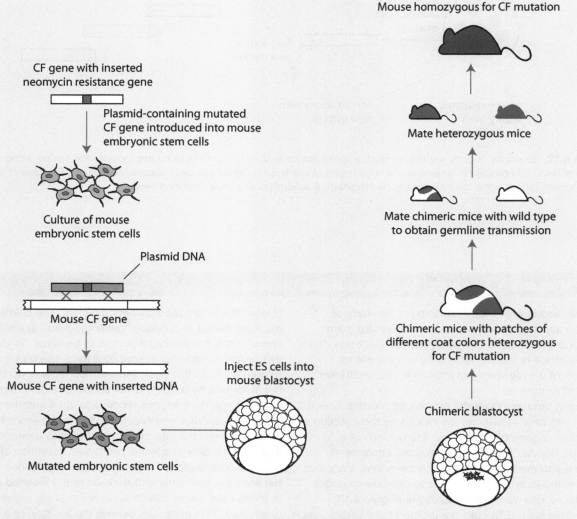

Figure 4.13 Creation of mouse model for cystic fibrosis by targeted knockout. The mutated *CFTR* gene is introduced into mouse embryonic stem cells. The mutant gene recombines with the homologous normal gene, disrupting the mouse gene. The embryonic stem cells are injected into blastocysts, which then grow into chimeric mice. Mating of the chimeric mice produces homozygous animals with the mutant *CFTR* gene. (Sources: Dorin *et al*. 1992; Snouwaert *et al*. 1992.)

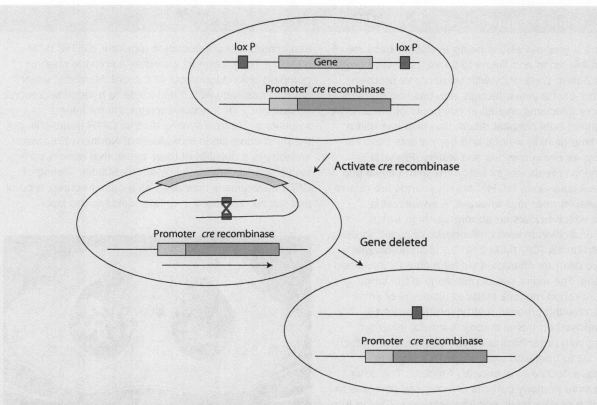

Figure 4.14 Conditional gene knockout. A normal gene is replaced by a copy that is flanked by loxP sites, which are repeated sequences. A separate gene, cre recombinase, is inserted elsewhere adjacent to a specific promoter. When the cre recombinase is activated, recombination between the loxP sites results in removal of the gene. The promoter might be inducible by administration of a hormone or chemical, in which case timing of the knockout is under control. Alternatively, it might be a tissue-specific promoter, in which case knockout will occur only in specific tissues.

cystic fibrosis (MIM 219700) (Clinical Snapshot 4.2), and neurofibromatosis type 1 (MIM 162200). This success continues to the present day, but the rate of success has been vastly increased thanks to the tools now provided by the completion of the Human Genome Project.

The Human Genome

The Human Genome Project was a large-scale international collaboration that began in the 1990s. The project benefited from major advances in sequencing technology that occurred over the ensuing decade. The culmination of the project, the completion of the human genome sequence, has placed major resources in the hands of the genetics community, and simultaneously raised major questions for the public, such as the issues discussed in Ethical Implications 4.1.

Sequencing the Human Genome

The basic approach for sequencing the human genome began with cloning of fragments of human DNA in large insert vectors such as YACs or BACs. These were assembled as overlapping "tiles" or contigs, which covered the entire genome (Figure 4.16). The location of these contigs could be referenced to a set of genetic markers that had been mapped along the human genome every million base pairs or so. With most of the genome covered by contigs of cloned sequence, it remained to use automated, high-speed sequencers to generate sequence data and assemble a sequence for each chromosome. As the process of sequencing contigs proceeded, another approach was introduced by a private company. This was based on "shotgun sequencing," in which fragments were sequenced at random. A computer was used to recognize overlaps in the fragments and to assemble them into contigs. This approach also made use of information about contig sequences available through the public effort.

The "first draft" of the human genome sequence was announced jointly by the public and private teams in June 2000. Over the ensuing several years, the sequence has been refined, filling in gaps and resolving areas of uncertainty. In truth, not every base of the genome has been sequenced, and the genome may never be completely sequenced. Some areas

Emily is a 2-year-old who is being evaluated because of frequent infections and failure to thrive. She was born after a full-term pregnancy with no neonatal problems. During the past 2 years, though, she has had frequent respiratory infections, including two bouts of pneumonia that required brief hospitalization. She also has had a difficult time gaining weight, and her parents describe her stools as being copious and watery. Physical examination reveals weight below the third centile and a lack of subcutaneous fat. Her breath sounds are coarse with scattered rales and wheezes. A sweat test is ordered, which reveals an abnormally high sweat sodium and chloride levels, diagnostic of cystic fibrosis.

Cystic fibrosis (CF) (MIM 219700) is an autosomal recessive disorder characterized by markedly thickened secretions. The major site of pathology is the lung, where thickened mucous leads to blockage of small airways, creating chronic obstruction (Figure 4.15). Superimposed on this is chronic bacterial infection, including with organisms such as *Pseudomonas*, which are difficult to treat with antibiotics. This leads to progressive decline in pulmonary function. The other major feature in many patients is malabsorption, due to obstruction of pancreatic enzyme secretion. This, in turn, causes poor weight gain.

Cystic fibrosis is diagnosed by analysis of sweat for sodium and chloride levels, which are abnormally high in affected individuals. There is no definitive treatment that will reverse the physiological problems of cystic fibrosis, but there are approaches to management that can markedly improve survival and quality of life. The pulmonary symptoms are treated with antibiotics and chest physical therapy (pounding on the chest) to loosen secretions. Inhaled medications are available that can further break up the thick mucus. Malabsorption can be effectively treated by ingestion of pancreatic enzymes. With a carefully designed and supervised program, survival of individuals with CF now is often into the fourth decade of life.

The gene responsible for CF was identified by positional cloning. It is located on chromosome 7 and encodes a protein known as the cystic fibrosis

transmembrane conductance regulator (CFTR) (MIM 602421). The protein functions as a chloride channel, pumping chloride ions out of the cell. Normally, water diffuses passively with the chloride to hydrate secretions, so lack of CFTR function explains the thickened secretions. There are many distinct *CFTR* mutations, but the most common in individuals of Northern European ancestry is a deletion of three bases that removes a single phenylalanine, designed Phe508del. Testing of *CFTR* mutations is now used as a carrier screen, a point that will be discussed in greater detail in this book.

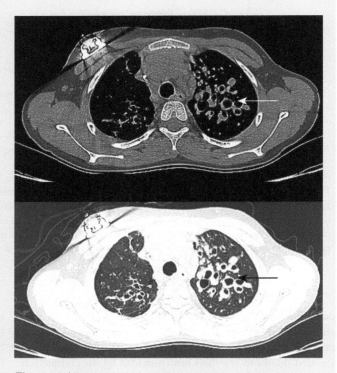

Figure 4.15 Sagittal CT sections through the thorax of a CF patient (mediastinal windows above; lung windows below). Note prominent bronchiectasis with pooling of airway secretions (most notable in the left upper lobe, arrow), with relative sparing of the alveolar compartment. Forced expiratory volume (FEV1) for this patient was 4.5% of predicted. (Courtesy of Dr. J. P. Clancy, Children's Hospital, Birmingham, Alabama.)

consist of large stretches of repeated sequences that are difficult to work with and unlikely to yield much information. The entire sequence can be viewed on the Internet using one of a number of genome browsers (Sources of Information 4.1).

Genome Organization

Before the Human Genome Project, a commonly heard estimate for the total number of genes was 100 000. This was a rough calculation based on there being approximately 3 billion base pairs of DNA and an average gene consisting of about 30 000 base pairs. The actual number of genes turns out to be around 23 000, however. Although this is not markedly more than the number of genes in "lower" organisms, such as the mouse or fruit fly, gene complexity is greater in humans. That is, individual genes consist of a larger number of domains and individual genes may encode multiple versions of a protein due to alternative splicing (see Chapter 1).

Protein-encoding sequences comprise about 1.5% of the genome. Collectively, this is referred to as the exome (i.e., sequences represented in exons). Another group of genes encodes RNA that does not get translated into protein. This includes transfer and ribosomal RNAs (tRNAs and rRNAs, respectively), RNA molecules that are involved in the mRNA splicing process, and RNAs involved in gene regulation. In addition, there are **pseudogenes**, which are inactive versions of genes (Figure 4.17). Some of these arose through gene duplication events, with one copy having subsequently acquired mutations that rendered the gene inactive. Other pseudogenes have resulted from reverse transcription of processed mRNAs and subsequent insertion of the cDNA copy back into the genome (processed pseudogenes).

At least 50% of the human genome consists of repeated sequences, which can be grouped into several classes (Figure 4.18). **Simple sequence repeats** consist of multiple copies of a short sequence, for example di-, tri-, or tetranucleotide repeats. Variable number tandem repeats consist of a 14–100 base pair block repeated tens or hundreds of times. There are blocks of repeated sequences clustered at the centromeric and subtelomeric regions of chromosomes that we will consider

further in Chapter 6. Upward of 5% of the genome consists of low-copy repeats (LCRs), also referred to as **segmental duplications**. A segmental duplication, as seen in Chapter 2, is defined as a set of sequences at least 1 kb in length with 95% or greater homology. Some segments can be hundreds of thousands of base pairs in length. Segmental duplications are not evenly distributed either along or among chromosomes. Some chromosomes are particularly rich in segmental duplications; as much as 25% of the Y chromosome consists of segmental duplications, for example. Segmental duplications are disproportionately located near centromeres and telomeres. In addition, it has become apparent that there is some degree of variation in the number of repeat units of some large duplicated segments. This is referred to as large-scale variation. It remains to be determined whether these variants have functional consequences, for example serving as risk factors in the occurrence of common disorders.

The final class of repeated sequences is **transposon-derived repeats**, of which there are four major types: long interspersed elements, short interspersed elements, long terminal repeat (LTR) retroposons, and DNA transposons. **Long interspersed elements (LINEs)** range from 6 to 8 kb; they include a

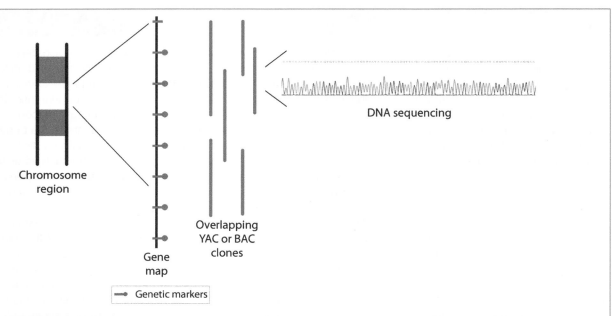

Figure 4.16 Human genome sequencing strategy. A set of large insert clones were aligned to the genome, referencing various mapped genetic markers. These segments were then sequenced, and the complete sequence pieced together from these contigs.

Sources of Information 4.1
Genome Browser

Human genome sequence information is regularly updated online. One of the most widely used portals of access to this information is the University of California, Santa Cruz (USCS) Genome Browser (genome.ucsc.edu). The browser permits searching by chromosomal region or by a specific gene. Multiple "tracks" of information can be visualized, and specific tracks selected or deselected to focus the view on needed information. A large amount of information can be seen, including known or inferred genes, interspecies homologies, repeated sequences, methylation, polymorphic markers, and many other features. No registration is required and no fee is charged for access to the site.

promoter site for RNA polymerase II and encode two proteins, one of which is a reverse transcriptase, which copies RNA into DNA. The LINE sequence is transcribed into RNA, which then moves to the cytoplasm where the two proteins are translated. These then bind to the RNA, which moves back to the nucleus, where it is reverse transcribed into DNA, which in turn may reinsert itself into the genome. In many cases, the reverse transcription does not copy the entire sequence, pro-

ducing a LINE insert that remains inert. There are approximately 850 000 LINE sequences in a human genome, comprising approximately 21% of the genome. **Short interspersed elements (SINEs)** are 100–400 bp in length and have an RNA polymerase III promoter, mostly derived from tRNA genes. SINE sequences do not encode protein, but can use the LINE reverse transcriptase to copy their RNA into DNA and insert into the genome. A human genome contains about 1.5 million SINE sequences, comprising approximately 13% of the genome. **LTR retroposons** consist of retroviral-like elements. These include the LTR elements required to support transcription and the two characteristic genes of the retrovirus, *gag* and *pol* (the reverse transcriptase). Reverse transcription of these elements occurs in the cytoplasm, with the DNA copy then being transported to the nucleus, where insertion occurs. Insertion of incomplete retrovirus-like elements results in many nonfunctional partial sequences in the genome. There are approximately 450 000 copies of retroviral-like elements in the human genome, comprising approximately 8%. **DNA transposons** are similar to the transposable genetic elements found in bacteria. These encode an enzyme, transposase, which can cut the transposon out of the genome and then reinsert it at other sites. There are approximately 300 000 transposons in the human genome, comprising approximately 3% of the base sequence. Transposable genetic elements have been viewed as parasitic sequences within the genome, although there is evidence that some may play a role in regulation of protein translation. Transposable elements also have been important

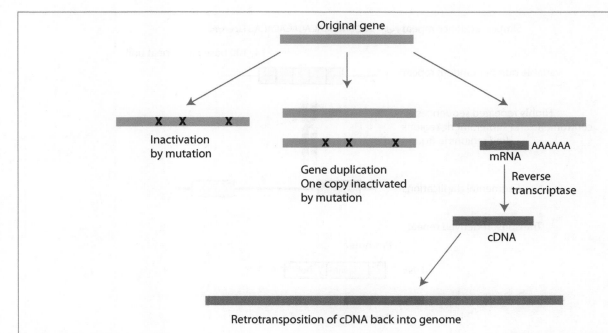

Figure 4.17 Three routes toward formation of a pseudogene. On the left, a gene accumulates mutations that prevent its expression. In the middle, the gene is duplicated. One copy accumulates mutations and becomes inactive, whereas the other remains active. On the right, the gene is transcribed into mRNA, and the mRNA is then copied into cDNA by reverse transcriptase encoded by a LINE sequence, which is then reinserted into the genome. The inserted sequence has had its introns removed and has no promoter, so it is not expressed. It is referred to as a processed pseudogene.

in evolution, leading to creation of new genes. Most of the transposable elements in the human genome are currently inactive, but there are examples of gene mutations that have been attributed to transposition into a gene, disrupting its function.

Genomics, Bioinformatics, and Systems Biology

The sequencing of the genome has spawned a set of new approaches to biological investigation. We will briefly consider three here: genomics, bioinformatics, and systems biology.

Genomics involves the study of large sets of genes, or gene products, up to and including the entire genome, or the entire set of transcripts (the **transcriptome**) or proteins (the **proteome**). Genomics relies on high-throughput, automated approaches, such as the gene chip, in which thousands to hundreds of thousands of DNA sequences can be affixed to spots on a glass chip and used to detect the presence of homologous sequences in a test sample (Methods 4.3). Many variations on this approach have been developed, and are used to rapidly detect sequence variants in a large number of samples or to characterize the entire set of transcribed genes in a particular tissue sample. The cost of DNA sequencing has plummeted in the years since the first human genome was sequenced. The technology is continually advancing; cur-

rently approaches based on massively parallel sequencing, referred to as next-generation sequencing (Methods 4.4), are making it possible to sequence individual genomes (Hot Topic 4.1).

Bioinformatics involves the use of computers to catalog and analyze large sets of biological data. Bioinformatic approaches have been applied to the human genome sequence to help identify genes or control elements. One particularly valuable tool is the comparison of sequences among different species. A major effort is underway to sequence the genomes of a wide variety of prokaryotic and eukaryotic organisms. Aside from providing information on the evolution of these species, such sequence comparisons help to identify functional regions that have been conserved through evolution.

Systems biology takes an integrated approach to the study of complex biological phenomena. Genes, gene products, proteins, and metabolites do not act in isolation, but interact with one another to form an integrated network. Systems biology involves an effort to understand how these networks are structured and how perturbations of a component of the network affect the whole. Much of the scientific effort of the past century, including the sequencing of the genome, can be seen as a reductionist approach aimed at identification of the individual components of biological systems. The task of systems biology is to put these pieces back together to obtain

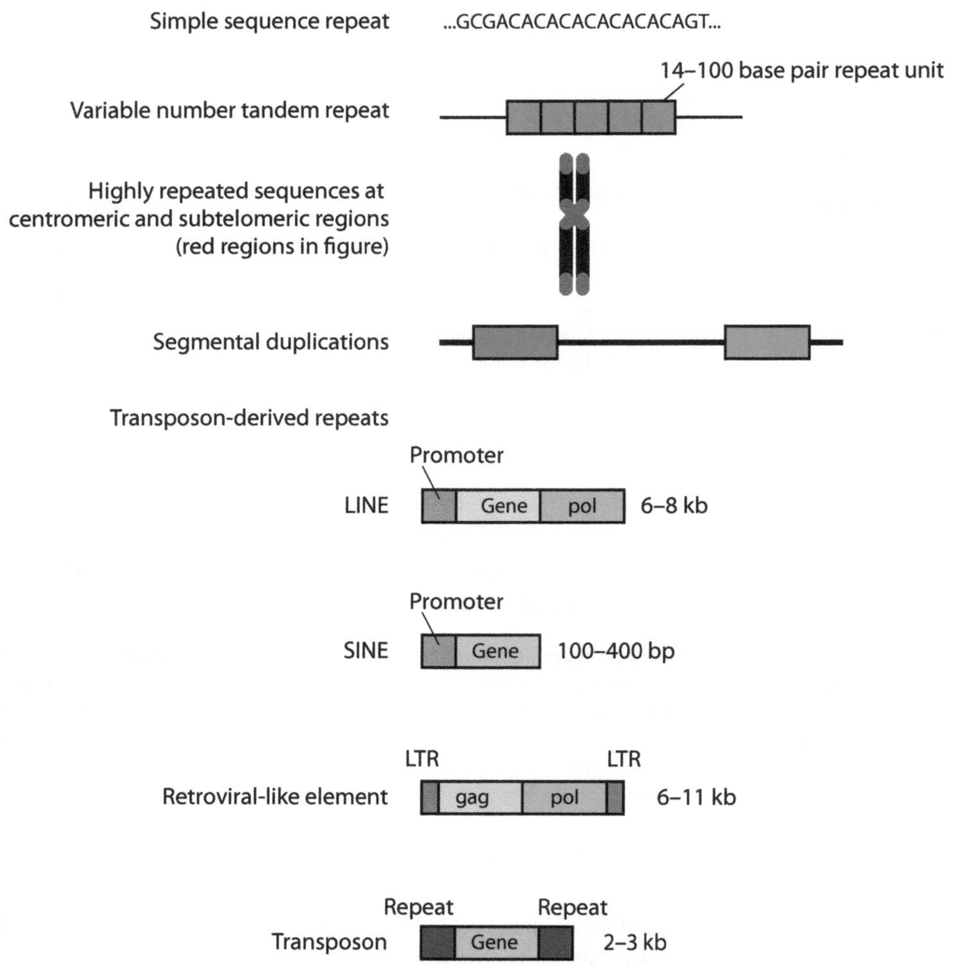

Simple sequence repeat ...GCGACACACACACACACAGT...

14–100 base pair repeat unit

Variable number tandem repeat

Highly repeated sequences at
centromeric and subtelomeric regions
(red regions in figure)

Segmental duplications

Transposon-derived repeats

Promoter

LINE | Gene | pol | 6–8 kb

Promoter

SINE | Gene | 100–400 bp

LTR   LTR

Retroviral-like element | gag | pol | 6–11 kb

Repeat   Repeat

Transposon | Gene | 2–3 kb

Figure 4.18 Various types of repeated sequences in the human genome. Simple sequence repeats consist of a small number of base pairs repeated multiple times (in this case, C–A repeated seven times). Variable-number tandem repeats consist of 14–100 base blocks of DNA repeated multiple times. Very highly repeated sequences tend to be localized near the centromeres and telomeres of each chromosome. Segmental duplications are blocks of DNA from 1 kb to hundreds of kb repeated at multiple sites; homology to blocks of repeated DNA need not be perfect. Four types of transposon-derived repeats are LINE sequences, SINE sequences, retroviral-like elements, and transposons. LINES are 6–8 kb in length and consist of a promoter sequence, a gene, and a gene that encodes reverse transcriptase (*pol*). SINES are 100–400 bp in length and consist of a promoter and single gene. Retroviral-like elements are 6–11 kb in length and consist of the *gag* and *pol* genes flanked by long terminal repeats (LTRs). Transposons are 2–3 kb and consist of a repeated sequence flanking a gene that encodes an enzyme required to transpose the element from place to place in the genome (*transposase*).

an understanding of how they function as a whole to make a living organism.

Conclusion

The success of the Human Genome Project has advanced medical genetics, and medicine in general, to a genomic level of analysis. It has opened the door to the detailed study of the inner workings of the cell, as well as the ways in which cells communicate with one another and with the environ-

ment. Mysteries of development and physiology are coming to be solved at a rapid pace. There remains the daunting task of putting all this information together to unravel what might be called the "wiring diagram" of the organism. This will keep at least a generation of biologists – and other scientists in fields such as computer science, physics, and chemistry – busy for a long time. Over the coming years, medical practice will be transformed as the underpinnings of health and disease increasingly come to light through this effort.

✓ Methods 4.3   Gene Chips

Genetic studies have historically focused on genes one at a time, but tools are now at hand that permit wider scale studies of the structure and function of large sets of genes simultaneously. One of the key technologies used in this effort is the gene chip. The basic principle (Figure 4.19) is that specific DNA sequences, either fragments isolated from a cell or synthetic oligonucleotides, can be fixed in place at a specific site on a glass chip. The sequences are attached using a photochemical reaction and an automated system, making it possible to create arrays with hundreds of

thousands of sequences. The DNA on the chip can correspond with genomic sequences, or can be homologous to RNA sequences and used to probe gene expression. The principle is the same, regardless. DNA to be tested (cDNA in the case of analysis of gene expression) is labeled with a colored fluorescent probe and hybridized with the DNA on the chip. Wherever there is homology, a spot will fluoresce, indicating hybridization. We will explore the use of DNA chips in analysis of copy number variations and gene expression in other chapters of this book.

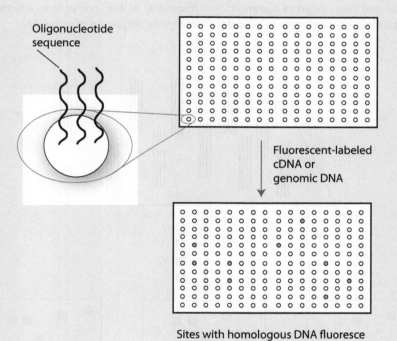

Oligonucleotide sequence

Fluorescent-labeled cDNA or genomic DNA

Sites with homologous DNA fluoresce

Figure 4.19 A microarray consists of thousands of tiny spots into which a specific DNA sequence is attached by a photochemical reaction. DNA from a test source is labeled with a fluorescent color and hybridized to DNA on the chip. Spots that contain homologous DNA will glow with the color of the label. If the identity of the DNA in each well is known, the identity of homologous DNA that hybridizes is identified accordingly.

✓ Methods 4.4 Next-Generation Sequencing

The human genome was sequenced one fragment at a time, which is why the project took many years and cost hundreds of millions of dollars. Technological advances in DNA sequencing have advanced dramatically since that time, and now make it possible to sequence a complete human genome in a matter of hours to days. There are many approaches to doing this, collectively referred to as next-generation sequencing. Most of the current approaches involve simultaneous sequencing of billions of DNA segments, known as massively parallel sequencing. One approach is illustrated in Figure 4.20. DNA fragments are attached to a solid substrate and amplified, leading to "tufts" of DNA segments. These are rendered single stranded and sequenced (a common primer is attached to each fragment before it is bound to the substrate). Fluorescently labeled nucleotides, with each nucleotide having a different color, are added that are blocked so that DNA synthesis stops after that base is incorporated. After incorporation of a base, a photograph is taken of the fragments, allowing the specific base incorporated into each tuft to be identified. The added base is then unblocked chemically, allowing the next base to bind, and another photograph is taken. Although the approach may be used to sequence only 100 or so bases, comprising the length of a fragment attached to the substrate, the entire genome may be represented in various regions of the substrate. A DNA sequence from these billions of 100 or so base pair fragments is then computationally assembled, yielding a complete sequence very quickly.

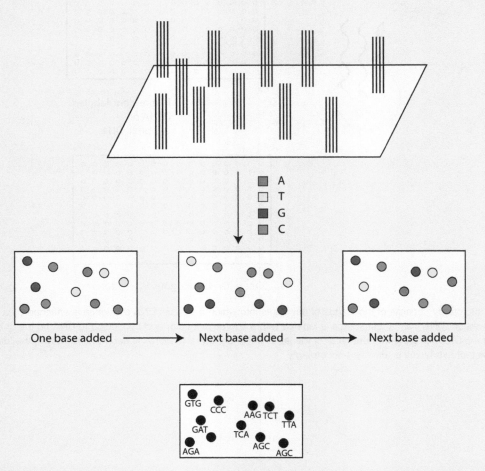

Figure 4.20 Diagram illustrating one approach to massively parallel sequencing. DNA fragments are linked to a common primer sequence, amplified, rendered single stranded, and bound to a solid substrate. DNA is copied off the templates using blocked bases, each labeled with a different color. Bases are incorporated one at a time, since the synthesis reaction stops after each base until the base is chemically unblocked. Each time, the fluorescent signal at each site is photographed, allowing the DNA sequence to be put together for billions of short fragments. The resulting sequence for three bases is shown at the bottom.

ⓘ Hot Topic 4.1 Genome Sequencing

The rapidly declining cost of DNA sequencing has opened the door toward sequencing entire genomes for medical purposes. At present, the rationale is usually to identify the genetic basis for a rare Mendelian disorder, though some people have had their genomes sequenced to satisfy personal curiosity and/or identify risk of future disease. Gene identification through DNA sequencing has made it possible to find genes that underlie extremely rare disorders that would not be possible to study using the approach of genetic linkage and positional cloning. One paper, published in 2010, accomplished this for a rare autosomal recessive form of Charcot–Marie–Tooth disease (an inherited peripheral neuropathy) (Lupski *et al*. 2010). The cost of whole-genome sequencing in 2010 was still tens of thousands of dollars, but an alternative that has been successful in a few cases is to focus sequencing on the 1.5% of the genome that encodes protein (the exome). Exons are "captured" by hybridization with DNA known to correspond with exons and then sequencing using next-generation technology. In 2013 this costs less than a thousand dollars, and the vast majority of genetic disorders have been found to be due to mutations in exons. The first published report of success using this approach was for identification of the gene involved in a rare developmental disorder called Miller syndrome (Eng *et al*. 2010). The number of disorders approached in this way is rapidly increasing, to a point where it may be more cost-effective than the linkage–positional cloning approach. Whole-genome sequencing currently remains an experimental approach and produces a vast amount of data; some data may be medically useful but, at present, most are of unknown significance. In 2008 James Watson's DNA was sequenced, revealing, among other things, heterozygosity for several autosomal recessive disorders (Wheeler *et al*. 2008). An approach to genetic counseling of individuals based on whole-genome analysis was published in 2010 (Ashley *et al*. 2010). We will explore the clinical utility of genome sequencing elsewhere in this book.

REFERENCES

Ashley EA, *et al*. 2010, "Clinical assessment incorporating a personal genome", *Lancet*, vol. 375, pp. 1525–35.

Dorin JR, *et al*. 1991, "Cystic fibrosis in the mouse by targeted insertional mutagenesis", *Nature*, vol. 359, pp. 211–15.

Eng SB, *et al*. 2010, "Exome sequencing identifies the cause of a Mendelian disorder", *Nature Genetics*, vol. 42, pp. 30–5.

Kwon BS, Haq AK, Pomerantz SH, Halaban R 1987, "Isolation and sequence of a cDNA clone from human tyrosinase that maps at the mouse c-albino locus", *Proceedings of the National Academy of Sciences of the USA*, vol. 84, pp. 74.73–7.

Lupski J, *et al*. 2010, "Whole-genome sequencing in a patient with Charcot–Marie–Tooth neuropathy", *New England Journal of Medicine*, vol. 362, pp. 1181–91.

Snouwaert JN, *et al*. 1992, "An animal model for cystic fibrosis made by gene targeting", *Science*, vol. 257, pp. 1083–8.

Wheeler DA, *et al*. 2008, "The complete genome of an individual by massively parallel sequencing", *Nature*, vol. 452, pp. 872–6.

FURTHER READING

Alberts B, Johnson A, Lewis J, Raff M, Roberts K, Walter P 2007, *Molecular biology of the cell*, 5th edn, Garland Science, New York.

Krebs JE, Goldstein, ES, Kilpatrick ST 2009, *Lewin's genes X*, Jones & Bartlett, Sudbury, MA.

Lander ES, *et al*. 2001, "Initial sequencing and analysis of the human genome", *Nature*, vol. 4, pp. 860–921.

Lodish H, Berk A, Kaiser CA, Krieger M, Scott MP, Bretscher A, Ploegh H, Matsudaira P 2007, *Molecular cell biology*, 6th edn, Freeman, New York.

Venter JC, *et al*. 2001, "The sequence of the human genome", *Science*, vol. 291, pp. 1304–51.

Find interactive self-test questions and additional resources for this chapter at **www.korfgenetics.com**.

Self-Assessment

Review Questions

4.1 If DNA from a genomic library were inserted into bacteria as part of a lambda phage expression vector, would you expect that a functional gene product would be obtained?

4.2 A fully penetrant autosomal dominant disorder is linked to a marker gene A, with alleles 1 and 4. Which of the following children is recombinant (shaded symbols are affected individuals)?

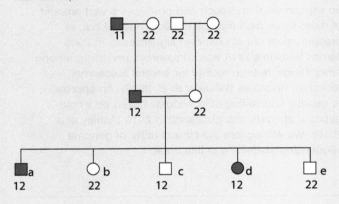

4.3 You are performing a linkage study with a marker that you think might represent the gene for a specific trait. At $\theta = 0$, the lod score is $-\infty$. What does this tell you about your hypothesis that the marker locus is the disease gene?

4.4 How does having the complete gene sequence facilitate the process of positional cloning?

4.5 What would be the expected consequence if a LINE sequence were to insert itself into an exon of a gene?

CHAPTER 5
Multifactorial Inheritance

Introduction

The best-studied genetic traits are not necessarily the ones responsible for the greatest worldwide burden of genetic disease. Single-gene disorders tend to be sharply defined traits, for which the genetic contribution lies close to the surface. These were the first disorders to be recognized as inherited and the first to be studied at the biochemical and then molecular levels. Genes do not function in isolation, however, nor is a human a closed system isolated from its environment. Therefore, it should be no surprise that among the most common and important of genetic traits are those that are determined by combinations of multiple genes and their interactions with the environment. This is referred to as multifactorial inheritance. In this chapter we will explore the concept of multifactorial inheritance and see how new genomic tools are being used to determine the genetic contributions to common disorders.

Key Points

- Multifactorial traits are determined by a combination of genetic and nongenetic factors. Evidence that genes contribute to a trait includes familial clustering, monozygotic twin concordance, and studies of heritability.
- Two models of multifactorial inheritance are the additive polygenic model and the threshold model.
- Most common disorders include at least some genetic component. The identification of these genes is a major goal of current research in human genetics.
- Genes that contribute to multifactorial disorders can be identified using single-nucleotide polymorphisms (SNPs) in association studies or transmission disequilibrium studies.

Human Genetics and Genomics, Fourth Edition. Bruce R. Korf and Mira B. Irons.
© 2013 John Wiley & Sons, Ltd. Published 2013 by John Wiley & Sons, Ltd.

Concept of Multifactorial Inheritance

The concept of **multifactorial inheritance** arose from the observation that there are traits that tend to cluster within families, yet are not transmitted in accordance with Mendel's laws as dominant or recessive traits. Examples include congenital anomalies, such as cleft lip or palate, spina bifida, and pyloric stenosis. They also include relatively common disorders, such as hypertension and diabetes mellitus. In this section we will look at the evidence for a genetic contribution to such traits, and at models of multifactorial inheritance.

Evidence for Multifactorial Inheritance

There are many lines of evidence that support the contribution of genes toward the determination of multifactorial traits. The major approaches used are family analysis, twin studies, and, for quantitative traits, studies of heritability.

Geneticists measure familial clustering with a variable λ, which is the ratio of the frequency of the trait in relatives divided by its frequency in the general population. This can be easily measured by looking at the frequency of the trait among siblings as compared with the general population, in which case the variable is λ_s. For an autosomal recessive trait the frequency in siblings is expected to be ¼, and for an autosomal dominant it will be ½. The value of λ_s will depend on the population frequency of the disorder. For the autosomal recessive disorder cystic fibrosis in the Northern European population, λ_s is $(0.25)/(0.0004) = 625$; for the dominant disorder Huntington disease, λ_s is $(0.5)/(0.0001) = 5000$. For the congenital anomaly pyloric stenosis (see Table 5.1), λ_s is $(0.032)/(0.002) = 16$. The expected values for λ_s for dominant, recessive, and multifactorial traits are as follows:

$$\text{Autosomal dominant } \lambda_s = \frac{1/2}{x} = \frac{1}{2x}$$

$$\text{Autosomal recessive } \lambda_s = \frac{1/4}{x} = \frac{1}{4x}$$

$$\text{Multifactorial } \lambda_s = \frac{1}{\sqrt{x}}$$

where x is the population frequency of the trait.

Multifactorial traits have also been studied by analysis of the segregation of these traits through families. Computer models are generated that assume the role of one or more genes, exerting dominant or recessive inheritance, with various levels of penetrance and factoring in interactions with the environment. Data from families then are evaluated, and the relative likelihood that observed data fit with the various models is determined. This **complex segregation analysis** has been used to discern the genetic contribution to a number of common phenotypic traits.

Twin studies involve comparison of the rate of concordance for a trait in monozygotic (identical) twins as compared with the concordance rate in full siblings. **Monozygotic twins** are formed as the result of cleavage of the early embryo into two embryos. These embryos are derived from a single fertilization event, so they are genetically identical. One would expect full concordance in monozygotic twins for a trait that is entirely determined by genes. This is indeed the case for fully penetrant, monogenic traits, for example the disorders cystic fibrosis or sickle cell anemia. Monozygotic twins will not be fully concordant for a multifactorial trait, since factors other than their shared genes, such as environmental exposures, may also play a role. In general, the greater the rate of concordance among identical twins as compared with full siblings, the greater the genetic contribution to the trait (Table 5.2).

Another approach, which applies to quantitative traits such as height or blood pressure, is to estimate the **heritability** of a trait (Methods 5.1). The term was coined by geneticists who were measuring genetic and environmental contributions to measurable traits in plants and animals. The variance in such a trait can be partitioned into that which is contributed by genetic factors, environmental factors, covariance between the two, and measurement variance. Genetic factors in turn can

Table 5.1 Empirical data on recurrence risk of selected congenital anomalies in first-degree relatives.

Anomaly	Population incidence	Recurrence risk (%)
Cleft lip ± cleft palate	1/1000	4.9
Congenital dislocation of hip	1/1000	3.5
Pyloric stenosis	1/500	3.2
Club foot	1/1000	2–8

Table 5.2 Concordance rate for common congenital anomalies in identical and nonidentical twins.

Trait	Identical twins (%)	Concordance Full siblings (%)
Cleft lip and palate	40	5
Pyloric stenosis	22	4
Clubfoot	32	3
Congenital dislocation of hip	33	4

Source: Smith and Aase (1970).

Methods 5.1 Heritability Concept and Estimation of Heritability from Phenotypic Correlation in Family Members

$$V_P = \overbrace{V_A + V_D}^{\text{Genetic variance}} + \overbrace{V_E + V_I}^{\text{Environmental variance}}$$

$$+ \text{Cov}_{GE} + \overbrace{V_M}^{\text{Measurement variance}}$$

V_A = additive genetic variance
V_D = deviation due to dominance and epistasis
V_E = environmental variance
V_I = interaction variance
V_G = $V_A + V_D$
Cov_{GE} = covariance of genetics and environment

Heritability in narrow sense $h^2 = V_A/V_P$
Heritability in broad sense $h^2 = V_G/V_P$

Relationship	Heritability
Monozygotic twins	$h^2 = r$
Sib–sib or dizygotic twins	$h^2 = 2r$
One parent–one offspring	$h^2 = 2r$
Midparent–offspring	$h^2 = r/\sqrt{0.5} = r/0.7071$
First cousins	$h^2 = 8r$

r = Correlation coefficient for quantitatively measurable trait.

be subdivided into those that represent additive effects of multiple genes and those that reflect interactions between genes. Environmental factors can be similarly partitioned. Heritability is defined as the proportion of variance contributed by genetic factors, and is traditionally considered in two forms: "heritability in the narrow sense" focuses on only the additive genetic factors, whereas "heritability in the broad sense" looks at all genetic factors, whether additive or interactive. For human traits we are usually interested in any genetic contribution, whether additive or interactive, and therefore focus on the latter.

Heritability can be estimated by looking at the degree of correlation of a trait in family members with different degrees of relationship. Heritability can be directly estimated from the concordance rate in monozygotic twins. Full sibs (including nonidentical, or dizygotic, twins) will share about half their genes, so heritability is estimated at twice the correlation between them. Other values for estimating heritability from the phenotypic correlation of family members are shown in Methods 5.1.

Models of Multifactorial Inheritance

The simplest model of multifactorial inheritance assumes the action of multiple genes, but not environmental factors. This is referred to as **polygenic inheritance**. As an example, consider a hypothetical genetic system in which two separate loci are involved in determining final adult height (Figure 5.1). There are two alleles at each locus, one dominant, which adds 2 cm to final height, and the other recessive, which adds nothing. Suppose that a person with the genotype aabb would be 150 cm tall. Someone with all dominant alleles would then measure 158 cm. A person with the genotype AaBb would be 154 cm, as would a person with the genotype aaBB. The effects of these genes, then, are additive with respect to height. If alleles are equally distributed, the additive model predicts a normal distribution of the quantitative trait in the population.

Many of the traits that are subject to multifactorial inheritance are quantitative, such as height and blood pressure. It is relatively easy to see how additive effects of multiple genes or environmental factors could determine the values of such traits. Other traits, particularly congenital malformations, are less easy to explain by the additive polygenic model. Such all-or-nothing traits are better explained by the **threshold model** of multifactorial inheritance.

The threshold model assumes that there is a "liability" toward development of a disorder that is normally distributed in the general population (Figure 5.2). This liability is composed of contributions from both genetic and environmental factors that can lead to expression of the trait. Individuals will have more or less liability toward the trait, depending on how many of the predisposing genes they have inherited and the degree to which they are exposed to the relevant environmental factors. Up to a point, they will not display signs of the trait. When a threshold of liability is crossed, however, the trait appears. Some will exceed the threshold because of having many genetic risk factors and little environmental risk, whereas in others the major contribution to liability may be environmental but, once the threshold is reached, the effect is the same.

An interesting observation has been made in some multifactorial disorders that is explained by the threshold model. Some disorders display a sex predilection, affecting either males or females more often. Neural tube defects, for example, tend to

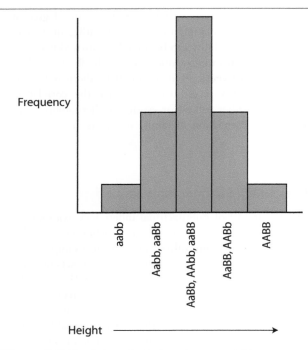

Figure 5.1 Simple hypothetical two-locus model for inheritance of height. The dominant alleles each add 2 cm to the height and are assumed to be equally distributed in the population, with the frequency of each allele being 0.5. According to this model, 1 in 16 individuals will have the genotype aabb and be the shortest. Likewise, 1 in 16 will be AABB and be tallest. One-fourth will have a single dominant allele or a single recessive allele. The majority will be of average height, having two dominant alleles. Note that, according to this model, it is the number of dominant alleles that determines height, not the specific combination (i.e., AaBb and AAbb give the same height).

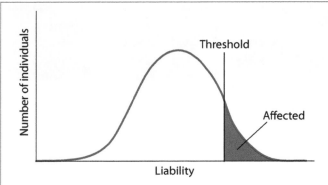

Figure 5.2 Threshold model for multifactorial inheritance. There is a liability toward the trait that consists of a combination of genetic and nongenetic factors and is normally distributed in the population. The trait is expressed only in individuals whose liability exceeds a threshold.

occur more often in females. Another example is pyloric stenosis (Clinical Snapshot 5.1), which is more common in males. The recurrence risk of pyloric stenosis is higher for families in which the **proband** is female than where the proband is male. The reason is that a female, being more rarely affected, is presumed to require a greater liability for the threshold to be crossed (Figure 5.4). A couple having a daughter with pyloric stenosis is likely to transmit a greater number of genes predisposing to the disorder and therefore has a higher recurrence risk than those who have had a son with the disorder. Recurrence, by the way, is more likely to occur in a son than in a daughter, as the male would require less liability to cross the threshold.

The threshold model is based on statistical analysis of the clustering of traits in families. The notion of genetic liability may seem vague. What is really going on? The answer is mostly unknown, as there are few multifactorial traits in which the

contributing genetic factors have been identified. It is believed that genetic liability is accounted for by alleles at one or more loci that individually are unable to cause a distinctive phenotype. The phenotype emerges only if an individual has some critical combination of alleles at these loci. Sometimes this is sufficient to produce the phenotype, and at other times it just leads to susceptibility to an otherwise harmless environmental agent.

Genetics of Common Disease

Much of the progress in medical genetics during the past 50 years has applied to relatively rare, single-gene or chromosomal disorders. In contrast, progress in understanding the genetic contribution to conditions that are the cause of more common diseases, such as cardiovascular disease, diabetes, and cancer, has been much slower. This is a consequence of the enormous complexity of these common disorders as compared to rarer conditions that result from mutations in single genes. Only recently have the tools of molecular genetics begun to penetrate more complex disorders.

There is substantial evidence that most, if not all, common disorders have a genetic component. The evidence is gathered from many of the approaches described earlier in this chapter – the disorders tend to cluster in families, there is increased concordance in identical twins, and so on. In rare instances, families may display single-gene Mendelian inheritance of a trait such as hypertension, diabetes, or Alzheimer disease. Aside from these exceptional cases, though, it is believed that the common forms of these disorders are the combined result of both genetic and environmental factors, and that there are multiple genetic factors, each of which may contribute only

Clinical Snapshot 5.1   Pyloric Stenosis

James is a 20-day-old infant seen in the emergency room for persistent vomiting. He was born after a full-term, uncomplicated pregnancy. He has been breast-fed and seemed to feed well, but he has been spitting up a lot of his feeds from the first day. During the last 24 hours, however, he has been vomiting everything he has been fed, sometimes very forcefully. During this time he has become increasingly sleepy, and now shows little interest in feeding. Examination reveals a lethargic baby with a depressed anterior fontanelle and no tears when crying. A small mass is palpated in the left upper quadrant of the abdomen. Blood studies reveal low chloride and potassium and a metabolic alkalosis. A diagnosis of pyloric stenosis is confirmed by ultrasound, and James is taken to surgery for a laparoscopic pyloroplasty. He is discharged from the hospital 2 days later.

Pyloric stenosis is due to hyperplasia of the muscles at the pylorus of the stomach and causes obstruction to gastric emptying (Figure 5.3). Infants present in the early weeks of life with recurrent vomiting, dehydration, and electrolyte imbalance due to loss of hydrochloric acid from the stomach and excretion of potassium and retention of hydrogen ions in the kidney. Surgical incision of the obstructing muscles is curative. Pyloric stenosis occurs in 2–4 per 1000 children with a 4:1 prevalence of affected males to affected females. It tends to cluster in families, with an increased risk among siblings or offspring of affected individuals. Inheritance is

multifactorial, and recently several different genetic susceptibility loci have been identified that may act as candidate genes for pyloric stenosis (MIM 179010). One of these, TRPC6 (MIM 603652), belongs to a family of canonical transient receptor potential (TRPC) cation channel genes implicated in smooth muscle control and hypertrophy. Because of the male predominance, recurrence risk is higher in boys than girls. If the proband is female, however, the recurrence risk is higher than if the proband is male.

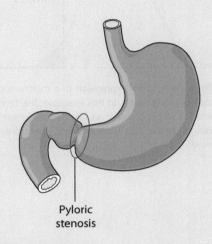

Figure 5.3 Pyloric stenosis.

modest increments of liability toward the condition. The major challenge is to define which genes these are, and how they make their contributions. We will explore the approaches currently in use to dissect the genetics of common disorders elsewhere in this book.

Genetic Association Studies

In spite of major success in the identification of genes involved in rare disorders, study of the genes involved in common disorders has been a much more difficult challenge. As we have seen, most common disorders have multifactorial etiology, with a combination of multiple genes interacting with the environment at the basis of pathogenesis. One approach to the study of genetic factors in common disorders relies on large population studies, looking for genetic variants that are associated with an increased risk of disease. In its simplest form, this is done using the **case–control study** (Table 5.3). A set of individuals who display the phenotype under study (cases) are

compared with a group who are matched as closely as possible, but who do not have the phenotype (controls) (Hot Topic 5.1). Genetic studies are then done to determine whether there is a significant difference in the frequency of a genetic trait between cases and controls. An odds ratio calculation is done, comparing the frequency of the trait in cases versus controls. An odds ratio greater than 1 indicates that the genetic variant is positively associated with the disorder; a value less than 1 indicates a protective association.

What kinds of genetic traits can be tested in an association study? For many years, relatively few genetic markers were available. Some of the most impressive progress involved the study of association with alleles in the human lymphocyte antigen (HLA) locus on chromosome 6 (Figure 5.5). The HLA locus is a region that includes multiple, highly polymorphic genes that are involved in regulation of the immune response. Specific alleles have been found to be associated with a variety of disorders, most of which involve an aberration in the immune response (Table 5.4). An example is a form of arthritis

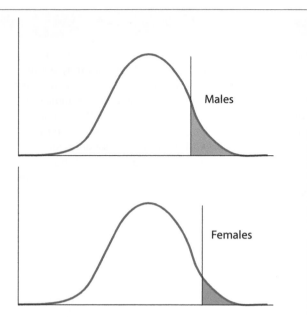

Figure 5.4 The threshold for expression of a multifactorial trait may differ in males and females. In this example, the threshold is higher for females. A couple with an affected daughter can be assumed to have a greater overall liability and, therefore, a higher recurrence risk.

Table 5.3 Hypothetical case–control study testing the hypothesis that allele 2 of a single-nucleotide polymorphism is associated with asthma.

	Asthma	No asthma
Allele 2 present	300	100
Allele 2 not present	700	900

Note: The polymorphism consists of a C (allele 1) or an A (allele 2) at one site in a gene of interest. Genotype is tested in 1000 people with asthma and 1000 controls. In this example, allele 2 is present (either homozygous or heterozygous) in cases with asthma more often than in controls. Odds ratio of asthma given allele 2 vs. not having allele 2 is 300/100 ÷ 700/900 = 3.86.

called ankylosing spondylitis (MIM 106300). Individuals with the HLA-B27 allele have a 20- to 30-fold relative risk of having this disorder. Success has also been achieved in Alzheimer disease, where association has been found with one of the apolipoprotein E alleles (Clinical Snapshot 5.2).

Hot Topic 5.1 Large-Cohort Studies

The ability to carry out a case–control study is dependent on access to a large cohort affected with the phenotype of interest. Ideally, cases will come from a single homogeneous population, thus minimizing the likelihood that different genetic risk factors are acting in different individuals. The phenotype needs to be defined as precisely as possible. Common disorders, such as diabetes or hypertension, can be the ultimate outcome of a number of distinct pathological processes. Diabetes, for example, may result from an autoimmune process or insulin resistance due to obesity. All cases in an association study should be similar in terms of the origin of their disease. This may be aided by "subphenotyping" – identifying cases through use of a test rather than a broad phenotypic categorization. In diabetes, for example, this could be a test for β-cell antibodies, insuring that all cases have an autoimmune cause of their disease.

These various restrictions create challenges in the assembly of large groups of cases. To facilitate that process, several large, prospective cohort studies have been launched. In the United Kingdom, a project called Biobank (www.ukbiobank.ac.uk) will follow a cohort of 500 000 adults for up to 30 years, tracking health status and obtaining blood and urine samples. In Iceland a private company, deCODE Genetics (www.decode.com), has established a database and DNA bank that will track the health status for thousands of Icelanders. The goal is to identify genes that contribute to the risk of common diseases and then to develop pharmaceuticals based on knowledge of the disease pathophysiology. Another study of tens of thousands individuals has been underway in Estonia (www.geenivaramu.ee). Many private companies in the United States have established independent tissue banks and patient databases.

In recent years, the major focus has been on SNPs, many of which reside within the coding sequence of genes. Case–control studies using SNPs are designed to determine whether a specific genotype is found more commonly in cases or controls. Initially, genetic association studies were conducted using SNPs in **candidate gene**s. These candidates consisted of genes that were predicted to be associated with disease based on knowledge of pathophysiology. There were some notable suc-

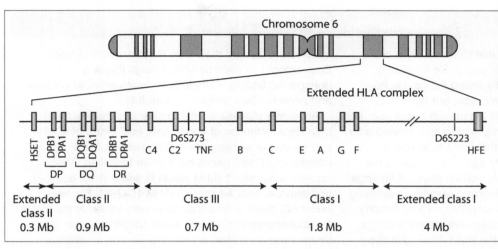

Figure 5.5 HLA locus. (Redrawn from Undlien DE, Lie BA, Thorsby E. Trends in Genetics 17:93, copyright 2001 with permission from Elsevier.)

Table 5.4 HLA–disease associations.

Disorder	Antigen	Relative risk
Ankylosing spondylitis	B27	69.1
Juvenile rheumatoid arthritis	B27	3.9
	DR8	3.6
Ulcerative colitis	B5	3.8
Psoriasis	Cw6	7.5
Multiple sclerosis	DR2	6.0
Narcolepsy	DR2	130.0
Source: Carpenter (1994).		

cesses with this approach, but it remained greatly limited, since only genes of already known relationship to disease could be tested.

The major breakthrough in the genetic analysis of common disease came when it became possible to do **genome-wide association studies (GWAS)**, that is, to study genetic variants across the genome, looking for any that display association with disease. The major obstacle to doing GWAS was the cost of genotyping, which made genotyping thousands of markers across the genome in thousands of cases and controls prohibitively expensive. Two advances in the past several years have overcome this obstacle. Firstly, the cost of genotyping has decreased dramatically; high-throughput genotyping approaches now permit testing for a fraction of a cent per genotype. Secondly, it was found that the human genome consists of blocks of DNA that have been inherited as intact haplotypes over very long periods of human evolution (Figure 5.7). These haplotype blocks were characterized in various

human populations through the HapMap Project (see Sources of Information 5.1), which then identified "tag SNPs" that could be tested on blocks of DNA from 10 to 20 kb in length, significantly reducing the number of SNPs that required testing to achieve genome-wide coverage. It is now possible to test SNPs several thousand bases apart at low cost, making it possible to identify associations with no prior assumption about plausible candidates.

GWAS have revealed hundreds of examples of association of SNPs with common disorders. These studies have been done in many large patient cohorts, and, for the most part, different studies have implicated the same set of genetic markers as being associated with a particular disease. It is important to realize that these genetic associations do not necessarily indicate that a particular gene is etiologically involved in a condition. The association is an indication of linkage disequilibrium with a disease trait, and could be explained by the genetic marker itself either being involved in disease pathogenesis, or being in linkage disequilibrium with another gene that is the true etiological agent.

In spite of the success of the GWAS approach, only a small proportion of the genetic contribution to most common disorders, as measured by approaches such as heritability estimation or twin studies, has been accounted for by SNP associations discovered to date. For example, in type 2 diabetes, it has been estimated that <10% of the heritability is accounted for by SNPs found to be associated with the condition. This indicates that the GWAS studies are missing a large proportion of the genetic factors that contribute to heritability. The assumption that underlies the GWAS approach is that common variants present in 1–5% of the population account for the genetic contribution to common disease. It is possible that this assumption is incorrect, and that much of the "missing heritability" is accounted for by very rare variants that are difficult to detect even in large case–control studies. It is also possible that SNPs

Clinical Snapshot 5.2   Alzheimer Disease

Sid is 70 years old, and it is clear to his family that his mental capacities have been slipping. He frequently forgets things and is constantly losing things. He has good memory for events of long ago, but does not seem to remember things said to him just hours ago. He often loses his way and recently had to stop driving after a minor accident. Sid denies that there is anything wrong with him, but reluctantly agrees to a visit to his doctor. His examination reveals normal physical findings, but poor recent memory. A magnetic resonance imaging (MRI) scan is done, which reveals only cortical atrophy. Blood tests are done, with mostly unrevealing findings, although he is found to have the ε3/ε4 ApoE genotype. A clinical diagnosis of Alzheimer disease is made.

Alzheimer disease (AD) is a common form of progressive dementia, with over 4 million people in the United States thought to be affected. It presents with memory loss and confusion and may include language problems, poor judgment, agitation, and hallucinations as it progresses. There are no distinct physical manifestations, and diagnosis is established clinically. Brain atrophy is seen by MRI, though this is a nonspecific finding. Pathology includes amyloid plaques and neurofibrillary tangles (Figure 5.6).

Alzheimer disease is an example of a multifactorial trait. Rare instances of early-onset (<65 years of age) AD can be due to single-gene autosomal dominant inheritance. Three genes have been identified. These encode presenilin 1 (MIM 104311) and 2 (MIM 600759) and amyloid beta A4 protein (MIM 104760). For late-onset AD, there is an association with alleles at the locus for apolipoprotein E (ApoE) (MIM 107741). There are three common alleles, ε2, ε3, and ε4. The ε4 allele is found in individuals with Alzheimer disease about three times as often as in controls. However, the allele is also found in controls, and many with AD do not have the ε4 allele. Therefore, testing for ε4 does not diagnose AD; in an individual with a history of the disorder, however, ApoE testing can provide another bit of evidence in support of the diagnosis.

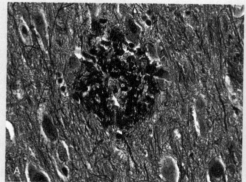 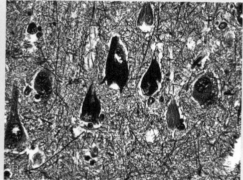

Figure 5.6 Amyloid plaque (A) and neurofibrillary tangles (B) in a section of brain from an individual with Alzheimer disease. (Courtesy of Dr. Steven Carroll, University of Alabama at Birmingham.)

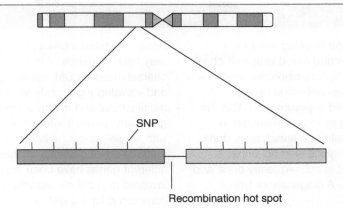

Figure 5.7 Haplotype blocks of single-nucleotide polymorphisms (SNPs). The genome is organized into 10–20 kb blocks that are transmitted more or less intact from generation to generation, separated by "hot spots" where recombination is most likely to occur. SNPs within a block tend to be in linkage disequilibrium with one another; therefore, a single SNP ("tag SNP") can be used as a marker for the entire group within a block.

🔍 Sources of Information 5.1
HapMap (www.hapmap.org)

The HapMap is a catalog of common genetic variants available in the public domain developed to help researchers identify genes associated with human disease. The information contained in the HapMap is derived from the DNA of 270 individuals of African, Asian, and European ancestry and is the product of a multinational collaboration, the International HapMap Project. The catalog describes what the variants are, where they reside in the human genome, and what the frequency of specific variants is in certain populations. The HapMap takes advantage of the fact that genetic variants that are located close to each other are often inherited together. The ability to study common haplotypes instead of single SNPs allows researchers to more easily narrow the search for genes associated with specific medical conditions.

are not the only kinds of variants that are associated with common disease; copy number variants, for example, may also contribute to risk of common disorders, and so far have not been thoroughly explored for disease association. Finally, it is possible that heritability has been overestimated for some

common disorders, and GWAS studies are giving a more accurate assessment of the genetic contribution to these conditions.

These approaches are beginning to bear fruit by revealing genetic variants that are associated with common disorders (Clinical Snapshot 5.3). We are also increasingly learning about important previously unknown factors that will increase our knowledge of the molecular determinants of human disease (Hot Topic 5.2). We will explore the progress in one area elsewhere in this book when we consider risk assessment for common disorders (Ethical Implications 5.1).

Conclusion

Understanding the genetic contribution to common disorders is one of the major goals in genetics and medicine. It is widely anticipated that this will yield new approaches to prevention through early identification of individuals at risk. It will also produce new insights into pathophysiology that may be translated into new approaches to prevention and treatment. It is likely that insights into the genetics of common disorders will occur gradually, one disorder at a time. It is through this effort, however, that genetics will exert its maximal effect on the day-to-day practice of medicine.

Clinical Snapshot 5.3   Diabetes Mellitus

Don is a 55-year-old man who is being seen for a routine physical examination and blood pressure check. He has a history of chronic hypertension, for which he is on medication. His physical examination reveals moderate obesity and a blood pressure of 150/88. He has mild hypertensive changes in his retinal blood vessels. As part of his evaluation, a urinalysis is done that reveals the presence of glucose in his urine. A blood glucose measurement is subsequently done and is also found to be elevated. A diagnosis of type 2 diabetes mellitus is made.

Diabetes mellitus (DM) is a disorder of glucose metabolism. Ordinarily, glucose uptake into cells is mediated by insulin, a peptide hormone synthesized in β cells of the pancreas and secreted in response to a rise in blood sugar. Individuals with DM either fail to produce insulin in normal quantities or have a deficient responsiveness.

There are two major types of DM, types 1 and 2. Type 1 DM tends to have onset in childhood and is due to autoimmune destruction of β cells. It is a multifactorial trait with both genetic and environmental components. The major genetic factor is linked to the HLA locus on chromosome 6. Several specific HLA gene alleles are associated with type 1 DM in different populations. In addition, there is a VNTR polymorphism near the 5′ end of the insulin gene that also is a risk factor (Figure 5.8).

Type 2 DM is most often an adult-onset disorder and is usually associated with decreased responsiveness to insulin. Affected individuals are also usually obese and may have evidence of metabolic syndrome, which is characterized by DM, insulin resistance, hypertension, and elevated triglyceride levels. Type 2 DM is also multifactorial and is characterized by gene–gene and gene–environment interactions. There are rare families with single-gene inheritance of an entity referred to as maturity-onset diabetes of youth (MODY). A variety of different genes have been implicated, including genes involved in β-cell development or insulin secretion. More commonly, type 2 DM occurs sporadically. Association studies have been done to identify genes that contribute to risk and have revealed that numerous genes have been implicated that exhibit variable penetrance. One gene, peroxisome proliferator-activated receptor-gamma (PPARG) (MIM 601487), has been shown in multiple studies to have an allele that is associated with type 2 DM, though having the allele conveys only a very small increase in relative risk. Susceptibility to insulin resistance has been associated with polymorphisms of many other genes, including the K121Q polymorphism in exon 4 of the ENPP1 gene (MIM 173335.0006). A haplotype defined with SNPs from this gene, including K121Q, is associated with obesity, glucose intolerance, and type 2 DM. It is likely that multiple genes are involved in the etiology of type 2 DM, with different combinations involved in different individuals.

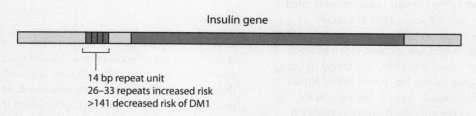

Insulin gene

14 bp repeat unit
26–33 repeats increased risk
>141 decreased risk of DM1

Figure 5.8 A tandem repeat polymorphism 5′ to the insulin gene that conveys risk of type 1 diabetes mellitus, with smaller repeat numbers conveying increased risk.

? Ethical Implications 5.1 Predictive Testing

Should predictive testing based on genetic association be offered as part of routine clinical care? Although it is widely anticipated that this will be done at some point, there are few examples in current practice. There are several cautions that should be observed in the clinical application of predictive tests by genetic association.

1. Tests based on genetic association are not diagnostic tests. The test result will indicate relative risk for a disorder, not whether the disorder is currently present or someday will be present. Many individuals with the allele that is associated with disease will never become symptomatic.
2. Tests based on genetic association cannot exclude disease. Although having a specific allele may increase the relative risk of a disorder, not having the allele does not mean that an individual will not develop the condition.
3. Relative risk of disease in individuals of a specified genotype can differ in different populations, as can the frequency of any specific allele. Data that are relevant to the population from which a particular patient is derived should be used to assess relative risks when possible.
4. There can be significant risks associated with predictive tests. These include stigmatization, anxiety, and the possibility of loss or denial of employment and/or health, disability, or life insurance. Laws to protect against such discrimination vary from state to state in the United States.
5. There may be limited benefit associated with predictive tests, particularly if there is no means of prevention of the occurrence of the disorder.

REFERENCES

Carpenter CB 1994, 'The major histocompatibility gene complex', in K Isselbacher, G Braunwald, J Wilson, *et al.* (eds.), *Harrison's Principles of Internal Medicine*, 13th edn, McGraw-Hill, New York.

Smith DW, Aase JM 1970, 'Polygenic inheritance of certain common malformations', *Journal of Pediatrics*, vol. 76, pp. 653–9.

Undlien DE, Lie BA, Thorsby E 2001, 'HLA complex genes in type 1 diabetes and other autoimmune diseases: which genes are involved?', *Trends in Genetics*, vol. 17, pp. 93–101.

Manolio T, Collins FS, Cox NJ, *et al.* 2010. Finding the missing heritability of complex diseases. *Nature*, vol. 461, pp. 747–753.

FURTHER READING

General References

Cardon LR, Abecasis GR 2003, 'Using haplotype blocks to map human complex trait loci', *Trends in Genetics*, vol. 19, pp. 135–40.

Glazier AM, Nadeau JH, Aitman TJ 2002, 'Finding genes that underlie complex traits', *Science*, vol. 298, pp. 2345–9.

Newton-Cheh C, Hirschhorn JN 2005, 'Genetic association studies of complex traits: design and analysis issues', *Mutation Research*, vol. 573, pp. 54–69.

Clinical Snapshot 5.1 Alzheimer Disease

St George-Hyslop PH, Petit A 2005, 'Molecular biology and genetics of Alzheimer's disease', *Comptes rendus biologies*, vol. 328, pp. 119–30.

Clinical Snapshot 5.2 Diabetes

Barroso I 2005, 'Genetics of type 2 diabetes', *Diabetic Medicine*, vol. 22, pp. 517–35.

Rewers M, Norris J, Dabelea D 2004, 'Epidemiology of type 1 diabetes mellitus', *Advances in Experimental Medicine and Biology*, vol. 552, pp. 219–46.

Ethics 5.1 Predictive Testing

Evans JP, Skrzynia C, Burke W 2001, 'The complexities of predictive genetic testing', *British Medical Journal*, vol. 522, pp. 1052–6.

Hot Topic 5.1 Large Cohort Studies

Cambon-Thomsen A 2004, 'The social and ethical issues of post-genomic human biobanks', *Nature Reviews Genetics*, vol. 5, pp. 866–73.

Collins FS 2004, 'The case for a US prospective cohort study of genes and environment', *Nature*, vol. 429, pp. 475–7.

Hot Topic 5.2 The Dark Side of the Genome

Costa FF 2005, 'Non-coding RNAs: new players in eukaryotic biology', *Gene*, vol. 357, pp. 83–94.

Michalak P 2006, 'RNA world: the dark matter of evolutionary genomics', *Journal of Evolutionary Biology*, vol. 19, pp. 1768–74.

Find interactive self-test questions and additional resources for this chapter at **www.korfgenetics.com**.

Self-Assessment

Review Questions

5.1   A pair of identical twins is found not to be concordant for a phenotypic trait. Does this mean that the trait is not genetically determined?

5.2   A couple have a son affected with a multifactorial trait that occurs more often in females than males. For their next child, is it more likely that a son or daughter would be affected?

5.3   A case–control study shows that a particular SNP allele is associated with a 2.3-fold increased odds of disease. What does this imply about the relationship of the SNP to the disease?

5.4   Your father, who is being treated for hypercholesterolemia, hears about the availability of direct-to-consumer genetic testing and sends a saliva specimen to the company. His report indicates that his risk for coronary artery disease is lower than that of other men his age. Should he stop taking his cholesterol-lowering medication?

5.5   How does the haplotype map facilitate whole-genome analysis for association of SNPs with common disorders?

CHAPTER 6
Cell Division and Chromosomes

Introduction

If each of the 23 000 or so genes were independently replicated and assorted to daughter cells, the process of cell replication would be hopelessly chaotic. In fact the process is highly organized, with the genome packaged into 23 pairs of chromosomes, which are replicated, line up in the cell, and split into strands that segregate to the daughter cells. In this chapter, we will focus on this process from multiple points of view. Firstly, we will explore mitosis and meiosis and see how the cell cycle is regulated so that DNA replication and cell division are coordinated. Secondly, we will look at the structure of chromosomes and how the genome is packaged. Finally, we will look at the techniques used to study chromosomes and at the major types of chromosomal abnormalities.

Human Genetics and Genomics, Fourth Edition. Bruce R. Korf and Mira B. Irons.
© 2013 John Wiley & Sons, Ltd. Published 2013 by John Wiley & Sons, Ltd.

Key Points

- The cell cycle is a highly regulated process that consists of four phases: G1, G2, S, and M.
- Somatic cell division is the process of mitosis, where an equal copy of the nuclear genome is distributed to each daughter cell. Germ cells are formed by the process of meiosis, which reduces chromosome number to the haploid state and also provides an opportunity for genetic recombination.
- Mitotic chromosomes are highly condensed structures, which include recognizable landmarks.
- Analysis of chromosomes can be performed by collecting dividing cells in culture, swelling the cells in hypotonic saline, fixing the chromosomes onto slides, and staining them with a variety of special stains.
- The technique of fluorescence in situ hybridization (FISH) can be used to detect small deletions or identify chromosomes involved in complex rearrangements.
- Genomic microarrays permit the detection of deletions or duplications at high resolution.
- Abnormalities of chromosome number or structure underlie many human developmental disorders and cancer.
- The presence of one or more extra complete chromosome sets is referred to as polyploidy, and usually is lethal.
- Aneuploidy is the presence of a non-integral number of the haploid set. A number of aneuploidy syndromes have been characterized.
- Structural abnormalities include deletions, duplications, inversions, rings, and translocations.
- Individuals who are balanced translocation or inversion carriers are at risk of having offspring with chromosomal imbalance.
- Microdeletion syndromes consist of deletion of multiple, contiguous genes, and are best detected using FISH or genomic microarrays.
- Uniparental disomy or deletion can underlie specific syndromes associated with deficiency in imprinted genes.

Cell Division

Cell division is fundamental to the growth and propagation of all living organisms. In eukaryotes, somatic cell division involves division of the nuclear contents (**mitosis**) and the cytoplasm (**cytokinesis**). Germ cells undergo a specialized form of cell division called **meiosis**. Meiosis results in production of haploid gametes and also provides the opportunity for genetic recombination.

The Cell Cycle

Rapidly dividing cells have a relatively constant interval between successive rounds of cell division. This interval is marked by sets of events known as the cell cycle (Figure 6.1). Following the end of mitosis, the cell enters the **G1 phase** (gap 1), which is a time when genes are transcribed and translated. Next is the **S phase**, when DNA replication occurs. Following S is the **G2 phase** (gap 2), an interval during which the cell prepares for the **M phase**, mitosis. The timing of the events in the cell cycle is regulated by a set of proteins called **cyclins**, which are expressed at specific points in the cycle, as their name implies. Cyclins interact with and activate **cyclin-dependent kinases (Cdk proteins)**, enabling them to phosphorylate other proteins required to proceed through the cell cycle. The cell commits to division at the restriction point, at which time Cyclin D accumulates and interacts with Cdks 4 and 6. This

leads to phophorylation of the Rb protein, which releases transcription factors from inhibition, in turn leading to synthesis of Cyclins A and E, which interact with Cdk2 to initiate DNA synthesis. Upon completion of the S phase, mitotic phase cyclins (A and B) accumulate, eventually triggering mitosis.

Entry into the cell cycle at the restriction point occurs in response to mitogenic stimuli, typically proteins that bind to cell surface receptors and set off a cascade of events that culminate in stimulation of transcription of Cyclin D. There are two checkpoints at which the presence of DNA damage inhibits the cell cycle, one at the restriction point and one at the S–G2 boundary. **Checkpoint proteins** are involved in pausing the cell cycle to repair DNA damage. DNA damage stimulates the proteins ATM (ataxia telangiectasia mutated) and ATR (ATM and Rad3-related), which leads to activation of the transcription factor p53. p53 stimulates transcription of p21, which binds to and inhibits G1–S/Cdk and S–Cdk complexes, preventing further DNA replication until damage is repaired. ATM and ATR also activate proteins that inhibit M cyclins, preventing a cell with DNA damage from entering mitosis. If the DNA damage is too extensive to repair, p53 initiates programmed cell death, called **apoptosis**. As is seen in Chapter 9, many of the proteins involved in regulation of the cell cycle are associated with initiation or progression of cancer or with disorders that lead to increased risk of cancer.

Figure 6.1 Proteins, referred to as cyclins, bind with specific cyclin-dependent kinases (CDKs), which phosphorylate specific proteins to initiate the events of G1, S, G2, and M.

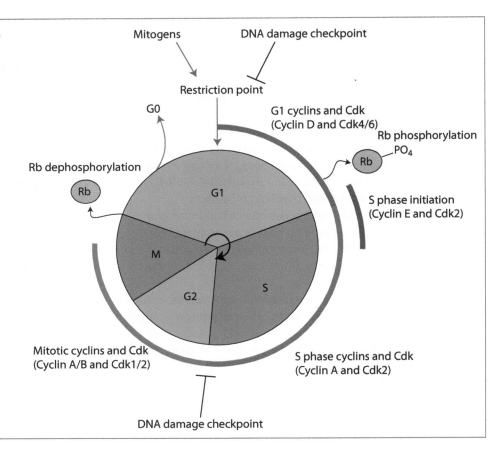

Mitosis and Meiosis

The process of mitosis consists of four phases: **prophase**, **metaphase**, **anaphase**, and **telophase** (Figure 6.2). DNA replication has already occurred during the S phase, so at the start of mitosis the chromosomes consist of two DNA strands, **chromatids**, joined together at the primary constriction, or **centromere** (Figure 6.3). During prophase, the chromosomes begin to condense and the nuclear membrane breaks down. The chromosomes are maximally compacted in metaphase, at which point they are lined up at the center of the cell and spindle fibers extend from centrioles at the two poles of the mitotic figure, connecting to a protein complex known as the kinetochore, located at the centromere. The two chromatids separate at anaphase and move toward the poles. Mitosis is completed at telophase with the formation of two new nuclear membranes, and daughter cells separate by a process of cytokinesis.

Meiosis begins in oocytes during fetal life, whereas in males it begins for a particular spermatogonial cell sometime after puberty. Meiosis is preceded by a round of DNA replication, so at the outset there are 46 chromosomes, each of which has replicated to consist of two chromatids, just as for mitosis. Two rounds of cell division occur during the process of meiosis (Figure 6.4). In the first, homologous chromosomes pair intimately and may undergo genetic recombination. The pairing is precise and involves formation of a protein structure called the **synaptonemal complex**. Recombination events always involve exchange between two DNA strands and result in a reshuffling of alleles on the recombined chromosomes (see Figure 6.4). In females, chromosome pairing begins during fetal life and continues until a particular oocyte is readied for ovulation, which is years to decades later. In males, the entire process of meiosis takes place over a period of several days. In either case, the first meiotic division is completed as the homologous chromosomes separate to either pole and two daughter cells result. In oogenesis, one of the daughter cells will become the egg, whereas the other is a smaller cell referred to as the first polar body. The daughter cells now contain a single copy of each chromosome, although each chromosomes consists of two chromatids. The cells then undergo a second round of division resembling mitosis but without a preceding round of DNA replication. In the male this results in four spermatids, which subsequently mature into spermatozoa. In the female

Stage		Chromosome Number	DNA Content
Interphase	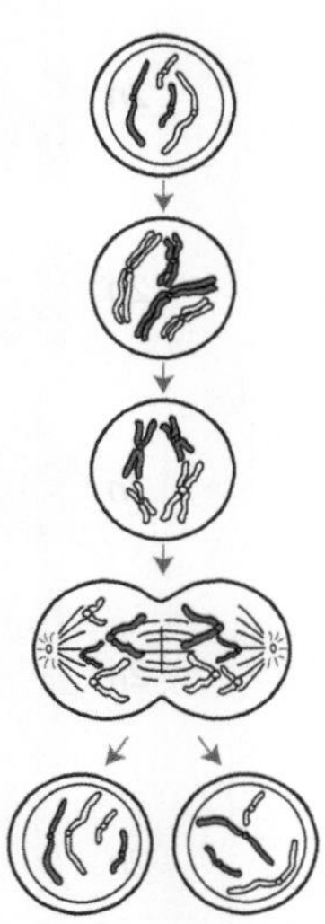	2n	2c
Prophase		2n	4c
Metaphase		2n	4c
Anaphase		2n	4c
Telophase		2n	2c

Figure 6.2 The process of mitosis. The replicated chromosomes condense during prophase, at which time the nuclear membrane breaks down. Chromosomes line up on the spindle at metaphase, and chromatids separate to the two daughter cells at anaphase. Chromosome content is indicated as diploid (2n) adjacent to each figure, and DNA content as two copies of each autosomal gene (2c) or four copies (4c).

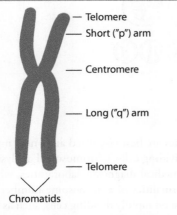

- Telomere
- Short ("p") arm
- Centromere
- Long ("q") arm
- Telomere

Chromatids

Figure 6.3 Major chromosome landmarks shown in a replicated metaphase chromosome.

membrane, formation of the spindle, and alignment of chromosomes on the spindle. The sister chromatids are held together at the centromere by the cohesin protein complex. Chromosome separation is triggered by activity of the anaphase protein complex (APC), which stimulates inactivation of mitotic cyclin and enzymatic cleavage of cohesion at the centromeres. Several genetic disorders are associated with mutations in the genes that encode cohesin proteins, including Cornelia de Lange syndrome (MIM 122470), Roberts syndrome (MIM 268300), and SC Phocomelia syndrome (MIM 269000). Spindle microtubules function as motors, propelling the sister chromatids (or chromosomes, in the case of meiosis) toward the spindle poles.

Chromosomes

The human karyotype consists of 22 pairs of nonsex chromosomes (**autosomes**) and two **sex chromosomes**, XX for females and XY for males. Each chromosome consists of a single continuous DNA strand, encoding from a few hundred to several thousand genes. Study of both normal and abnormal chromosome structure has provided valuable tools for analysis of human developmental disorders and cancer.

Chromosome Structure and Analysis

Chromosomes undergo a cycle of condensation and decondensation through the cell cycle. Chromosomes are maximally decompacted during interphase, and achieve maximal compaction during the metaphase stage of mitosis, just prior to the

the second meiotic division occurs at the time of fertilization and results in a second polar body and a fertilized egg. Meiosis fulfills two crucial roles. Firstly, it reduces the chromosome set to the haploid number, so that upon fertilization a diploid number is restored. Secondly, it allows for genetic recombination.

The various steps of both mitosis and meiosis are, like the cell cycle, highly regulated processes. Mitotic cyclin–Cdk complexes are involved in directing the dissolution of the nuclear

Figure 6.4 Process of meiosis. Homologous chromosomes pair during the first meiotic prophase and separate in the first division. Chromatids then separate during the second meiotic division to form four haploid germ cells. Chromosome content is indicated as diploid (2n) or haploid (n) adjacent to each figure, and DNA content as two copies of each autosomal gene (2c), four copies (4c), or one copy (c).

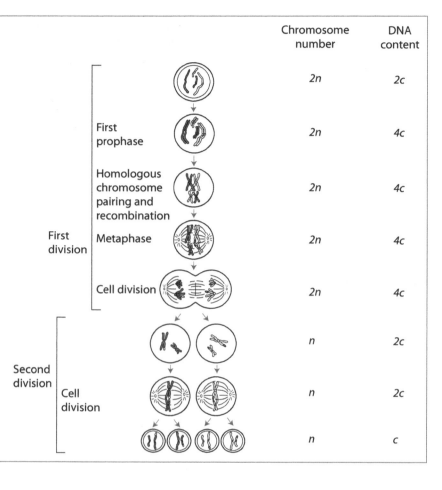

	Chromosome number	DNA content
	2n	2c
First prophase	2n	4c
Homologous chromosome pairing and recombination	2n	4c
Metaphase	2n	4c
Cell division	2n	4c
	n	2c
Cell division	n	2c
	n	c

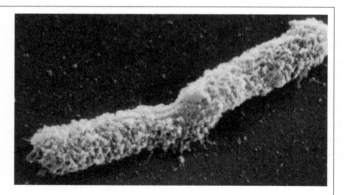

Figure 6.5 Scanning electron micrograph of mitotic chromosome, showing loops of chromatin fibers.

separation of sister chromosomes to the two daughter cells. We discussed the structure of chromatin in Chapter 1. The metaphase chromosome consists of loops of chromatin (Figure 6.5) compacted by binding to protein structures called condensins. The overall condensation is about 10 000- to 20 000-fold relative to the "naked" DNA double helix.

Chromosomes are best visualized at or near maximum condensation in dividing cells. Chromosomal analysis is routinely performed in medical diagnostic laboratories, where it is used to detect abnormalities of chromosome number or structure. Analysis is done on rapidly dividing cells, such as bone marrow or cancer cells, or on cells grown in culture (Methods 6.1). Special staining techniques are used to reveal fine structural features of chromosomes (Figure 6.7) that facilitate identification of each chromosome and reveal structural abnormalities.

Chromosomes are classified according to size and position of the centromere into a standard array referred to as the karyotype. The centromere divides most chromosomes into a long arm (designed the **q arm**, or "q") and a short arm (designated the **p arm**, or "p," for petit). Chromosomes are classified as **metacentric** (centromere in the center), **submetacentric** (centromere displaced to one end), or **acrocentric** (centromere near one end of the chromosome) (Methods 6.2). The acrocentric chromosomes are 13, 14, 15, 21, and 22. The short arms of these chromosomes consist of DNA that encodes ribosomal RNA. These regions often remain decondensed, forming stalks, with small knobs at the end referred to as satellites.

✓ Methods 6.1 Chromosomal Analysis

The major source of cells used for clinical cytogenetics is peripheral blood T lymphocytes, which are stimulated to divide in culture by the lectin phytohemagglutinin. Cells are collected at metaphase by treatment with a spindle inhibitor such as colchicine. They are then swollen with hypotonic saline to facilitate cell membrane disruption and spread the chromosomes, fixed onto microscope slides, and stained (Figure 6.6). It was the discovery of hypotonic treatment in 1956 that ushered in the era of clinical cytogenetics. Prior to that,

chromosomes appeared clumped within the nucleus and could not easily be distinguished from one another. The normal human chromosome number at that time was thought to be 48. Soon after the introduction of hypotonic treatment, the correct number of 46 was determined. The use of peripheral blood cultures greatly simplified the collection of dividing cells for analysis. In 1959, the first human chromosome abnormality, trisomy 21, responsible for Down syndrome, was described.

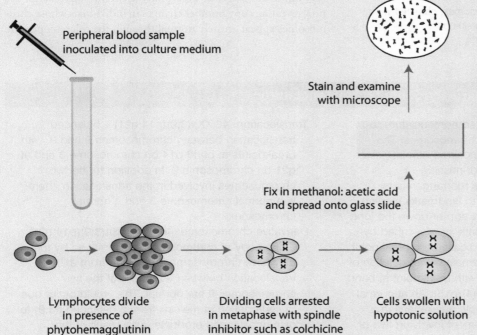

Figure 6.6 Process of analysis of mitotic chromosomes from peripheral blood. Whole blood is inoculated into a culture containing the lectin **phytohemagglutinin**, which stimulates the division of T cells. After 3 days in culture, the cells are swollen in hypotonic saline, fixed onto glass slides, stained, and examined through the microscope.

Peripheral blood sample inoculated into culture medium

Stain and examine with microscope

Fix in methanol: acetic acid and spread onto glass slide

Lymphocytes divide in presence of phytohemagglutinin

Dividing cells arrested in metaphase with spindle inhibitor such as colchicine

Cells swollen with hypotonic solution

The centromeres are surrounded by blocks of highly repeated DNA sequences (Figure 6.8). A major component is referred to as **alpha-satellite DNA**, which consists of thousands of copies of a 171 bp repeat. (Do not confuse this use of the term "satellite" with the acrocentric chromosome satellites also described in this section. Satellite DNA is so-called because it consists of a highly repeated sequence that separates from the main mass of DNA by density gradient centrifugation to form a distinct band, referred to as a "satellite.") This region remains highly compacted throughout the cell cycle. The telomeres consist of 10–15 kb of a repeat unit GGGTTA, with repeated sequences extending for 100–300 kb inside of this region (see Chapter 1). **Interspersed repeated sequences** account for the chromosome-banding patterns obtained with special stains.

Interspersed repeated sequences are short DNA segments that are scattered throughout the genome. As described in Chapter 4, two major types are called short interspersed elements (SINEs) and long interspersed elements (LINEs). SINE sequences are GC rich and tend to be found in gene-rich areas, whereas LINEs are AT rich and are found in gene-poor regions (Figure 6.9). Chromosome banding reflects differences in protein binding and chromatin condensation, which is greater in AT-rich, gene-poor regions.

Molecular Cytogenetics

Methods of chromosomal analysis for clinical diagnosis have evolved steadily since the 1950s. Initially it was possible to

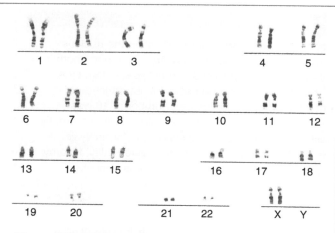

Figure 6.7 G-banded human chromosomes, obtained with trypsin treatment followed by Giemsa staining.

identify only gross abnormalities such as an extra or missing chromosome or major structural rearrangements. The introduction of chromosome banding in the late 1960s permitted smaller and subtler changes to be identified. Beginning in the 1990s, molecular tools began to be introduced that extended the resolution of detection to submicroscopic levels. **Fluorescence** in situ **hybridization (FISH)** (Methods 6.3) permitted detection of deletions or duplications of about a million base pairs. The approach led to the discovery of a group of disorders associated with microdeletion or microduplication that were previously not recognized to be due to chromosomal changes. Most recently, techniques of comparative genomic hybridization and use of genomic microarrays (Methods 6.4) have permitted detection of copy number changes down to a few hundred thousand base pairs. Genomic approaches are now revealing copy number changes in individuals whose chromosomes appear entirely normal through the microscope. The

---

✓ Methods 6.2 Standard Cytogenetic Nomenclature

Cytogeneticists use a standardized nomenclature to describe normal and abnormal chromosomes. The nomenclature includes the chromosome number, sex chromosome constitution, extra or missing chromosomes, and chromosome rearrangements. Bands are numbered according to landmarks starting from the centromere up the short arm or down the long arm. Chromosomal rearrangements are described by noting the rearrangement and indicating the breakpoint or breakpoints. For example, a female with a deletion of the short arm of chromosome 4 with breakpoint at band p15 has the karyotype 46,XX,del(4)(p15). An abnormal chromosome generated by multiple aberrations in a single chromosome or rearrangement involving two or more chromosomes is defined as a derivative chromosome. An abnormal chromosome that cannot be identified is defined as a marker chromosome.

I.   Normal karyotype
     Male: 46,XY
     Female: 46,XX
II. Aneuploidy
     Female with Down syndrome: 47,XX,+21
     Male with trisomy 18: 47,XY,+18
     Turner syndrome: 45,X
     Klinefelter syndrome: 47,XXY
III. Rearrangements
     Deletion: 46,XX,del(4)(p15)
     Inversion: 46,XY,inv(2)(p12q12) – inversion of
        chromosome 2 with breakpoints at p12
        and q12
     Ring: 46,XY,r(13) – male with ring chromosome 13

Translocation: 46,XX,t(3;9)(p14;q21) – balanced translocation between chromosomes 3 and 9, with breakpoints at band p14 on chromosome 3 and at q21 on chromosome 9. In addition to the two chromosomes involved in the translocation, there is a normal chromosome 3 and a normal chromosome 9.
Derivative chromosome: 46,XY,der(3)t(3;9)(p14;q21) – one copy of chromosome 3 is replaced by the derivative chromosome 3 resulting from a translocation between 3 and 9, but the two chromosomes 9 are normal. This would occur due to segregation at meiosis from a balanced t(3;9) to give unbalanced products. As a result of this unbalanced translocation, the patient is monosomic for part of chromosome 3 (3p14→p terminal) and trisomic for part of chromosome 9 (9q21→q terminal).
IV. FISH results
     ish del(22)(q11.2q11.2)(TUPLE1–) – metaphase FISH analysis using the TUPLE1 probe demonstrating a microdeletion in chromosome 22 at band q11.2 in the DiGeorge syndrome and velocardiofacial syndrome region
V.   Cytogenomic array result
     arr 22q11.21(17,274,835-19,835,417)x1 – Cytogenomic array analysis demonstrating an interstitial deletion in the proximal region of the long (q) arm of chromosome 22 between linear genomic positions 17,274,835 and 19,835,417 bp (NCBI36/hg18) in the DiGeorge syndrome and velocardiofacial syndrome region

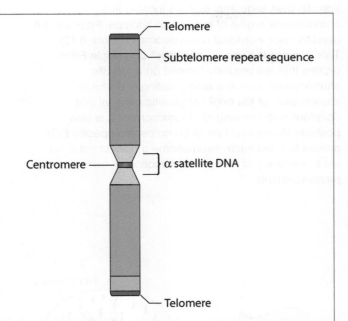

Figure 6.8 Diagram showing the major types of repeated DNA on a chromosome. Satellite DNA flanks the centromeric region. Subtelomere repeated DNA occurs just proximal to the two telomeres. Not drawn to scale.

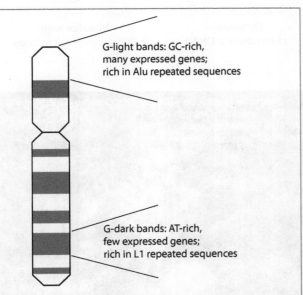

Figure 6.9 G-light bands are GC rich and contain SINEs such as Alu repeats. G-dark bands are AT rich and contain LINE sequences, such as L1.

high sensitivity of this approach has made it the first-line technique for diagnostic study of individuals with congenital anomalies or developmental impairment. The approach will detect unbalanced rearrangements but will miss balanced changes, making analysis with the microscope still necessary in some cases. Indications for chromosomal analysis and choice of approach are discussed at the end of this chapter.

Chromosome Abnormalities

The ability to examine human chromosomes in readily accessible tissues, such as peripheral blood, led to the discovery of innumerable examples of abnormalities of chromosome number or structure. These abnormalities tend to occur in two settings: individuals with congenital anomalies and/or developmental impairment, and in somatic cells obtained from malignant tissue. We will explore cancer cytogenetics in detail in Chapter 8; here we will take a closer look at chromosomal abnormalities and their developmental consequences. Three main types of chromosomal abnormalities will be considered: polyploidy, aneuploidy, and chromosomal rearrangements. We will also consider the cytogenetic consequences of imprinting disorders.

Polyploidy

The normal diploid number of chromosomes arises by fertilization of a haploid egg by a haploid sperm. **Polyploidy** represents the occurrence of one or more entire extra sets of chromosomes. **Triploidy** is the presence of 69 chromosomes, three haploid sets; and **tetraploidy** is 92 chromosomes, four sets. Polyploidy is generally not compatible with survival. Most polyploid embryos spontaneously miscarry. Rare triploid fetuses survive to live birth, though the condition is associated with severe congenital anomalies and virtually all of the infants die. Triploidy results from aberrant fertilization events, including fertilization by two sperm (dispermy), or fusion of a polar body with the egg cell, producing a diploid ovum that results in triploidy upon fertilization.

Aneuploidy

The term **aneuploidy** refers to the presence of a non-integral multiple of the haploid number of chromosomes, usually one chromosome more or less than the diploid number due to **trisomy** (an extra chromosome) or **monosomy** (a single copy of a particular chromosome). The first human chromosomal abnormality to be recognized was trisomy 21, which results in Down syndrome. **Down syndrome** is a well-recognized clinical condition (Clinical Snapshot 6.1). It was relatively easy to recognize trisomy in the early days of cytogenetic testing, since it requires only a count of chromosomes, not an analysis of fine structure for subtle changes.

The recognition of trisomy 21 in 1959 was the first of a series of studies of other syndromes that, like Down syndrome, have fairly consistent clinical features yet usually occur

The principle of FISH is illustrated in Figure 6.10. DNA on the microscope slide is separated into single strands, but the strands remain in position on the fixed chromosomes. A purified DNA sequence is labeled with a fluorescent dye and also separated into single strands. A solution of this labeled "probe" DNA is then placed on the slide. Wherever the probe DNA finds homologous chromosomal DNA a stable double helix will form. The sites of binding of probe DNA to the fixed chromosomes can be visualized by fluorescence microscopy.

FISH enables detection of the deletion of small chromosome regions (Figure 6.11). This is usually accomplished using FISH probes corresponding to specific DNA segments that are located in a chromosome region of interest. In addition, FISH can be used to paint individual chromosomes (Figure 6.12). This requires the use of "cocktails" of multiple FISH probes that are uniquely located on a specific chromosome. Chromosome painting is useful in identification of the origin of genetic material that contributes to rearranged chromosomes. It is now possible to use cocktails of chromosome-specific FISH probes to paint each chromosome a distinct color, an aid in the study of complex chromosomal rearrangements.

Figure 6.10 Fluorescence *in situ* hybridization (FISH). Metaphase chromosomes are fixed onto slides, and DNA is separated into single strands. A single-stranded, fluorescent-labeled DNA "probe" binds to homologous DNA on the slide, and sites of binding visualized by fluorescence microscopy.

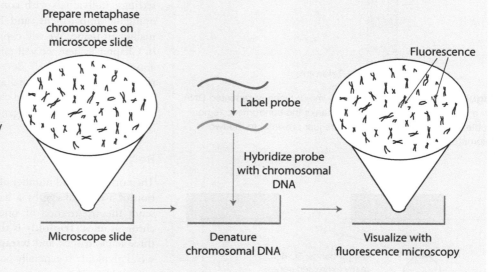

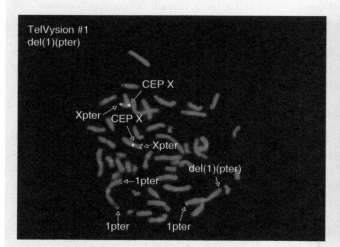

Figure 6.11 Deletion of subtelomeric sequences from one copy of chromosome 1pter (the terminal region of the short arm of chromosome 1). The deleted chromosome is at the lower right, and the normal homolog is to the left. The centromeric region of the X (CEP X) and the terminal short arm of the X (Xpter) are also labeled, as indicated.

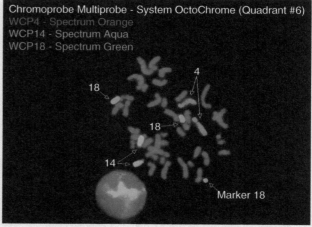

Figure 6.12 Chromosome painting identifies a marker chromosome as being derived from chromosome 18 (lower right). Whole-chromosome paints are shown for chromosomes 4, 14, and 18.

The resolution of FISH is limited by the requirement of light microscopic analysis to detect hybridization and the use of relatively large probes to generate sufficient fluorescence to be visible. The smallest rearrangements that can be seen are in the range of 1 million base pairs. The use of genomic microarrays (referred to as cytogenomics) has vastly increased the resolution of analysis. A genomic microarray consists of tens to hundreds of thousands of DNA sequences permanently attached to a solid substrate, each sequence corresponding to a specific region of chromosomal DNA. Hybridization of a test sequence, as from a patient, is used to test for deletion or duplication of corresponding sequences in the test DNA. Two methods of detection are used.

Comparative genomic hybridization (CGH) involves competition of the test sequences with a reference sample for hybridization to sequences on the microarray (Figure 6.13). The test and reference DNA samples are fragmented into small segments and each is fluorescently labeled with a different color, usually red and green. The two colors combine to make yellow if there is equal hybridization of a sequence to its homologue on the array. If there is duplication of the test sequence, its color will dominate on the corresponding spot in the array; if there is deletion of the test sequence, the reference DNA color will be seen on the spot. Computer analysis of all the spots in the array will reveal deleted or duplicated segments. The second method involves quantitative analysis of hybridization of a test sample to the microarray; no reference sample is used. Deletions or duplications are detected as decreased or increased hybridization signals over background. The resolution of genomic analysis is limited by the size of the fragments attached to the array. Any individual segment may appear duplicated or deleted due to "noise" in the system, but

true copy number changes are inferred when signals from multiple contiguous sequences are found to be abnormal (Figure 6.14). The major challenge with interpretation of genomic microarrays is not whether copy number changes are truly present, but whether these changes are clinically significant (see Hot Topic 6.1).

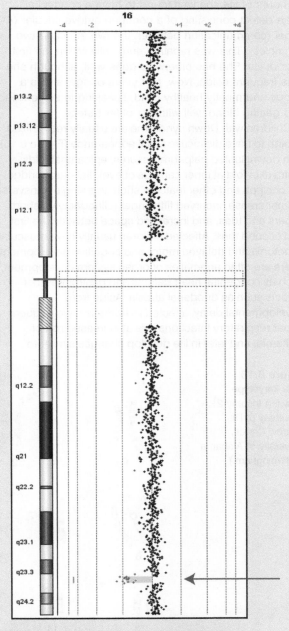

Figure 6.14 Comparative genomic hybridization demonstrating deletion of small region on the long arm of chromosome 16 (arrow). Each dot represents the difference in test versus reference hybridization at a specific oligonucleotide. Most are centered at "0," indicating approximately equal fluorescence. The deletion is indicated by numerous contiguous oligonucleotides where the test hybridization is deficient by 1 copy ("−W1") compared with reference. (Courtesy of Dr. Fady Mikhail, University of Alabama at Birmingham.)

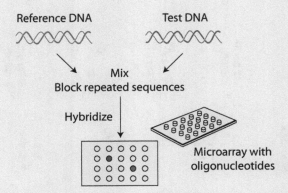

Figure 6.13 Comparative genomic hybridization. The test sample is labeled with red fluorescence, and the reference with green. The two are mixed together and hybridized with DNA oligonucleotides bound to a microarray. Equal hybridization produces a yellow signal; excess test (due to duplication) results in red, whereas excess reference (due to test DNA deletion) results in a green signal.

👁 Clinical Snapshot 6.1 Down Syndrome

Laura was born after a full-term, uncomplicated pregnancy. Both her parents were 30 years old. No prenatal genetic studies were done. Laura was noted by the obstetrician to have features of Down syndrome at birth. Her neonatal course was at first uneventful, but at 48 hours of life she was found to have a congenital heart defect consisting of a common atrioventricular (AV) canal (communication between the two atria and two ventricles). This was repaired surgically within the first year of life. She has otherwise done well, although she gets frequent colds. Now, at 4 years of age, she is a happy and mostly healthy child, speaking in sentences, and getting along well with her older sister.

Children with Down syndrome are usually recognized at birth to have distinctive facial appearance (Figure 6.15) with downslanted palpebral fissures, epicanthal folds (extra skin fold at inner canthus of eye), flat nasal bridge, flat occiput, and other features such as a single transverse palmar crease, incurved fifth finger (clinodactyly), short fingers and toes, and increased space between the first and second toes. Affected children usually have muscular hypotonia and delayed motor and cognitive development. There are often anomalies of organ system development, such as congenital heart defects and gastrointestinal defects such as duodenal atresia. Aside from developmental delay, affected individuals have frequent upper respiratory infections, are at increased risk of leukemia, and later in life develop changes similar to

those of Alzheimer disease. Although there are individual differences for any of these features, the general similarity of the constellation of signs and symptoms led to the recognition of a common underlying cause, trisomy 21 (Figure 6.16).

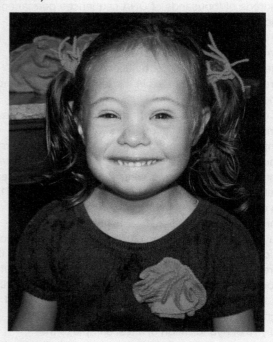

Figure 6.15 Child with Down syndrome.

Figure 6.16
Male karyotype showing trisomy 21. (Courtesy of Dr. Andrew Carroll, University of Alabama at Birmingham.)

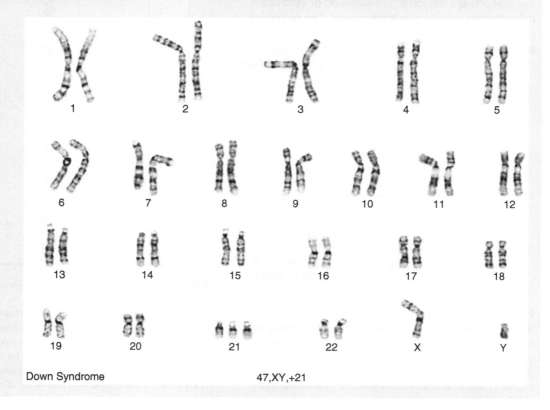

Down Syndrome   47,XY,+21

Table 6.1 Major chromosome aneuploidy syndromes compatible with live birth.

Syndrome	Karyotype	Major features
Patau syndrome	Trisomy 13	Cleft lip and palate, severe central nervous system anomaly, polydactyly, and renal anomalies
Edwards syndrome	Trisomy 18	Low birth weight, central nervous system anomalies, and heart defects
Down syndrome	Trisomy 21	Hypotonia, characteristic facial features, developmental delay, and heart defects
Turner syndrome	Monosomy X	Short stature, amenorrhea, lack of secondary sexual development, and infertility
Klinefelter syndrome	XXY	Small tests, infertility, tall stature, and learning problems
Triple X	XXX	Learning disabilities; no major physical anomalies
XYY	XYY	Learning and behavioral problems

sporadically. Two other autosomal trisomy syndromes were quickly identified: Patau syndrome due to trisomy 13 and Edwards syndrome due to trisomy 18 (Table 6.1). None of the other autosomal trisomies is compatible with live birth, and no autosomal monosomy is. Chromosomal studies of early spontaneous abortions have revealed a high frequency of aneuploidy, usually trisomy, involving any of the chromosomes. Sex chromosome aneuploidy is more readily tolerated. X chromosome monosomy, designated 45,X, produces the phenotype of Turner syndrome (Clinical Snapshot 6.2). Monosomy for the Y is lethal. Having additional X or Y chromosomes is compatible with survival, though specific phenotypes occur as a consequence.

Aneuploidy results from an error in meiosis or mitosis called **nondisjunction** (Figure 6.18). Meiotic nondisjunction during the first division results in both homologous chromosomes going to the same gamete. If the nondisjunction occurs in the second meiotic division, two identical chromatids go to the same gamete. Mitotic nondisjunction occurs during somatic cell division and results in mosaicism, assuming that it occurs after the first cleavage. The coexistence of a chromosomally normal cell line with an aneuploid line can ameliorate the developmental effects of trisomy. This permits survival of some fetuses with mosaic trisomy for chromosomes that would not be compatible with survival if all cells were affected. The relative proportion of trisomic and nontrisomic cells depends, in part, on when in the course of cell division the nondisjunction occurred, but also in part on the relative rate of growth and survival of the two cell lines.

Nondisjunction appears to occur most often in the first meiotic division in females. Hence, most individuals with trisomy 21 have two maternal chromosomes 21 and one paternal. Causes of nondisjunction are, for the most part, unknown. The only risk factor so far recognized is advanced maternal age. Risk of having a child with aneuploidy rises sharply with maternal age after about 35 years (Figure 6.19). Genetic factors may also play a role, since there are rare families with apparent clustering of instances of aneuploidy. Couples at increased risk of having a child with trisomy can be offered prenatal testing (Ethical Implications 6.1). We will explore the application of prenatal diagnosis elsewhere in this book.

The phenotypic effects of chromosomal imbalance are presumed to result from abnormal levels of gene expression. Increased levels of transcription have been demonstrated for chromosome 21 genes in cells from individuals with Down syndrome. It is likely that some genes will be more vulnerable to disruption of function by dosage effects than others. There are more than 200 genes on chromosome 21, so it should not be a surprise that a complex phenotype results from trisomy 21. What may be more surprising is that the phenotype is as reproducible as it is with this large degree of genetic imbalance. Studies are underway to identify the genes that are critical to particular phenotypes in Down syndrome, using mouse models of Down syndrome as well as studying the phenotypes in persons who have trisomy for small regions of chromosome 21 due to chromosomal rearrangements. This is narrowing the search for genes that contribute to various clinical features, and may eventually uncover pathogenetic mechanisms that may suggest therapeutic approaches to improve quality of life for those with the condition.

Structural Abnormalities

Chromosomal rearrangements can involve single chromosomes or an exchange of material between chromosomes (Figure 6.20). A piece of a chromosome may be lost by deletion or may be duplicated. The former results in monosomy for a group of genes, and the latter in trisomy for the genes. Chromosome segments also can be inverted – flipped 180 degrees from their normal orientation. If no material is gained or lost, the changes probably will have no phenotypic impact. In some cases, a gene may be disrupted by the chromosome breakage involved in the inversion, but there are vast regions of genetically inert material between groups of genes, so

👁 Clinical Snapshot 6.2 Turner Syndrome

Vanessa is a 15 year old who is referred for evaluation of delayed puberty. She has been healthy, but is increasingly frustrated that she has not begun any of the signs of puberty, including breast enlargement or menstruation. This is a significant social problem, as her friends at school are changing whereas she is not. Examination reveals that she is 4 feet 11 inches tall, which is short for members of her family. She has a webbed neck and prepubertal pattern of sexual maturation. A chromosomal analysis is sent, and she is found to have a 45,X karyotype consistent with Turner syndrome.

Turner syndrome is the only chromosomal monosomy syndrome compatible with live birth. Most conceptuses with the 45,X karyotype miscarry, but some make it to term and can survive for a long period thereafter. Individuals with Turner syndrome have a female phenotype. At birth they may have swollen hands and feet due to an inadequately developed lymphatic system. *In utero*, they can have massive edema, especially around the base of the neck. This stretches the skin in this region and is responsible for the webbed neck seen later in life. There may be internal malformations, especially coarctation of the aorta and renal anomalies such as horseshoe kidney. Intelligence is usually normal, but cognitive problems, including learning disabilities and difficulties with visuospatial perception, are common. Affected girls tend to be short and do not develop female secondary sex characteristics. Their ovaries degenerate into fibrous streaks and produce neither estrogen nor oocytes.

The principal karyotypic finding in Turner syndrome is a single X chromosome. Some affected girls have two Xs, including one normal and one rearranged X chromosome. The rearrangement often is a deletion, usually of the short arm, or may be an isochromosome (Figure 6.17), usually for the long arms. Some are mosaics, with one cell line having 46 chromosomes with a rearranged X or Y and the other 45 chromosomes without the rearranged X.

Turner syndrome is only one of several sex chromosome abnormalities. Females with three or more X chromosomes tend to have developmental delay as the principal phenotype. The presence of a Y chromosome confers a male phenotype. Individuals who are mosaic for a rearranged Y and a 45,X cell line may have a testis on one side and a streak gonad on the other, referred to as mixed-gonadal dysgenesis. Males with two or more X chromosomes plus a Y have Klinefelter syndrome. This consists of atrophic testes with azoospermia, some degree of female secondary sex characteristics, and learning problems.

Figure 6.17

Karyotype from a woman with Turner syndrome showing one normal X chromosome and an isochromosome for the long arm of the X (arrows). (Courtesy of Dr. Andrew Carroll, University of Alabama at Birmingham.)

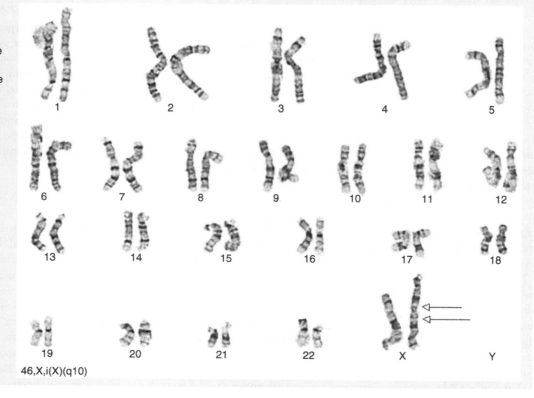

46,X,i(X)(q10)

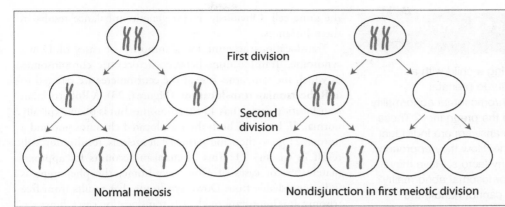

Figure 6.18 Normal meiosis (left), and first-division meiotic nondisjunction (right).

First division

Second division

Normal meiosis

Nondisjunction in first meiotic division

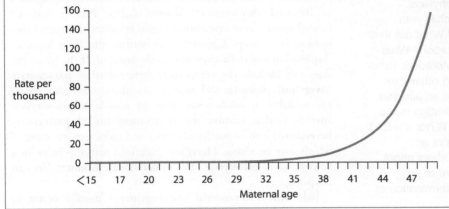

Figure 6.19 Increase in the risk of nondisjunction resulting in trisomy 21 with advanced maternal age.

Rate per thousand

Maternal age

usually these breaks cause no phenotype. As will be seen in this chapter, however, such breaks can lead to unbalanced chromosomes after crossing over in meiosis. Another intrachromosomal rearrangement is formation of a **ring chromosome**. This arises from breakage of the two ends and their subsequent fusion into a ring structure. There may be phenotypic consequences from deletion of chromatin from the two ends and also from mitotic instability of rings, resulting in trisomic or monosomic cells. **Isochromosomes** represent duplications of either the short or long arms due to misdivision of the centromere.

Translocation involves the exchange of material between chromosomes (Figure 6.21). Usually, translocations arise as reciprocal exchanges. If no material is lost or gained, the translocation is said to be balanced. Balanced translocations – and inversions, for that matter – are occasionally found as variants in the general population. It is estimated that approximately 0.2% of individuals carry an asymptomatic chromosomal rearrangement. If one comes to medical attention, it is usually as

a consequence of the generation of unbalanced gametes during meiosis, leading to spontaneous abortion or the birth of a child with congenital anomalies. Most, if not all, translocations are reciprocal. Balanced reciprocal translocations can spawn gametes with genetic imbalance due to aberrant segregation during meiosis.

Meiotic pairing between chromosomes involved in a balanced translocation requires a complex association of four chromosomes – the two involved in the exchange and the two homologues (Figure 6.22). When first anaphase occurs, these chromosomes can separate in several ways. If the two normal homologues go to one cell and the two involved in the exchange go to another, the resulting gametes will be genetically balanced – either normal or having both rearranged chromosomes. Genetic imbalance will result, however, if germ cells get one normal chromosome and one rearranged chromosome. The translocation complex can also segregate so that three chromosomes go to one cell and only one to the other. Rarely, all four chromosomes can go to

Should a couple at risk of having a child with a chromosomal abnormality undergo prenatal diagnosis? If they do, and a chromosomal abnormality is found, should they continue the pregnancy? These are difficult questions, and the answers are individual matters for the couple to decide. How they approach the questions depends on many factors. Have they already had a child with a chromosomal abnormality? If so, they might feel that they cannot handle the challenge of having another. But they also might experience guilt if they terminate the pregnancy, feeling that it is a refutation of the value of their previous affected child. Do they have experience with the care of a child with a chromosomal abnormality? Do they understand the challenges – physical, emotional, and financial – of raising a child with special needs, and are they prepared? What are their personal and religious views about abortion? What about other members of their family? Moreover, there are reasons to undergo prenatal testing other than consideration of possible termination of an affected pregnancy. Some couples embark on testing in the hope of being reassured that the fetus is not affected and only begin to face the implications of an abnormal result after it has occurred. Others might wish to be tested to prepare for the care of an affected child and would not consider termination of pregnancy.

The tradition in prenatal genetic counseling is to provide information and support in a nondirective manner. This means that the counselor does not advise the couple to take a specific course of action (i.e., to have prenatal testing or not, or to continue an affected pregnancy or not). Genetic counselors are trained to present all options in a neutral manner, and to support the couple whatever decision they make. The counselor tries to avoid letting his or her personal views influence the decision.

Is it possible to give truly nondirective counseling? Although a counselor might try to provide information in a neutral way, subtle matters of emphasis or body language might communicate bias toward a particular course of action. Genetic counselors endeavor to recognize and minimize the impact of such bias. Nondirective counseling is not the norm in other areas of medical care. Patients usually expect a health professional to provide advice on the best course of action, for example choice of medication. As we will see in this book, nondirective counseling may be difficult in other areas of genetics, such as when presenting care options for a treatable disorder.

the same cell. Obviously, major genetic imbalance results in these instances.

Translocations account for a minority of cases of Down syndrome. Translocations between acrocentric chromosomes in which the long arms fuse at the centromeres are referred to as **Robertsonian translocation**s (Figure 6.23). A Robertsonian translocation carrier has 45 chromosomes but is phenotypically normal. If, however, both the translocated chromosome and a normal 21 go to the same germ cell at meiosis, fertilization will result in trisomy 21. This mechanism accounts for approximately 5% of cases of Down syndrome; the phenotype is indistinguishable from Down syndrome that results from free trisomy. It is important to identify translocation cases, however, because a carrier is at risk of having additional offspring with trisomy. Robertsonian translocations can be present in many members of a family, all of whom are at risk of having children with Down syndrome.

Genetic imbalance can also result from meiotic segregation of inverted chromosomes (Figure 6.24). Pairing between homologues where one chromosome is inverted requires formation of a loop. Crossing over within the loop leads to duplication and deficiency of genetic material. If the inversion does not include the centromere (referred to as **paracentric inversion**), dicentric and acentric chromosomes result. These are unstable at mitosis and lead to nonviable phenotypes. Inversions that involve the centromere (called **pericentric inversions**) lead to partial trisomies and monosomies, some of which may be viable. Here, too, balanced rearrangement in a carrier can predispose to unbalanced products in an offspring.

Balanced chromosomal rearrangements usually come to attention through a child who has the rearrangement in an unbalanced form. Sometimes it is discovered when chromosomal analysis is done as part of an evaluation for recurrent miscarriage. Once found, other relatives may be tested to determine whether they also carry the rearrangement. Carriers are provided with genetic counseling, and prenatal diagnosis can be offered.

Chromosome deletion syndromes also affect gene dosage. Deletion of large segments or of entire chromosomes usually is poorly tolerated. Except for 45,X Turner syndrome, there are no other whole-chromosome monosomy syndromes compatible with live birth. Smaller deletions, as well as small duplications, may result in recognizable syndromes. It is believed that complex phenotypes result from simultaneous deletion or duplication of a group of genes, each of which is responsible for a specific developmental process. The exact phenotype may vary according to the extent of the rearrangement and which genes are deleted or duplicated. Although the larger chromosome copy number changes are readily identified by standard cytogenetic analysis, deletions of fewer than a million base pairs or so cannot be resolved with the light microscope. Cytological detection of very small changes requires the use of FISH (Methods 6.3) or cytogenomic analysis (Methods 6.4). Many microdeletion and microduplication syndromes have been defined (Table

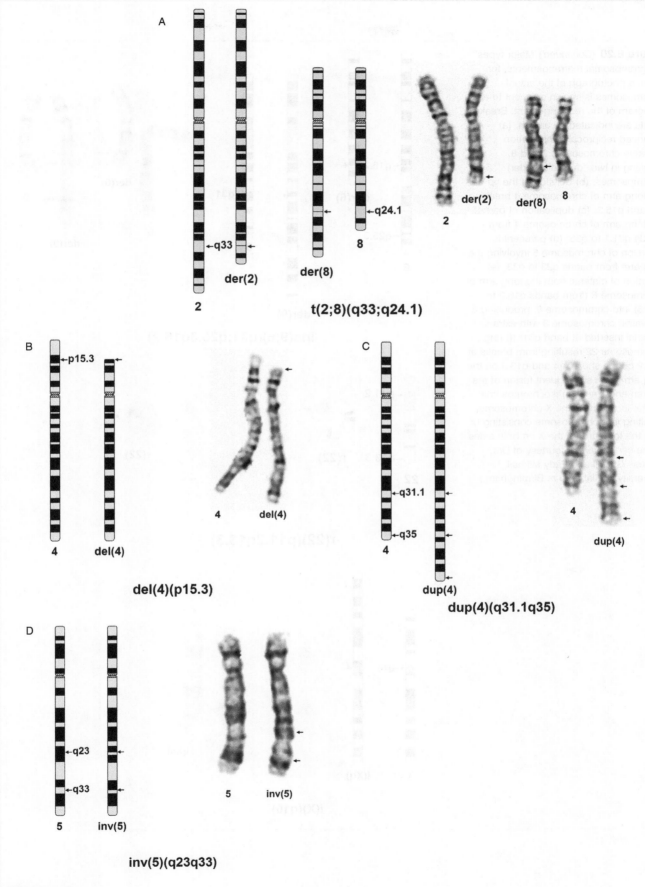

Figure 6.20

Figure 6.20 (*Continued*) Major types of chromosomal rearrangements; for each, a photograph of the actual chromosomes is shown adjacent to an ideogram of the rearrangement. Break points are indicated by arrows. (a) Balanced reciprocal translocation between chromosomes 2 and 8, resulting in two "derivative" (der) chromosomes; (b) deletion of the tip of the long arm of chromosome 4 breaking at band p15.3; (c) duplication of part of the long arm of chromosome 4 from bands q31.1 to q35; (d) paracentric inversion of chromosome 5 involving the long arm from bands q23 to q33; (e) insertion of material from the long arm of chromosome 6 (from bands q16.2 to q25.3) into chromosome 9, producing a derivative chromosome 9 with extra material inserted at band q31; (f) ring chromosome 22 resulting from breaks at p11.2 on the short arm and q13.3 on the long arm, with subsequent fusion of the broken ends; and (g) isochromosome for the long arm of the X chromosome, resulting in a chromosome consisting of only the long arm of the X on both sides of the centromere. (Courtesy of Drs. Andrew Carroll and Fady Mikhail, University of Alabama at Birmingham.)

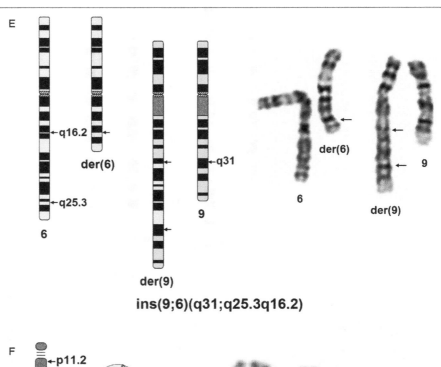

ins(9;6)(q31;q25.3q16.2)

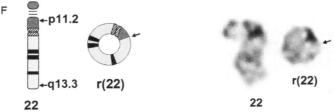

r(22)(p11.2q13.3)

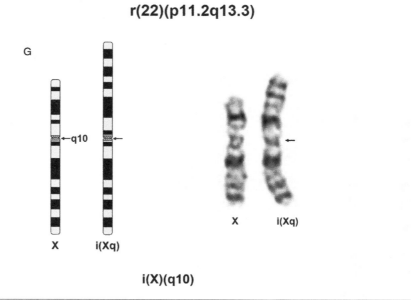

i(X)(q10)

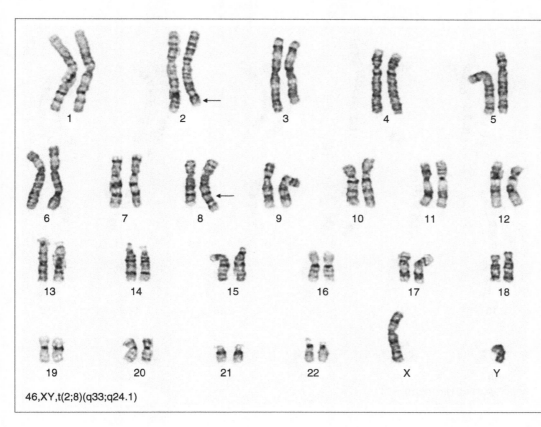

Figure 6.21 Balanced reciprocal translocation between the long arms of chromosomes 2 and 8. Breakpoints are shown by the arrows. (Courtesy of Dr. Andrew Carroll, University of Alabama at Birmingham.)

46,XY,t(2;8)(q33;q24.1)

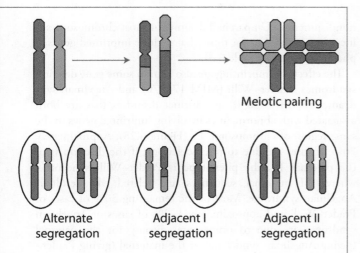

Meiotic pairing

Alternate segregation

Adjacent I segregation

Adjacent II segregation

Figure 6.22 Segregation of balanced reciprocal translocation in meiosis. Alternate segregation results in production of normal or balanced chromosomes. Separation of homologous centromeres (adjacent I) or nonhomologous centromeres (adjacent II) results in production of gametes with unbalanced chromosomes.

6.2; Clinical Snapshot 6.3). Although the phenotypes of these different syndromes are distinct, the deleted or duplicated regions are typically flanked by repeated sequences, suggesting that unequal crossing over or nonhomologous recombination is a common mechanism (see Chapter 2).

Imprinting and Chromosomal Abnormalities

The phenomenon of genomic imprinting has been described in Chapters 1 and 3. We have seen that there are certain genes that are expressed only from the maternal or paternal copy and that this can result in complex patterns of inheritance of single-gene disorders. Imprinting has also been found to have a role in determining the phenotype in individuals with certain chromosomal abnormalities.

The effects of imprinting in humans first came to light through studies of rare individuals affected with the autosomal recessive disorder cystic fibrosis who had, in addition, severe growth and developmental delay. They were found to have inherited the cystic fibrosis gene mutation – along with other genes on chromosome 7 – from just one parent (Figure 6.27). This is referred to as **uniparental disomy**. Uniparental disomy can arise by a number of mechanisms. A disomic egg could be fertilized by a nullisomic sperm; a monosomic zygote could duplicate the single chromosome to become disomic; or a trisomic zygote could lose one extra chromosome due to

Figure 6.23
Robertsonian translocation between chromosomes 14 and 21 (arrow) resulting in trisomy 21. (Courtesy of Dr. Andrew Carroll, University of Alabama at Birmingham.)

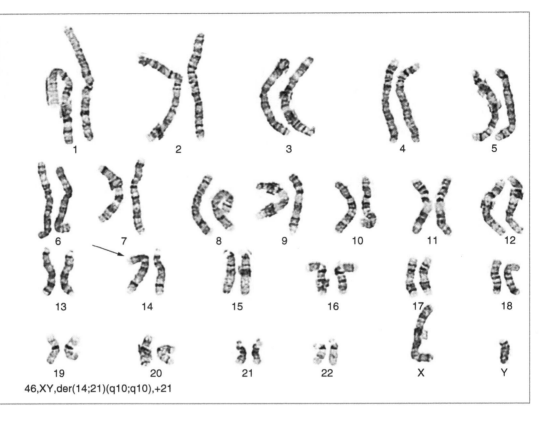

46,XY,der(14;21)(q10;q10),+21

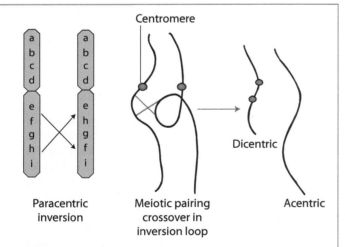

Paracentric inversion

Meiotic pairing crossover in inversion loop

Dicentric

Acentric

Centromere

Figure 6.24 Crossing over within an inversion loop of a paracentric inversion results in production of dicentric and acentric chromosomes. If the inversion is pericentric, deletion and deficiency chromosome products result.

nondisjunction. Uniparental disomy for most chromosomes is inconsequential, but for those that include imprinted genes, a phenotype results (Table 6.3).

The effects of imprinting are also seen in some gene deletion syndromes. Prader–Willi (MIM 176270) and Angelman syndromes (MIM 105830) are distinct disorders that are both associated with abnormalities involving imprinted genes in the same region of chromosome 15 (Figure 6.28). Approximately 70% of cases are due to microdeletions; if the deletion is of the paternal 15, the phenotype is Prader–Willi syndrome, whereas if maternal sequences are deleted, the result is Angelman syndrome. Most of the remaining 30% of cases of Prader–Willi and approximately 1–2% of cases of Angelman syndrome are due to uniparental disomy for the paternal (giving Angelman syndrome) or the maternal (giving Prader–Willi syndrome) copy of 15. Uniparental disomy is more common in Prader–Willi than in Angelman syndrome because trisomy 15 more commonly occurs due to maternal nondisjunction, leading to Prader–Willi syndrome through loss of the paternal 15 via a trisomy rescue mechanism (see Figure 6.27). There are imprinted genes in this region, some of which are expressed on the paternal and some on the maternal 15. One such gene, designated *UBE3A* (MIM 601623), is mutated in some patients with Angelman syndrome. The critical region

Table 6.2 Some chromosome microdeletion or microduplication syndromes.

Syndrome	Major features	Chromosome region
del (1p)	Intellectual disability, seizures, growth delay, and dysmorphic features	1p36
Williams	Characteristic facies, intellectual disability, supravalvar aortic stenosis, and neonatal hypercalcaemia	7q11.23 (elastin locus)
Langer–Giedion	Exostoses, abnormal facies, and intellectual disability	8q24.1
WAGR	Wilms' tumor, aniridia, genitourinary dysplasia, and intellectual disability	11p13
Retinoblastoma/ID	Retinoblastoma and intellectual disability	13q14
Prader–Willi	Hypotonia, obesity, and intellectual disability	15q12 (paternal deletion)
Angelman	Seizures, abnormal movements, and intellectual disability	15q12 (maternal deletion)
α-thalassemia/MR	α-thalassemia and intellectual disability	16p13.3
Rubenstein–Taybi	Microcephaly, characteristic facies, and intellectual disability	16p13.3
Smith–Magenis	Intellectual disability, characteristic facies, sleep disturbance, behavioral problems, and obesity	17p11.2
Miller–Dieker	Lissencephaly and characteristic facies	17p13.3
Charcot–Marie–Tooth	Peripheral neuropathy	17p12 duplication
Hereditary neuropathy with susceptibility to pressure palsies	Neuropathy and pressure palsies	17p12 deletion
Alagille	Intrahepatic biliary atresia, peripheral pulmonic stenosis, and characteristic facies	20p11.23
Chromosome 22q deletion syndrome	Palatal anomalies, conotruncal cardiac anomalies, and thymic and parathyroid hypoplasia	22q11.2
Steroid sulfatase deficiency/Kallman	Ichthyosis and anosmia	Xp22.3

involved in Prader–Willi syndrome includes several imprinted genes, though the specific gene or genes involved in the pathogenesis are not yet known.

Indications for Chromosomal Analysis

Chromosomal analysis has long been used to search for a genetic etiology in individuals with multiple congenital anomalies or developmental impairment. Aside from those with recognizable syndromes such as Down syndrome or Turner syndrome, there are many who have smaller deletions or duplications of chromosomal material. Some of these also lead to recognizable phenotypes, but in many the phenotypes are more nondescript, and consist of impaired neurocognitive development with or without congenital anomalies. One

general rule is to obtain chromosomal studies for any person with two or more congenital anomalies or with unexplained severe developmental delay (along with testing for other possible causes of developmental impairment such as Fragile X syndrome). Couples with recurrent early-pregnancy miscarriage (two or more first-trimester spontaneous abortions) also may be offered chromosomal analysis, looking for a balanced rearrangement in one partner that would predispose to unbalanced karyotypes in an offspring. Cytogenomic analysis has changed the approach to genetic investigation of individuals with neurocognitive impairment, autism spectrum disorders, and congenital anomalies. Genomic microarray studies will detect any copy number change that would be seen by standard cytogenetics, and will detect many that would not be seen through the microscope. Distinguishing benign variants from

◉ Clinical Snapshot 6.3 22q11.2 Deletion Syndrome

Tess is a 4-year-old girl who is referred for a speech and language evaluation. She began to say single words well after her second birthday and still is not speaking in full sentences. Her enunciation is also poor, and her voice is nasal. She has had many upper respiratory infections and has been followed for a heart murmur. Examination by an otolaryngologist reveals velopharyngeal incompetence (lack of complete closure of the nasopharynx by the soft palate). A chromosome study is sent, and FISH reveals a deletion at chromosome 22q11.2. A diagnosis of 22q11.2 deletion syndrome is made.

Chromosome 22q11.2 deletion syndrome is a congenital anomaly syndrome consisting of palatal abnormalities, congenital heart defects, and facial anomalies (Figure 6.25). This constellation of anomalies reflects its other name, velocardiofacial syndrome. The palatal anomalies can include cleft palate, submucous cleft palate, and velopharyngeal incompetence. The latter causes nasality of the voice. The cardiac anomalies tend to involve the conotrucal region, that is, the root of the aorta and pulmonary artery. These include coarctation (constriction) of the aorta, tetralogy of Fallot (pulmonic stenosis, ventricular septal defect, abnormal placement of the aortic outlet, and left ventricular hypertrophy), and truncus arteriosis (common aorta and pulmonary vessel). Facial anomalies include narrow palpebral fissures and prominent nasal root. In addition, there may be decreased resistance to infection due to immunological anomalies because of underdevelopment of the thymus. The more severe instances are recognized at birth in a syndrome of congenital heart defects, hypoplasia of the parathyroids resulting in hypocalcemia, and thymic aplasia, referred to as DiGeorge syndrome. The chromosome 22q11.2 deletion is easily detected by FISH (Figure 6.26) or by cytogenomic analysis. In some cases, the deletion can be familial, giving rise to dominant transmission of the phenotype.

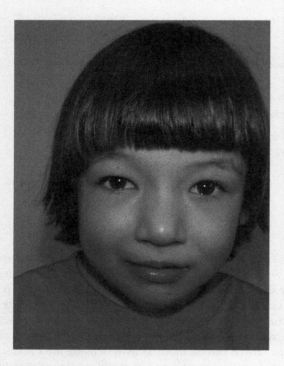

Figure 6.25 Child with chromosome 22q11.2 deletion syndrome. (Courtesy of Dr. Robert Shprintzen, SUNY Upstate Medical University, Syracuse, New York.)

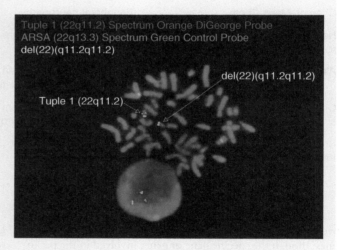

Figure 6.26 Detection of a submicroscopic deletion of chromosome 22q11.2 by FISH with two labeled probes. The control probe (ARSA, 22q13.3) binds to the end of chromosome 22, whereas the other probe (Tuple 1, 22q11.2) binds to a sequence in the region that is commonly deleted in individuals with chromosome 22q11.2 deletion syndrome. The chromosome at the right binds only with the ARSA probe, indicative of deletion of this region. (Courtesy of Dr. Andrew Carroll, University of Alabama at Birmingham.)

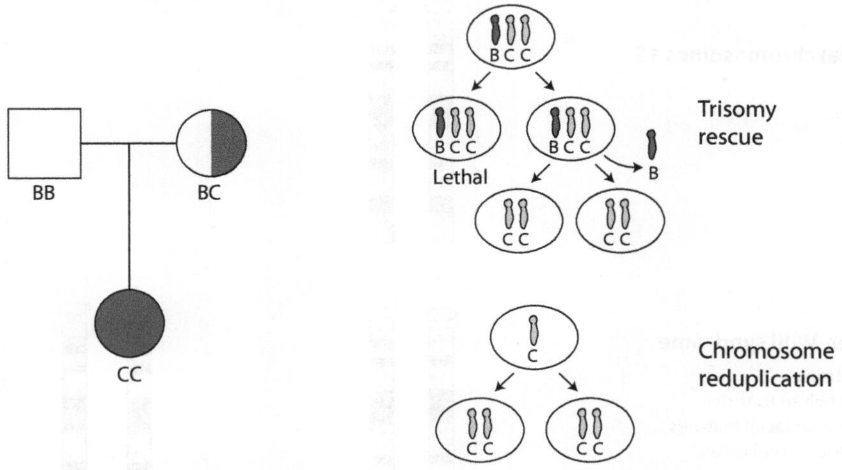

Figure 6.27 A child is homozygous for allele C, inherited from the mother, due to the phenomenon of uniparental disomy. This occurs by loss of the paternal chromosome, containing allele B, from a trisomic zygote.

Table 6.3 Some chromosomes implicated in clinical disorders due to uniparental disomy of the maternal or paternal chromosome or chromosome region.

Chromosome	Parent	Clinical effects
6	Paternal	Transient neonatal diabetes
7	Maternal	Russell–Silver syndrome
11	Paternal	Beckwith–Wiedemann syndrome
14	Paternal	Polyhydramnios, limb, chest, and abdominal wall defects, intellectual impairment
14	Maternal	Developmental impairment and bell-shaped thorax
15	Paternal	Prader–Willi syndrome
15	Maternal	Angelman syndrome
20	Paternal	Pseudohypoparathyroidism
20	Maternal	Impaired growth and development

clinically significant copy number changes requires careful assessment of genotypic changes in relation to phenotype (see Hot Topic 6.1; Sources of Information 6.1). Genomic micro-array analysis is now viewed as the first-line test in evaluation of congenital anomalies and neurocognitive disorders. It is important to remember, though, that only copy number variants are detected by this approach; detection of a structural rearrangement such as a balanced translocation or an inversion requires standard cytogenetic testing using the light microscope.

Conclusion

The ability to study chromosome number and structure helped to launch the discipline of medical genetics. Since then, advances have been made in prenatal diagnosis and the resolution of cytogenetic analysis has steadily improved. We are now seeing a convergence of cytological and molecular analysis, which is dramatically increasing the power of genetic testing, improving our ability to establish diagnoses and provide counseling to families.

Figure 6.28 Deletions and uniparental disomy involving chromosome 15 resulting in Prader–Willi or Angelman syndrome.

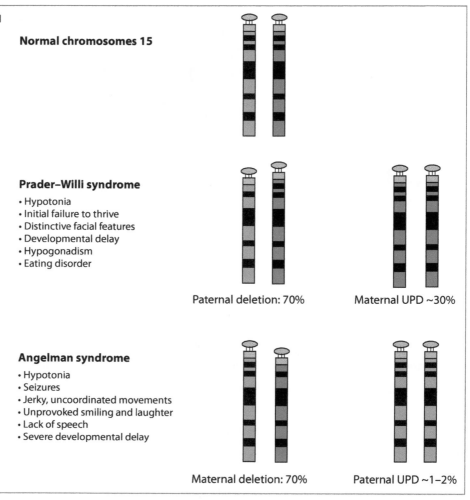

Normal chromosomes 15

Prader–Willi syndrome
- Hypotonia
- Initial failure to thrive
- Distinctive facial features
- Developmental delay
- Hypogonadism
- Eating disorder

Paternal deletion: 70%   Maternal UPD ~30%

Angelman syndrome
- Hypotonia
- Seizures
- Jerky, uncoordinated movements
- Unprovoked smiling and laughter
- Lack of speech
- Severe developmental delay

Maternal deletion: 70%   Paternal UPD ~1–2%

⚠ Hot Topic 6.1   Pathology Associated with Copy Number Variation

The use of genomic microarrays permits detection of copy number variants (CNVs) that previously would have escaped detection. How common are these variants, and how can we know whether a variant is pathological? Itsara *et al.* (2009) analyzed the frequency of copy number variants larger than 500 kb in 2500 apparently normal adults and performed a meta-analysis of CNVs reported in 12 500 individuals with autism spectrum disorders, mental retardation, and schizophrenia. They found an average of 3–7 variants per person, and an average of 540 kb of CNV per person, with no population-specific differences. Many CNVs were found to occur repeatedly in the neurologically impaired individuals, implicating these as pathological. Girirajan *et*

al. (2010) published a detailed study of one of these variants, a 520 kb microdeletion at 16p12.1. They found this CNV in 20 out of 11 873 cases of children with developmental delay compared with 2 out of 8450 controls. Most of the affected children had inherited the deletion from a parent who also had psychiatric problems, and 10 out of 42 cases had additional large CNVs. They proposed a "two-hit model" for neurodevelopmental disorders, in which the 16p12.1 deletion predisposes to neuropsychiatric symptoms, but the presence of a co-occurring CNV at another site leads to more severe developmental impairment, often accompanied by congenital anomalies.

Sources of Information 6.1   The DECIPHER Database

The increasing use of cytogenomic analysis to detect copy number variations has led to the discovery of innumerable novel deletions and duplications in phenotypically affected individuals. As noted in Hot Topic 6.1, the clinical significance of these is sometimes clear, other times not. Recognizing the need for clinicians and laboratory geneticists to share data on the phenotypic consequences of CNVs, the DECIPHER database was created in 2004 as part of a worldwide consortium. DECIPHER is an acronym for the Database of Chromosomal Imbalance and Phenotype in Humans Using Ensembl Resources. Both phenotypic data and data on the extent of the CNV are entered into the secure database, with full data entered only with patient consent and available only to members of the consortium. The genotypic data are referenced to the current version of the human genome sequence as recorded in the Ensembl database. Genes involved in the CNV, defined syndromes associated with CNVs in the region, and known imprinted genes are all indicated. The tool is used by cytogenetics laboratories and clinicians as an aid to interpretation of the clinical significance of CNVs, and also helps to annotate the genome with phenotypic information collected from consortium members.

REFERENCES

Girirajan S, Rosenfeld JA, Cooper GM, *et al.* 2010, "A recurrent 16p12.1 microdeletion supports a two-hit model for severe developmental delay", *Nature Genetics*, vol. 42, pp. 203–10.

Itsara A, Cooper G, *et al.* 2009, "Population Analysis of Large Copy Number Variants and Hotspots of Human Genetic Disease", *American Journal of Human Genetics*, vol. 84, pp. 148–61.

FURTHER READING

Babu A, Verma RS 1995, *Human chromosomes: principles and techniques*, McGraw-Hill, New York.

Ferguson-Smith MA 2008, "Cytogenetics and the evolution of medical genetics", *Genetics in Medicine*, vol. 10, pp. 553–9.

Kumar D 2008, "Disorders of genomic architecture", *Genomic Medicine*, vol. 2, pp. 69–76.

Miller DT *et al.* 2010, "Consensus statement: chromosomal microarray is a first-tier diagnostic test for individuals with developmental disabilities or congenital anomalies", *American Journal of Human Genetics*, vol. 86, pp. 749–64.

 Find interactive self-test questions and additional resources for this chapter at **www.korfgenetics.com**.

Self-Assessment

Review Questions

6.1   What would you expect to be the effect of a complete loss of p53 function?

6.2   At what point in meiosis do homologous centromeres separate? Do all homologous segments separate at this time?

6.3   A child with Down syndrome has the genotype 1,2,3 for a polymorphism on chromosome 21 that has alleles 1, 2, 3, and 4. His mother is 1,2 and father is 3,4. In which parent did nondisjunction occur, and did it occur in the first or second meiotic division?

6.4   Are pericentric or paracentric inversions most likely to be associated with the birth of a child with congenital anomalies? Is this more likely for a large or small inverted segment?

6.5   What kind of evidence would be required to determine whether a copy number change involving 250 kb of genomic DNA is clinically significant?

CHAPTER 7
Population Genetics

Introduction

So far we have considered genetic traits from the perspectives of the individual and the family. Some, like Down syndrome, are rare conditions that affect individuals throughout the world. Others, such as cystic fibrosis, are more prevalent in some populations than others. In this chapter, we will consider genetic traits from a different perspective – that of the population. Although genes act on individuals and flow through families, the forces that determine gene frequencies act at the level of populations. Study of these forces can have important implications for medicine. Firstly, we can understand why some populations appear to be singled out for particular genetic disorders and may be relatively free of others. Secondly, the principles of population genetics provide tools for calculating gene frequencies to use in genetic counseling. The frequency of carriers for recessive traits cannot be determined directly but can be calculated using a simple equation that is the cornerstone of population genetics. Population genetics helps us to understand the significance of genetic variation, and has provided the basis for the intersection of genetics with public health in the form of population screening programs (Sources of Information 7.1).

Human Genetics and Genomics, Fourth Edition. Bruce R. Korf and Mira B. Irons.
© 2013 John Wiley & Sons, Ltd. Published 2013 by John Wiley & Sons, Ltd.

Key Points

- The relationship between allele frequency and gene frequency is given by the Hardy–Weinberg equilibrium. In a two-allele system, if the frequency of the A allele is p and the a allele is q, then the genotype frequencies are given by p^2, 2pq, and q^2 for AA, Aa, and aa, respectively. These frequencies will remain stable from generation to generation, provided a set of assumptions are met, including no mutation, selection, or migration, and a large population size.
- Reduction of the ability of individuals with a specific genotype to reproduce constitutes selection. This can lead to a reduction of the frequency of the allele that is selected against. Eventually, an equilibrium may be reached between loss of the allele by selection and its replacement by new mutation.
- In some instances, selection may act against homozygotes for both alleles in a two-allele system. Heterozygotes may be favored, resulting in the two alleles being retained in the population. This constitutes a balanced polymorphism, and may result in the persistence of an otherwise deleterious allele.
- If a breeding population is small, there may be significant fluctuations in allele frequency from generation to generation, referred to as genetic drift.
- If a population goes through a "bottleneck" in which there are a small number of individuals, there can be major changes in allele frequency, including an increase in the frequency of a deleterious allele.

Sources of Information 7.1 Public Health Genetics

The power of genetics and genomics extends well beyond the care of individuals or families. There are profound implications for public health, with many initiatives already underway. Some of the areas of interest include:

- Programs for population screening, including carrier-screening programs and newborn-screening programs. The latter include screening for inborn errors of metabolism as well as conditions such as congenital deafness. Newborn-screening programs have traditionally been managed at a state level, but now there is discussion about bringing consistency to programs across different states in the United States.
- Quality assurance of genetic testing. As new genetic tests are developed, there is a need to track the

various pathogenic and nonpathogenic changes in genes. This will provide a dataset with which to judge the clinical significance of mutations found in the course of clinical testing.

- Prevention of common disorders. As genetic factors that contribute to common disorders come to light, it will be important to provide public education and access to testing to insure access to tests and appropriate counseling. The public health community also has a major interest in determining which tests are appropriate for use in screening and conducting studies to determine the efficacy of screening.

Information about topics in public health genetics and genetic epidemiology are tracked on a website, HuGEnet (www.cdc.gov/genomics/hugenet).

Hardy–Weinberg Equilibrium

The Hardy–Weinberg equilibrium provides the cornerstone for our understanding of population genetics. The concept was established in 1908 independently by the English mathematician G.H. Hardy and the German physician W. Weinberg. Their formulation states a simple relationship between the frequency of alleles at a genetic locus and the genotypes resulting from those alleles.

Consider a gene locus with alleles A and a. Let the frequency of A be designated by the variable p and the frequency of a by the variable q. If all alleles at this locus are either A or a, then

p + q = 1. The frequency of sperm or egg cells in the population carrying A or a will thus be p or q, respectively (Figure 7.1). If we assume that the union of germ cells carrying either A or a is entirely random, we can easily calculate the frequency of zygotes having the genotype AA, Aa, or aa. The frequency of AA will be p^2 and of aa will be q^2. The frequency of heterozygotes will be 2pq, reflecting that Aa individuals can arise in two ways: fusion of A-bearing sperm with a-bearing eggs, or vice versa (Methods 7.1).

The Hardy–Weinberg equilibrium depends on a number of assumptions. As already noted, mating must be random with respect to genotype. If there is preferential mating between AA

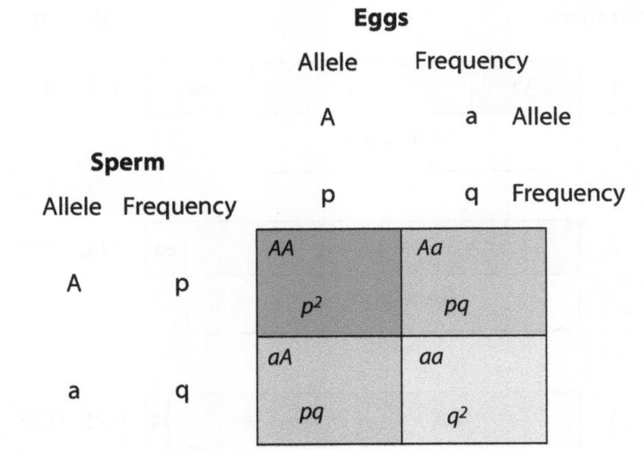

Eggs

	Allele	Frequency
	A	a	Allele

Sperm

Allele Frequency p q Frequency

		A (p)	a (q)
A	p	AA p^2	Aa pq
a	q	aA pq	aa q^2

Figure 7.1 The frequency of A-bearing sperm or eggs is p and of a-bearing sperm or eggs is q. Assuming that mating is random with respect to genotype, that there is no mutation from A to a or vice versa, that there is no migration in or out of the population, and that mating efficiency is equal for all genotypes, the frequency of the genotype AA is p^2, of Aa is 2pq, and of aa is q^2.

Methods 7.1 Derivation of the Hardy–Weinberg Equation

The Hardy–Weinberg equation can be easily derived algebraically. Start with a population in which the frequency of AA = x, Aa = y, and aa = z (i.e., the frequencies of the three genotypes are found to have values of x, y, and z, where $x + y + z = 1$). At this point, the frequency of A = p = $x + \frac{1}{2}y$ and the frequency of a = q = $z + \frac{1}{2}y$. We will show that, after one generation of random mating, the frequency of AA = p^2, Aa = 2pq, and aa = q^2.

First, let's consider all possible matings:

Mating type	Frequency	Outcome
AA × AA	x^2	All AA
AA × Aa	2xy	½ AA, ½ Aa
AA × aa	2xz	All Aa
Aa × Aa	y^2	¼ AA, ½ Aa, ¼ aa
Aa × aa	2yz	½ Aa, ½ aa
aa × aa	z^2	All aa

A mating type such as AA × Aa can occur in two ways: The male can be AA and the female Aa, or vice versa. Hence the frequency is 2xy (not xy).

Now let's tally the three genotypes in the next generation:

$$AA = x^2 + \tfrac{1}{2}(2xy) + \tfrac{1}{4}(y^2)$$
$$= (x + \tfrac{1}{2}y)^2 = p^2$$
$$Aa = \tfrac{1}{2}(2xy) + 2xz + \tfrac{1}{2}(y^2) + \tfrac{1}{2}(2yz)$$
$$= 2(x + \tfrac{1}{2}y)(z + \tfrac{1}{2}y) = 2pq$$
$$aa = \tfrac{1}{4}(y^2) + \tfrac{1}{2}(2yz) + z^2$$
$$= (z + \tfrac{1}{2}y)^2 = q^2$$

and AA individuals, for example, there will be more homozygous individuals and fewer heterozygotes. Also, the population is assumed to be very large, so statistical fluctuations will be negligible. Later we will explore the consequences of deviation from this assumption. There must be no mutation of A alleles into a, or a into A. Finally, individuals of all genotypes must be equally capable of reproduction (i.e., there must be no selection).

How is the Hardy–Weinberg equilibrium used to calculate carrier frequency of a recessive disorder? Consider the recessive condition cystic fibrosis. In this case, the A allele is the wild type and a is the cystic fibrosis mutation. The frequency of aa – that is, of individuals affected with cystic fibrosis – is 1 in 2500 in Northern European whites. Thus $q^2 = 1/2500$, and hence q = 1/50. Because p + q = 1, p must be 49/50. The carrier frequency, then, is 2pq = 2(49/50)(1/50) ≈ 1/25 in this population.

We are assuming, of course, that the cystic fibrosis gene obeys the assumptions of the Hardy–Weinberg equilibrium. The Northern European population is very large, large enough to minimize random statistical fluctuation (such as the chance that only noncarriers happen to bear children in one generation). Mating may not be entirely random with respect to genotype. Some cystic fibrosis carriers may meet one another because of their affected siblings, for example, and choose either to mate or not to mate, having been brought together because of genotype. For the most part, however, cystic fibrosis carriers are not aware of their carrier status.

Two other assumptions clearly are not fulfilled. The ability of individuals with cystic fibrosis to have offspring is definitely impaired. Males with cystic fibrosis usually are infertile. Females may be fertile, but reproduction is limited by the medical burden of the disorder. Many cystic fibrosis homozygotes therefore do not reproduce, which should cause loss of cystic fibrosis alleles in the population from one generation to the next. The rate of change of the frequency of the cystic fibrosis allele is very slow, however, as only 1 in 2500 individuals is subject to this negative selection. Most cystic fibrosis alleles exist in heterozygous carriers who are not subject to selection.

The Hardy–Weinberg equation also predicts that the gene frequencies will remain stable from generation to generation, provided that there is no mutation of A to a or of a to A, no migration of individuals to or from the population, random mating, and no selection. This may seem an obvious result: Under the assumptions of an "ideal" Hardy–Weinberg population, the alleles A and a have nowhere to go; they cannot leave or enter the population by migration, be lost by infertility, change by mutation, or dwindle by chance, so their stability is assured.

The Hardy–Weinberg equilibrium applies to X-linked traits as well as to autosomal traits. For an X-linked gene, males are hemizygous; the frequency of males with the genotype A is simply the frequency of the A allele, or p. Likewise, the frequency of males with the a genotype is q. Females can be AA, Aa, or aa, with the usual frequencies of p^2, $2pq$, and q^2, respectively.

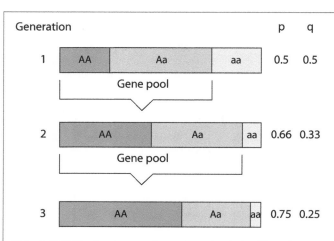

Figure 7.2 Decline in gene frequency after imposition of complete selection against the homozygous recessive individuals. Only AA and Aa individuals contribute to the gene pool. The frequency of a diminishes in each generation owing to lack of reproduction of aa individuals.

Deviations from the Hardy–Weinberg Equilibrium

The ideal Hardy–Weinberg population must fulfill several requirements that may not be met in real populations. In this section, we will explore the impact of deviators from these assumptions.

Selection

What happens if the ability to reproduce is not equal for individuals with various genotypes? To answer this, let us first consider the simple situation of a pair of alleles, A and a, with A dominant to a. Suppose that the frequency of both A and a is 0.5. If the population obeys the assumptions of the Hardy–Weinberg equation, we would expect these frequencies to remain stable over time. Approximately 25% of individuals would be AA, 50% Aa, and 25% aa.

Now suppose that aa individuals suddenly are rendered unable to reproduce. It doesn't matter how this happens: Those with the aa genotype might die before reproductive age or might be healthy but sterile. What matters is that they do not contribute to the gene pool of the next generation. Geneticists refer to this as a **lethal trait**, but it may be only the germ cells that die.

One might expect that this change would lead to a gradual loss of a alleles and corresponding increase in the proportion of A. In the first generation after imposition of selection, 25% of individuals are aa and are lost to the gene pool. Among the survivors, the 25% AA and 50% Aa, two-thirds of the alleles are A and one-third are a, so the frequency of a diminishes from 0.5 to 0.33. In the next generation, some aa homozygotes are produced through matings between heterozygotes, and the frequency of a will decrease again due to the inability of aa individuals to produce offspring. As the frequency of a diminishes, however, the proportion of heterozygotes also diminishes, so, with each generation there are fewer and fewer aa offspring to be subjected to selection (Figure 7.2). Therefore, the rate of decrease of the frequency of a slows. A graph of the

frequency of a as a function of time shows a rapid decline that approaches zero asymptotically (Figure 7.3). In an infinitely large population, a will approach, but will never reach, zero. In a real population, the day may come when there are very few Aa individuals who, by chance, happen not to produce any offspring with the a allele. At that point, the frequency of a becomes 0, and a is said to be extinguished and A fixed.

What if aa homozygotes are able to produce some offspring but do so less efficiently than AA or Aa individuals? The aa individuals are said to be selected against, or to have reduced **reproductive fitness**. The rate of decrease of the frequency of a will be slower, but the frequency will decrease nevertheless. The **coefficient of selection**, given by the variable s, is the proportion by which reproductive fitness is reduced by selection. Hence, a genotype associated with a coefficient of selection of 0.3 has a 30% reduction in ability to produce offspring compared with the general population. For a recessive trait where the homozygotes have a coefficient of selection of s, the loss of recessive alleles each generation is $2sq^2$ (for each homozygote who fails to reproduce, two recessive alleles are lost from the population). For a dominant, where the predominant affected genotype is the heterozygote (with a frequency of $2pq \approx 2p$ if $q \approx 1$), the proportion of lost alleles is $2ps$.

The frequency of allele under selection will continue to decline, albeit at a progressively slower rate, unless lost alleles are replaced by new mutation (Figure 7.4). Mutation rate per gamete per generation is denoted by μ. For a recessive, equilibrium is reached when $\mu = sq^2$; for dominant, $\mu = ps$. (The coefficient 2 factors out because each individual has two alleles

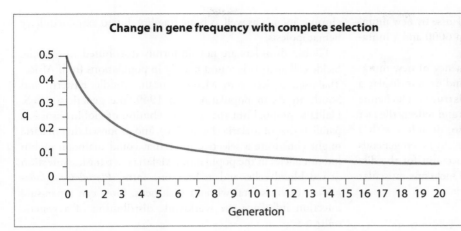

Figure 7.3 Graph of q as a function of generations after the imposition of complete selection, assuming that, at the start, p = q = 0.5. Note that the frequency decreases quickly at first, as there are many aa individuals. As the frequency of aa individuals declines, however, the rate of decrease in q also declines.

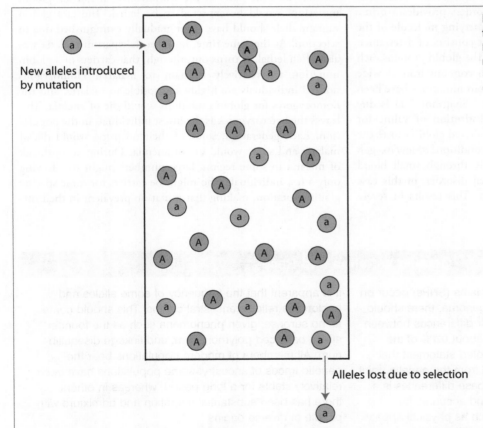

New alleles introduced by mutation

Alleles lost due to selection

Figure 7.4 Equilibrium in allele frequency is achieved when the alleles lost due to selection are replaced by new mutation.

that are subject to mutation in the germline in any cell, so for a recessive $2\mu = 2sq^2$ and for a dominant $2\mu = 2ps$.)

It is easy to find examples of genetic traits that are subject to selection. Consider Duchenne muscular dystrophy, an X-linked recessive trait that is lethal in males. In a given generation, the proportion of affected males is q and of heterozygous females is $2pq \approx 2q$. The proportion of mutant alleles lost in each generation is therefore $q/(q+2q) = 1/3$. At equilibrium, $\mu = q/3$. For the dominant disorder neurofibromatosis type 1, which occurs with a frequency of 1 in 3000 persons, approximately half of the cases in the world arise by new mutation. This predicts a gene frequency of 1 in 6000 and a mutation rate of 1 in 12 000.

Genetic disorders that have a high frequency of new mutation tend to occur throughout the world and do not display a racial, ethnic, or regional predilection. This is true for Duchenne muscular dystrophy and neurofibromatosis and reflects the fact that new mutations occur at random. Also, disorders with a high rate of new mutation tend to be genetically heterogeneous (i.e., a wide range of different mutations account for the disorder in different people, as is the case for Duchenne muscular dystrophy and neurofibromatosis).

Balanced Polymorphism

In contrast to Duchenne muscular dystrophy and neurofibromatosis, some genetic disorders exhibit a restricted geographical distribution (Ethical Implications 7.1). The worldwide distribution of globin disorders provides a prime example. Hemoglobin is the oxygen-carrying molecule of the red blood cell (RBC). In the adult it consists of a tetramer, with two α chains and two β chains. The globin proteins each bind a porphyrin heme group, which contains iron. A wide variety of genetic disorders due to globin mutations have been identified. Sickle cell anemia (Clinical Snapshot 7.1) is due to a specific β-globin mutation, substitution of valine for glutamic acid at the sixth codon. The altered globin causes the RBCs to assume a sickle shape under conditions of low oxygen tension, and these do not flow easily through small blood vessels. Thalassemia is another red cell disorder, in this case due to a deficient globin production. This results in severe chronic anemia as well as bone fragility due to extramedullary hematopoiesis.

Globin disorders are not uniformly distributed worldwide. Sickle cell anemia is found mainly in populations from Africa. Thalassemia occurs in Mediterranean, Middle Eastern, and Southeast Asian populations. In 1949, the geneticist J.B.S. Haldane pointed out that the distribution of globin disorders parallels that of malaria (Figure 7.6), and proposed that malaria might constitute a selective force that could maintain globin mutant alleles in the population. Malaria is a parasitic infection of red blood cells, and at least one form, *Plasmodium falciparum*, often is fatal without treatment. How can a parasitic infection influence the worldwide distribution of a genetic trait?

Haldane proposed that the frequency of globin disorders in malaria-endemic regions was due to a phenomenon of **balanced polymorphism**. If we look back in history, and to this day in some parts of the world, most, if not all, globin mutations would be expected to be lethal. The rare globin mutant allele should have been gradually extinguished due to selection. At the same time, however, falciparum malaria was also often lethal. It turns out, though, that carriers of a globin mutation are relatively resistant to malaria. Homozygous normal individuals are highly susceptible to malaria, and the homozygotes for globin mutations would die of anemia. This leaves the heterozygotes as the fittest individuals in the population. Each generation, some of their offspring would die of malaria and some would die of anemia. During an outbreak of malaria in some region, large numbers might die, leaving only a few individuals who might be carriers for some specific globin mutation, making that mutation prevalent in their off-

---

⑦ Ethical Implications 7.1 Genetic Variation and Race

Since single-nucleotide polymorphisms (SNPs) occur on average every 1000 bases in the genome, there should be approximately 3×10^6 base pair differences between any two persons. This represents about 0.1% of the genome, hence the commonly quoted statement that humans are about 99.9% identical from the genetic point of view. Of course, 3×10^6 single base differences is a large number in absolute terms, and accounts for phenotypic differences in traits such as physical appearance as well as differences in susceptibility to both rare and common disorders. It is also commonly pointed out that there are as many genetic differences within groups commonly identified as "races" as there are between such groups. What does this mean for the concept of "race"? Is there a biological basis for the notion?

It is indeed difficult to define in genetic terms what would constitute a "race" of people. If one looks at the distribution of allele frequencies in different populations,

it is apparent that the frequency of some alleles and haplotypes reflects ancestral origins. This should come as no surprise, given phenomena such as the founder effect, balanced polymorphism, and linkage disequilibrium. All members of modern populations bear the genetic traces of ancestry; some populations have been relatively stable for a long period, whereas in others there has been substantial migration and admixture with people of diverse origins.

Race is a social, political, and cultural concept. As we will see in this book, there are some instances where common categorizations of race are used as surrogates for genetic traits that are prevalent in groups of individuals who share ancestral origins. For the most part, the specific genes in question are not yet known. Stratification of the population by these categorizations may have some practical utility, but also risks confusion with a long and difficult political and cultural history.

👁 Clinical Snapshot 7.1 Sickle Cell Anemia

James is a 3-year-old African American boy who is brought to the emergency room with leg pain and fever. He has been exhibiting symptoms of a cold for the past few days, but today woke up with a fever of 39°C, crying, and complaining that his legs hurt. His parents explain that James has sickle cell anemia. His examination shows rhinorrhea, fever of 38.5°C, and dry mucous membranes. James is exquisitely sensitive to being touched, especially in his legs. There is no visible swelling or redness to his legs, however. He is admitted to the hospital and started on intravenous fluids, pain medications, and antibiotics.

Sickle cell anemia is an autosomal recessive disorder due to an amino acid substitution (valine for glutamic acid) in the β-globin gene. Adult hemoglobin consists of two α chains and two β chains. The sickle cell mutation causes the β chain to misfold, particularly under conditions of low oxygen tension. This causes the red blood cells to assume a sickle shape (Figure 7.5). Sickle cells do not pass readily through small blood vessels, which leads to tissue hypoxemia. Individuals with sickle cell anemia suffer from painful crises, due to hypoxemia of tissues such as bone. Chronic hypoxia in the spleen leads to gradual loss of splenic tissue, resulting in an increased risk of bacterial infection. For this reason, children with sickle cell anemia are treated with prophylactic antibiotics and are given intravenous antibiotics if there are signs of infection. The painful

crises are treated with hydration and pain medications, and resolve over a period of days.

Sickle cell anemia is particularly prevalent among people of sub-Saharan African descent. Approximately 1 in 500 African American births is affected. This calculates to a carrier frequency in this population of approximately 1 in 11 individuals. The mutation is also found in other parts of the world, including the Mediterranean region and the Middle East.

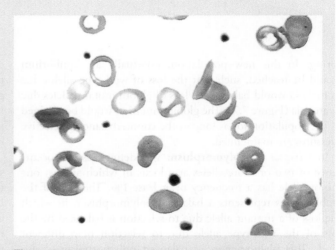

Figure 7.5 Photomicrograph of sickle cells. (Courtesy of Dr. Orah Platt, Children's Hospital, Boston.)

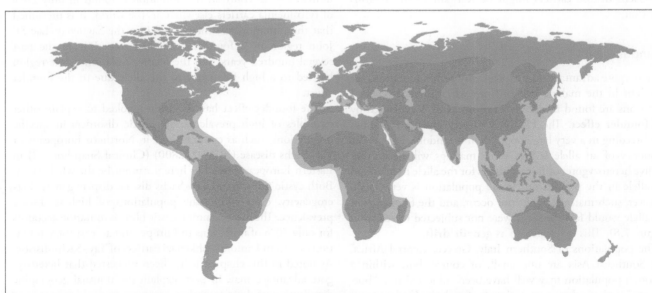

Figure 7.6 Worldwide distribution of thalassemia, paralleling the distribution of malaria (orange area).

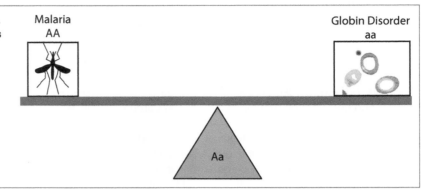

Figure 7.7 Concept of balanced polymorphism. Both the homozygous wild-type and homozygous mutant individuals are subjected to selection by malaria and anemia, respectively. The Aa individuals have the greatest reproductive fitness and serve as a reservoir for the a allele.

spring. In this new population, eventually an equilibrium would be reached, such that the loss of wild-type alleles due to malaria would balance the loss of globin mutant alleles due to anemia (Figure 7.7). The globin mutation would be retained in the population for as long as the counterbalancing selective pressures are maintained.

In Chapter 2, **polymorphism** was defined as the occurrence of two or more alleles at a locus in which at least one minor allele has a frequency of at least 1%. The case of the globin genes represents a balanced polymorphism, in which the loss of a mutant allele due to selection is balanced by the loss of the wild-type allele due to selection of a different kind. This phenomenon of balanced polymorphism – also known as heterozygote advantage – is well known in plants and other animals. Several other cases have been suggested for human populations. For example, it has been proposed that cystic fibrosis heterozygotes are resistant to cholera, a bacterial infection that causes a secretory diarrhea, and that Tay–Sachs disease carriers might be resistant to tuberculosis infection.

Founder Effect

Heterozygote advantage may explain why globin mutations are prevalent in the malaria belt but not why different types of mutations are found in different regions. This is explained by the **founder effect**. The Hardy–Weinberg equation assumes that breeding in a very large population is random. Even if the frequency of an allele is low, some matings will occur that involve heterozygotes or homozygotes for the allele to maintain the allele in the population. If the population is very small, however, such matings might not occur, and the frequency of the allele would fall even if it were not subjected to selection (Figure 7.8). This is referred to as **genetic drift**.

The populations of Southern Italy, Greece, Central Africa, and Southeast Asia are not small, of course, but, within a region, a population may well have been subjected to a "bottleneck," perhaps due to an outbreak of malaria. If a large part

of the breeding population succumbed to malaria and, among the few survivors, there was one individual with a specific globin mutation, that mutation would become more prevalent in the new population that formed in the region after the bottleneck (Figure 7.9). This illustrates the concept of founder effect.

A striking example of a founder effect has been demonstrated among French Canadians with tyrosinemia type I (MIM 276700), in which a single mutation in the enzyme fumarylacetoacetate hydrolase accounts for most cases. This disorder is an inborn error of tyrosine metabolism that leads to liver damage caused by buildup of toxic metabolites. It is rare around the world, but in the Saguenay–Lac St. John region of Quebec it affects 1 of every 1846 newborns, predicting a carrier frequency of 0.045, or nearly 1 in 22. Molecular analysis has revealed that one mutation – a splicing mutation in intron 12 – occurs in 90% of carriers in this region and therefore occurs in homozygous form in 81% of affected individuals. In contrast, this mutation is found in only 28% of tyrosinemia carriers elsewhere in the world. It is presumed that the mutation was introduced into the Saguenay–Lac St. John region by a founder individual sometime in the past several hundred years, and the relative isolation of the region has led to a high frequency of the allele due to the founder effect.

The founder effect has also been invoked to explain other examples of high prevalence of genetic disorders in specific populations, such as cystic fibrosis in Northern Europeans or Tay–Sachs disease (MIM 272800) (Clinical Snapshot 7.2) in Eastern European Jews, but here it cannot be the whole story. Both cystic fibrosis and Tay–Sachs disease display genetic heterogeneity, even within the populations of highest disease prevalence. The most common cystic fibrosis mutation accounts for only 70% of mutations in Europe, and at least three mutations are found among Ashkenazi carriers of Tay–Sachs disease. As noted in this chapter, it has been suggested that heterozygote advantage may, in part, explain the unusual geographic distribution of these mutations.

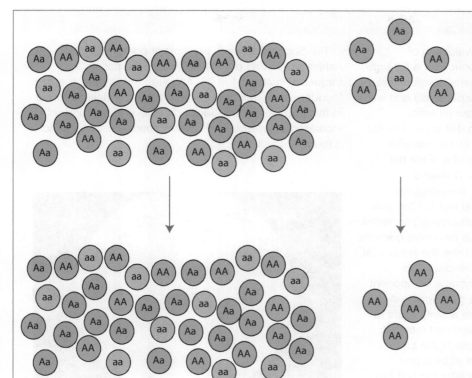

Figure 7.8 Concept of genetic drift. In a large population with random mating, large fluctuations of gene frequency are unlikely. In a small population, however, gene frequency can change dramatically from one generation to the next, if, for example, only the AA individuals participate in mating by chance.

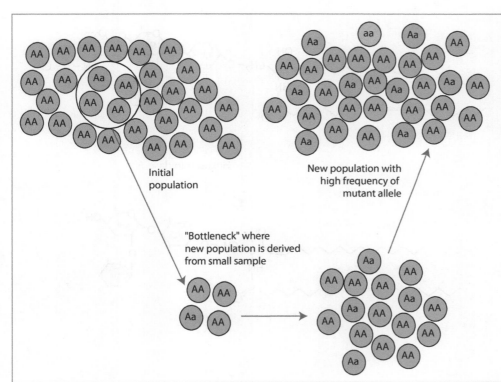

Initial population

New population with high frequency of mutant allele

"Bottleneck" where new population is derived from small sample

Figure 7.9 Founder effect. The frequency of the a allele is low in the initial population, but a small subset, in which one individual is Aa, is removed from the large population and founds a new population. The frequency of a is markedly higher in this new population, due to its relatively high frequency in the founders.

👁 Clinical Snapshot 7.2 Tay–Sachs Disease

Lewis is a 9-month-old referred for evaluation of developmental regression. He was born after a full-term, uncomplicated pregnancy, and his early development was normal. He had been smiling responsively and was able to get to sitting. Over the past few months, however, he has stopped doing both. He stares blankly much of the time now, lying in his crib. He has also become quite irritable. His physical exam is normal except for the lack of interactiveness. A dilated fundoscopic exam is done, however, revealing the cherry-red spot (Figure 7.10). A blood test is sent, and the clinical diagnosis of Tay–Sachs disease is confirmed.

Tay–Sachs disease is an autosomal recessive disorder due to mutation in the gene that encodes the lysosomal enzyme hexosaminidase A. Hexosaminidase A is required to break down the cell membrane component GM2 ganglioside (Figure 7.11). GM2 ganglioside is found in neurons, and lack of enzyme activity leads to engorgement of lysosomes with undigested material. This is toxic and leads to neuronal loss in the brain. Children with the disorder are normal at birth and achieve normal early milestones, but after the first few months of life begin to lose abilities and regress to the point of total dependency. Most die in the first 2 years of life due to aspiration pneumonia as a consequence of swallowing incoordination.

Tay–Sachs disease is particularly prevalent in the Ashkenazi Jewish population, where the carrier frequency is about 1 in 30. Although this is reflective of a founder effect, there are several distinct mutations found in this population. Tay–Sachs disease is also found with increased prevalence in French Canadians, also due to a founder effect.

Figure 7.10 Cherry-red spot from an infant with Tay–Sachs disease. (Courtesy of Dr. Robert Petersen, Children's Hospital, Boston.)

Figure 7.11
Hexosaminidase A catalyzes the removal of N-acetylgalactosamine from GM2 ganglioside.

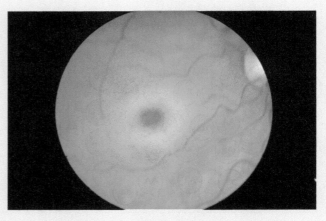

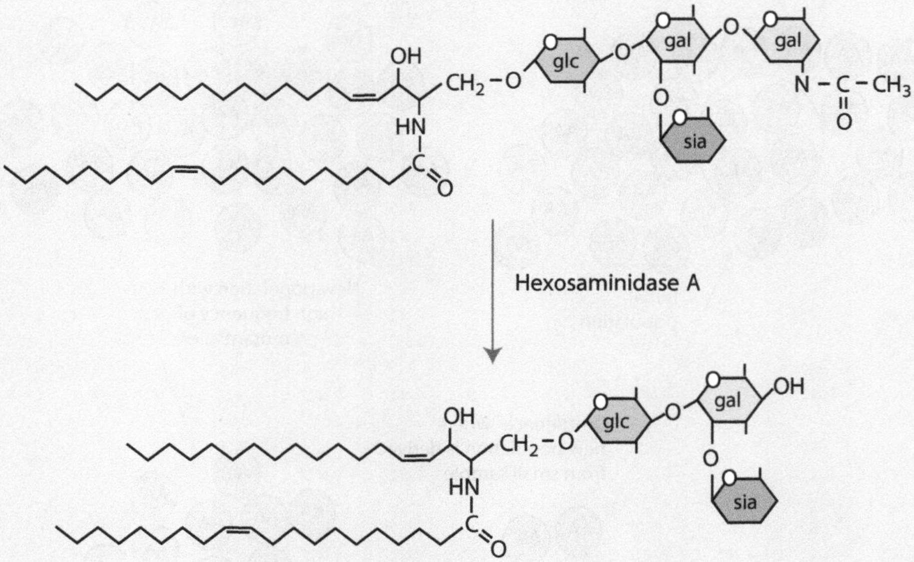

ⓘ Hot Topic 7.1 Carrier Testing

Couples in which both partners are carriers for an autosomal recessive trait usually learn this after the birth of an affected child. By the time a diagnosis is made, there may be other children conceived and even born, potentially with the same disorder. For several decades, carrier-screening programs have been in place in specific populations for disorders for which individuals are at increased risk. This includes screens for Tay-Sachs disease in the Ashkenazi Jewish and French Canadian populations, several other traits in Ashkenazi Jews, and globin disorders in those of African, Mediterranean, and Asian ancestry. The general approach has been to screen for traits known to be present at high frequency, for which a reliable carrier test is available, and where the natural history of the disorder is well known and is severe. The introduction of genomic technologies now makes it possible to test for hundreds – potentially thousands – of genetic traits at low cost; there is essentially no incremental cost to adding a test to a panel that already includes dozens or even hundreds. This has raised the question of whether DNA-based screening should be offered to couples regardless of ancestry, and also whether disorders of less clear natural history should be included. The argument in favor is that some couples will learn of risk for very rare but nevertheless devastating disorders that would otherwise not have been on a screening panel. The arguments against are that some of the mutations being tested are not of clear pathological significance, and the natural history of some rare disorders is not well known. Some companies are already offering such testing, in some cases as a direct-to-consumer test. Everyone, regardless of ancestry, is a carrier for one or more recessive conditions, often associated with severe phenotypes in the recessive state. Whether testing for a very large number of conditions, some severe and others less so, makes sense as a medical or public health procedure, and how individuals will be counseled regarding their risks, remains an unanswered question for future study.

Selective forces have undoubtedly acted on many other genetic traits in human history. Traits that are now considered deleterious may well have resulted in a selective advantage to heterozygotes at some point in time. If the same selective forces acted independently in different populations, there may be different mutations at the same locus that were subject to selection, accounting for genetic heterogeneity between populations and a founder effect within a population. These phenomena – heterozygote advantage, founder effect, and genetic heterogeneity – do not act in isolation but together represent some of the major forces that mold gene frequencies in populations.

Conclusion

Genetic variation is the engine of evolution, and it is also a major determinate of differences in human health and vulnerability to disease. The study of population genetics has provided insights into the reasons that specific human populations bear a disproportionate burden of specific genetic disorders. The medical implications include the need to consider ancestry in assessing individual risks of disease, and the establishment of population-wide carrier-screening programs (Hot Topic 7.1). We will explore both of these applications in the second half of this book.

FURTHER READING

Desnick RJ, Kaback MM 2001, "Future perspectives for Tay–Sachs disease", *Advances in Genetics*, vol. 44, pp. 349–56.

Foster MW, Sharp RR 2004, "Beyond race: towards a whole-genome perspective on human populations and genetic variation", *Nature Reviews Genetics*, vol. 5, pp. 790–6.

Khoury MJ, McCabe LL, McCabe ER 2003, "Population screening in the age of genomic medicine", *New England Journal of Medicine*, vol. 348, pp. 50–8.

Khoury MJ, Millikan R, Little J, Gwinn M 2004, "The emergence of epidemiology in the genomics age", *International Journal of Epidemiology*, vol. 33, pp. 936–44.

Piel FB, *et al.* 2010, "Global distribution of the sickle cell gene and geographical confirmation of the malaria hypothesis", *Nature Communications*, vol. 1, pp. 1–6.

 Find interactive self-test questions and additional resources for this chapter at **www.korfgenetics.com**.

Self-Assessment

Review Questions

7.1   A woman has a brother with an autosomal recessive condition, but she is unaffected. Her husband is not known to have a family history of the disorder. The population frequency of the disorder is 1:40 000. What is their risk of having an affected child?

7.2   Hemochromatosis is an autosomal recessive disorder in which iron accumulates in the body due to abnormal intestinal iron absorption. The prevalence of hemochromatosis is approximately 1:400 individuals in some Caucasian populations. Using the Hardy–Weinberg equation, what is the calculated carrier frequency? What is the risk of hemochromatosis in a child who has one affected parent, assuming that both come from a population with the frequency quoted here? It has been suggested that hemochromatosis carriers have an increased ability to absorb iron and thereby maintain adequate iron stores during times of famine. How might this explain the high prevalence of hemochromatosis?

7.3   You are asked to see a child with hereditary tyrosinemia, an autosomal recessive disorder of amino acid metabolism that causes liver failure. Both parents are of French Canadian ancestry, and come from a region of Quebec where 1:1600 newborns are affected with tyrosinemia. What is the carrier frequency of tyrosinemia in this region? You learn that 90% of mutations responsible for tyrosinemia in this population consist of the same single base change. This mutation is much less common elsewhere in the world. What is most likely to account for the high frequency of this mutation in a small region in Quebec?

7.4   A sudden wave of migration brings a large number of new individuals into a population. For an autosomal recessive trait, how long does it take for a new Hardy–Weinberg equilibrium to be reached, assuming that there is random mating between all members of the new population, including newcomers and original inhabitants?

7.5   Consider a locus with three alleles, a, b, and c, with frequencies of 0.2, 0.3, and 0.5, respectively. What is the frequency of bc heterozygotes in the population, assuming Hardy–Weinberg equilibrium?

CHAPTER 8
Cancer Genetics

Introduction

We have focused thus far on genetic traits present in cells throughout the body, owing either to inheritance from a parent or to new mutation. We have encountered instances in which genetic variation exists from cell to cell in an individual, owing to mosaicism for nuclear genetic traits or heteroplasmy for mitochondrial mutations. We now turn our attention to another form of somatic genetic variation, acquired genetic change leading to malignancy. Chromosomal changes in cancer cells were recognized early in the 20th century, and it was later found that environmental agents that cause cancer are also mutagenic. Families at high risk for specific cancers were recognized. All this suggested that genetic change might underlie the pathogenesis of malignancy, a hypothesis that has been overwhelmingly confirmed in recent years. It now is recognized that a tumor arises as a clonal growth, originating from genetic change in a single cell. The properties referred to as malignancy represent phenotypic features due to the accumulation of changes in multiple genes. The identification of such genes, referred to as tumor suppressor genes and oncogenes, has led to major advances in understanding cancer biology. This, in turn, has led to improvements in diagnostic techniques and the promise of improved methods of treatment for persons with cancer. It has also shed light on the mechanisms of normal cell growth and differentiation.

Key Points

- Several lines of evidence support the idea that cancer is the result of genetic changes in somatic cells.
- Two major types of genes that contribute to malignant change are tumor suppressor genes and oncogenes.
- Tumor suppressor genes contribute to transformation to cancer when both alleles are mutated. In some cases, one of the mutations is inherited, and the other acquired somatically.
- Oncogenes are normal cellular genes that, when activated by mutation, convey abnormal growth properties, contributing to malignancy.
- Oncogenes encode proteins that are involved in the signal transduction pathways involved in stimulation of cell growth; tumor suppressor genes encode proteins involved in regulation of growth.
- Epigenetic changes such as hyper- or hypomethylation and altered expression of microRNAs can contribute toward aberrant expression of tumor suppressor genes or oncogenes.
- Progression toward malignancy is a multistep process due to the gradual accumulation of genetic changes, including activation of oncogenes and loss of function of tumor suppressor genes.
- Knowledge of the molecular basis of cancer is being used to develop new methods of diagnosis and treatment.

Human Genetics and Genomics, Fourth Edition. Bruce R. Korf and Mira B. Irons.

Cancer Is a Genetic Disorder

A connection between cancer and genetics began to be suspected long before the existence of the gene was firmly established. The notion dates back to the early years of the 20th century and was articulated by the pathologist Theodor Boveri, who noticed abnormalities of the nucleus in cancer cells. Over the ensuing decades, four lines of evidence converged to demonstrate that cancer is a genetic disease. These were the observation of chromosomal anomalies in cancer, the existence of families in which risk of cancer is transmitted as a genetic trait, the fact that carcinogens also tend to be mutagens, and the occurrence of individuals with DNA repair deficiency syndromes who are at increased risk of cancer.

The chromosomal basis of malignancy dates back to Boveri's observation, but it received substantial support after it became possible to efficiently study mammalian chromosomes in the 1950s. It rapidly became clear that cancer cells often harbor multiple chromosomal rearrangements (Figure 8.1). Sometimes a particular type of cancer is associated with a specific rearrangement. This is the case in chronic myelogenous leukemia (CML), where a translocation between chromosomes 9 and 22 results in a foreshortened 22 referred to as the Philadelphia chromosome (Figure 8.2). The Philadelphia chromosome was used as a marker of CML long before the molecular basis for the rearrangement came to be understood (to be described in this chapter). Many other cancers have been found to be associated with specific chromosomal markers, and others are characterized by wide-scale chromosome abnormality without a reproducible pattern. Whatever the mechanism of these chromosomal changes, it is clear that alterations of chromosome structure are common in cancer, and presumably are involved in the etiology of the disease.

Familial clustering of cancer represents the second line of evidence. Cancer is common in the general population, so virtually everyone has a family history of cancer in some relative. Some families, however, seem to be singled out for an unusually high frequency of cancer, with the disease segregat-

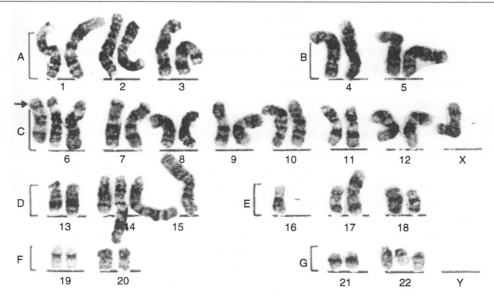

Figure 8.1 G-banded karyotype from retinoblastoma. Numerous chromosome abnormalities are present including isochromosome for the short arm of chromosome 6 (arrow). (Courtesy of Dr. Brenda Gallie, Hospital for Sick Children, Toronto.)

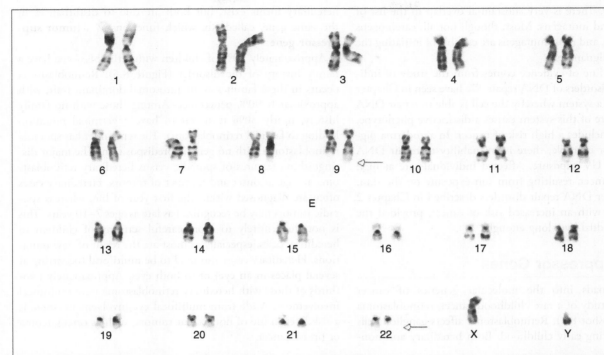

Figure 8.2 Karyotype showing the Philadelphia chromosome, consisting of a translocation between chromosomes 9 and 22 (arrows).

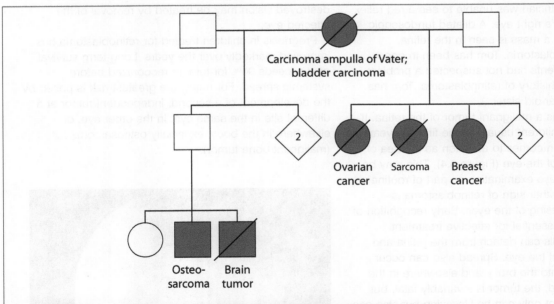

Carcinoma ampulla of Vater;
bladder carcinoma

Ovarian cancer   Sarcoma   Breast cancer

Osteo-sarcoma   Brain tumor

Figure 8.3 Pedigree of family with Li–Fraumeni syndrome. (Source: Malkin *et al.* 1990.)

ing in a Mendelian pattern. An example is Li–Fraumeni syndrome (MIM 151623) (Figure 8.3), where there is autosomal dominant transmission of risk for multiple forms of cancer. Other examples include various familial forms of colon cancer and breast and ovarian cancer. The fact that it is possible to

inherit a predisposition to malignancy as the sole phenotype suggests that genes must be involved in cancer etiology.

We have seen that various types of chemicals or radiation exposure can be mutagenic. Likewise, it has been known for many years that certain chemicals and radiation can predispose to malignancy. There is very substantial overlap in the list of carcinogens and mutagens. Most, though not all, carcinogens are mutagenic, and most mutagens are capable of initiating the growth of malignancies.

The fourth line of evidence comes from the study of individuals with disorders of DNA repair. We have seen in Chapter 2 that there is a system whereby the cell is able to repair DNA damage. Failure of this system causes a distinctive phenotype, which often includes a high risk of cancer. In xeroderma pigmentosum, for example, there is an inability to repair DNA damage from UV exposure. Affected individuals are at high risk of skin cancer, resulting from sun exposure on the skin. All of the other DNA repair disorders described in Chapter 2 are associated with an increased risk of cancer, provided the affected individual lives long enough.

Tumor Suppressor Genes

The first inroads into the molecular genetics of cancer involved the study of a rare childhood cancer, retinoblastoma (Clinical Snapshot 8.1). Retinoblastoma affects ganglion cells in the eye during early childhood. Both hereditary and non-hereditary forms exist, but both are due to disturbances in the same gene, called Rb, which functions as a **tumor suppressor gene**.

Approximately 10% of children with retinoblastoma have a family history of the disorder (Figure 8.5). Retinoblastoma occurs in these families as an autosomal dominant trait, with approximately 90% penetrance. Among those with no family history, nearly 30% turn out to have a germinal mutation leading to familial retinoblastoma. The remainder has sporadic retinoblastoma with no genetic predisposition. The major distinguishing features of sporadic versus hereditary retinoblastoma are age at onset and number of tumors. Hereditary cases often are diagnosed within the first year of life, whereas sporadic tumors may be recognized as late as ages 7–10 years. This is not due entirely to more careful scrutiny of children in hereditary cases, especially as most are the result of new mutations. Hereditary cases also tend to be multifocal (occurring at several places in an eye) or in both eyes. Approximately two-thirds of those with hereditary retinoblastoma have multifocal involvement. Aside from multifocal eye involvement, there is a risk later in life of non-ocular tumors, such as osteosarcoma or breast cancer.

👁 Clinical Snapshot 8.1   Retinoblastoma

Tom is a 2 year old referred by his pediatrician for an ophthalmological examination. The referral was set up because the pediatrician was unable to see a red reflex in the back of Tom's right eye. A dilated fundoscopic exam is done, and a mass is seen in the retina, indicative of retinoblastoma. Tom has been in good health, and his parents had not suspected a problem. There is no family history of retinoblastoma. Tom has one sibling, a 3-year-old sister.

Retinoblastoma is a malignant tumor of the retina. It occurs in young children, usually in the first few years of life. The tumor often comes to attention as an area of pallor at the back of the eye (Figure 8.4). This may be noticed during an eye examination as part of routine well-child care. Another sign of retinoblastoma is strabismus, or crossing of the eyes. Early recognition of retinoblastoma is essential for effective treatment. Retinoblastoma cells can detach from the retina and seed the vitreous of the eye. Spread also can occur back in the orbit, into the brain, and elsewhere in the body. Left untreated, the tumor is invariably fatal, but early recognition not only can be lifesaving but also can preserve vision. Treatment typically consists of radiation therapy, applied over several weeks. This usually is effective in dealing with tumors localized to the eye. Systemic chemotherapy is used if there is evidence of tumor spread. Other modes of treatment may be used for very small, intraocular tumors. These include photocoagulation (using light to burn the tumor cells through the lens of the eye), cryotherapy (freezing tumor cells through the eye), or implantation of radioactive substances into the eye. Advanced tumors that have destroyed vision may be treated by removal of the affected eye.

Prognosis in children treated for retinoblastoma has improved markedly over the years. Long-term survival now exceeds 90% for tumors recognized before systemic spread. For many, the greatest risk is posed by the development of a second, independent tumor at a different site in the same eye, in the other eye, or elsewhere in the body, especially osteosarcoma (malignant bone tumor).

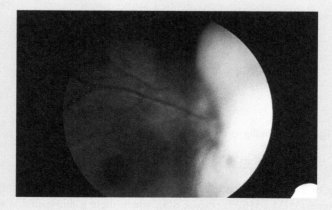

Figure 8.4 Photograph of retina in child with retinoblastoma. The white area on the right is the tumor. (Courtesy of Dr. Robert Petersen, Children's Hospital, Boston.)

In 1971, Alfred Knudson reviewed records of children with either unilateral or bilateral retinoblastoma. At the time retinoblastoma was first diagnosed, children who eventually developed bilateral tumors were younger than children whose tumors remained unilateral. The rate of diagnosis of bilateral cases increased exponentially with time, whereas the rate of diagnosis for unilateral cases increased much more slowly (Figure 8.6). Knudson proposed a model (Figure 8.7) in which retinoblastoma formation requires the occurrence of two separate mutation events in a retinal cell lineage. Individuals with hereditary retinoblastoma have inherited one of these mutations, and therefore all their retinal cells carry the mutation. Only one additional event needs to occur to produce a tumor. In contrast, sporadic retinoblastoma occurs only when two independent mutational events occur in the same cell lineage. This would be expected to be much rarer, and so age at onset is later and tumors are invariably unilateral. Knudson's hypothesis has come to be called the **two-hit hypothesis**. It has been the cornerstone for understanding hereditary predisposition to malignancy.

The molecular basis for the two-hit hypothesis was established with the cloning of a gene, now referred to as *RB1*, on chromosome 13 that was found to be involved in the first step in retinoblastoma carcinogenesis. One copy of the gene is mutated in all cells of individuals with hereditary retinoblastoma. In retinoblastoma tumors, however, both copies of the gene are mutated. Sometimes, one copy is deleted in the tumor, referred to as **loss of heterozygosity** (Figure 8.8). The copy that is lost is invariably the one inherited from the non-affected parent. At other times, that copy of the gene is not deleted, but is mutated. The net effect is that both copies of the gene are nonfunctional in tumor cells.

The retinoblastoma gene was the first of a series of genes to be identified that are associated with familial predisposition to cancer. Other examples are listed in Table 8.1. These syndromes are dominantly inherited. Tumors that occur in affected persons are seen also in the general population, but those with the hereditary form develop them earlier in life and often have multiple, independent cancers. The genes have come to be referred to as tumor suppressor genes. They behave in a recessive manner at the cellular level, so that both copies of the gene

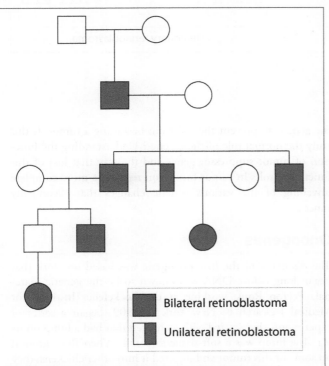

Figure 8.5 Pedigree showing dominant transmission of retinoblastoma. Some individuals have unilateral tumors, whereas others have bilateral retinoblastoma. The father of the youngest affected female is himself unaffected, indicative of nonpenetrance. (Source: Vogel 1979.)

Legend:
- ■ Bilateral retinoblastoma
- ◧ Unilateral retinoblastoma

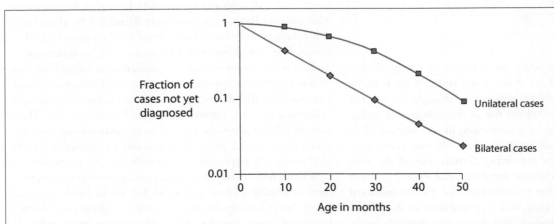

Figure 8.6 Graph of fraction of cases of retinoblastoma not yet diagnosed as a function of age for individuals who developed unilateral or bilateral retinoblastomas. The rate of accumulation of cases of bilateral retinoblastoma has increased exponentially, whereas the unilateral cases increased more slowly. (Source: Knudson 1971.)

Figure 8.7 Two-hit model. A tumor ensues when two "hits" have occurred in the same cell lineage that knocks out both copies of a gene. Two rare events must occur to produce a sporadic tumor. A person who is born with the first mutation, however, needs to acquire only one additional mutation to develop a tumor.

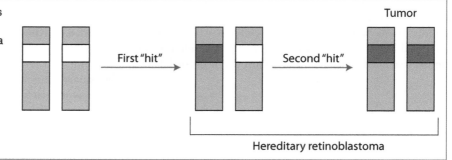

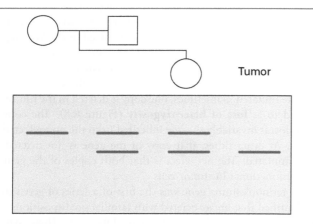

Figure 8.8 Loss of heterozygosity for polymorphic marker on chromosome 13. DNA from the mother, father, and daughter, as well as the daughter's retinoblastoma tumor, was analyzed for a polymorphism involving DNA sequence from chromosome 13q14, demonstrating two alleles of different size (producing an upper and lower band after gel electrophoresis). The mother is homozygous for the upper allele, and the father and affected daughter are heterozygous. DNA from the retinoblastoma, however, shows only the lower allele, indicating loss of the upper allele in the tumor.

must be inactivated in order for a tumor to occur. Within a family, however, they act as dominant traits. What is transmitted from generation to generation, though, is not the malignancy itself but rather the risk of development of malignancy. This is conveyed by transmission of one mutant allele at the tumor suppressor locus, so that only one event need occur – mutation of the remaining normal copy of the gene – for a cell to become a tumor. For these same tumors to occur in the general population requires two rare events: mutation of the first copy of the gene, and then mutation of the second copy in the same cell lineage. This does occur, but only rarely.

The term "tumor suppressor gene" is apt, though in one sense it is misleading. It implies that the normal function of the gene is to prevent the cell from becoming a tumor. Is this truly the normal role of these genes? Understanding the function of tumor suppressor genes and the way that loss of this function results in tumor formation requires a more complete unveiling of the various genetic changes that accompany cancer.

Oncogenes

The discovery of the first **oncogene** was based on work that began long before DNA was known to be the genetic material. Peyton Rous, working at the Rockefeller Institute for Medical Research in New York in 1909, began a series of experiments that started with a chicken that had a lump on its leg. The lump was a soft-tissue sarcoma. When Rous ground up some of this tumor and injected it into other chickens, they too developed sarcomas. The active agent was identified as a virus – in fact, a retrovirus – and was called Rous sarcoma virus. Decades later, it was found that of the four genes in this virus, one, referred to as *src*, is responsible for the transforming properties. When *src* is lost or mutated, the virus is no longer oncogenic.

By the 1980s, approximately 20 different retroviruses, each containing a distinct oncogene, were known to be associated with cancer. These oncogenes were identified by three-letter abbreviations and were usually named for the tumor types they caused (e.g., *erb-B* for erythroblastosis). The breakthrough in understanding nonretroviral malignancies was recognition that viral oncogenes are homologous with normal eukaryotic genes. For example, the viral *src* gene, or *v-src*, is homologous to a eukaryotic *src* gene, referred to as *c-src* (for cellular *src*). These normal cellular genes are referred to as **proto-oncogene**s. The overexpression of a proto-oncogene due to regulation by the viral genome is responsible for its transforming properties.

When a retrovirus containing an oncogene infects an animal, there is usually a latent period of 2–3 weeks before a tumor grows. Some retroviruses, however, are oncogenic with a longer latency of many months. When retroviruses infect cells, the viral RNA is copied into cDNA, and this cDNA copy of the viral genome integrates into the host cell genome. Longer

Table 8.1 Some tumor suppressor genes, associated syndromes resulting from germline mutations, and characteristic tumors.

Gene	Syndrome	Major tumors
APC	Familial adenomatosis polyposis	Bowel carcinoma
VHL	Von Hippel–Lindau syndrome	Hemangioblastoma, pheochromocytoma, and renal cell carcinoma
TP53	Li–Fraumeni syndrome	Soft tissue sarcoma, glioma, and leukemia
BRCA1/2	Familial breast and ovarian cancer syndrome	Breast, ovarian, pancreatic, prostate, and melanoma
NF1	Neurofibromatosis type 1	Neurofibroma, astrocytoma, sarcoma, and leukemia
NF2	Neurofibromatosis type 2	Schwanoma, meningioma, and ependymoma
Rb	Retinoblastoma	Retinoblastoma and osteosarcoma
TSC1/2	Tuberous sclerosis complex	Cortical hamartomas, renal angiomyolipoma, and cardiac rhabdomyoma
WT1	WAGR: Wilms' tumor, aniridia, genitourinary tract anomalies, and growth retardation	Wilms' tumor
P16	Familial melanoma	Melanoma
MSH2, MLH1, PMS1/2, and GTBP	Hereditary nonpolyposis colon cancer syndrome (Lynch syndrome)	Colon cancer and endometrial carcinoma
PTCH	Basal cell nevus syndrome	Basal cell carcinoma and medulloblastoma
MEN1	Multiple endocrine neoplasia 1	Islet cell adenoma, pituitary adenoma, and parathyroid adenoma
RET or MEN2	Multiple endocrine neoplasia 2	Pheochromocytoma and medullary thyroid carcinoma

latency retroviruses do not carry oncogenes. Examination of the DNA from tumors in infected animals, however, indicates that the virus has integrated, by chance, adjacent to a cellular proto-oncogene (Figure 8.9). This places the cellular gene under the influence of the active retroviral promoter, activating the proto-oncogene and causing a tumor. Rarely, an aberrant recombination event causes the cellular proto-oncogene to incorporate into the viral genome. This is how oncogenes are "captured" from the eukaryotic genome by retroviruses.

Not all proto-oncogenes were discovered from studies with retroviruses. Oncogenes exert a dominant effect – that is, overexpression of one copy contributes some transformed properties to the cell. An assay was developed whereby DNA was isolated from tumor cells, broken into pieces, and then introduced into nontransformed cells (Figure 8.10). In the presence of calcium phosphate, the isolated DNA is taken up into the

cells by a process known as **transfection**. Some DNA integrates into the recipient cell genome and is expressed. Using a mouse fibroblast cell line as recipient, it was found that transfection of tumor cell DNA resulted in isolation of fibroblast clones with some properties of transformation, such as ability to grow in soft agar. When human tumor cells were used as the donor, the transfected DNA could be identified in the mouse cells because of the presence of repeated sequences found in the human but not the mouse genome. It was found that the transforming genes corresponded in some cases with oncogenes already known to be involved in retroviral-mediated oncogenesis. Moreover, it was found that specific oncogenes tended to be involved in certain tumor types.

Oncogenes are normal cellular genes that, when their patterns of expression are changed, confer on the cell some neoplastic properties. There are many routes to oncogene

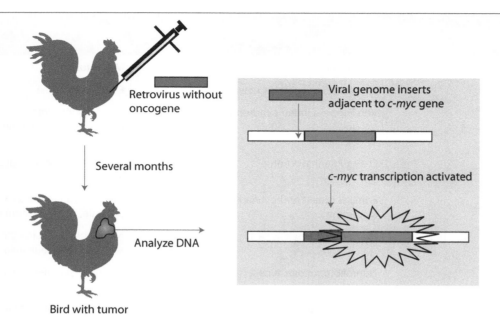

Figure 8.9 Insertion of avian leukemia retrovirus lacking an oncogene into a site in an avian genome adjacent to *c-myc* gene. Activation of *c-myc* transcription results in tumor formation.

activation. Some have already been mentioned – namely, incorporation into a virus or insertion of a retrovirus adjacent to a proto-oncogene. Most mechanisms do not rely on viruses, though. The most direct route to proto-oncogene activation is gene amplification, wherein a block of DNA, including an oncogene and some neighboring genes, is replicated tens or hundreds of times in the cell. This probably occurs by random errors of DNA replication but when it occurs a selective advantage is conferred on the cell, which proliferates faster than other cells in the tissue. Tumor cells with gene amplification contain tiny objects referred to as double minute chromatin bodies, which harbor the amplified DNA (Figure 8.11).

Another route to proto-oncogene activation is through chromosome rearrangement. This was first demonstrated in the Burkitt lymphoma tumor (Figure 8.12), which commonly includes a translocation between chromosomes 8 and 14. The breakpoint on chromosome 14 corresponds with the immunoglobulin heavy-chain locus, and that on chromosome 8 with a proto-oncogene, *c-myc*. The immunoglobulin heavy-chain gene tends to undergo rearrangement during the process of lymphocyte maturation and, on rare occasions, this rearrangement process goes awry. If an aberrant rearrangement juxtaposes the heavy-chain gene with the *myc* oncogene, altered expression of the oncogene ensues and contributes to tumor formation.

In most cases, activation of a proto-oncogene is not associated with a visible change in chromosome structure. The transforming gene isolated from transfection of DNA from bladder carcinoma cells is the *ras* oncogene, also a retroviral oncogene. In bladder carcinomas, the *ras* gene is found to be mutated, a single-base substitution leading to an altered amino acid. The mutations tend to occur at characteristic sites in the gene and lead to an altered protein that causes transformation of the cell.

Normal Roles of Tumor Suppressor Genes and Oncogenes

The discovery of oncogenes and tumor suppressor genes has revealed the major cast of characters responsible for the growth of neoplastic cells. It remains for the tools of molecular biology to reveal their roles. Although this story still is unfolding, major advances have been made.

Dominant proto-oncogenes sort into four classes of molecules, all of which are involved in the control of cell differentiation and proliferation (Figure 8.13). The first class encodes growth factors. The prototype is the proto-oncogene *c-sis*, which encodes the beta chain of platelet-derived growth factor. Such growth factors are able to stimulate the proliferation of certain types of cells. Overexpression, or expression of an aberrant protein, leads to enhanced cell proliferation. Tumor cells that secrete such factors and simultaneously respond to them are subject to autocrine growth control.

Growth factors must interact with membrane receptors to exert their activity, and growth factor receptors comprise the second class of proto-oncogene products. A mutation that renders a receptor active even in the absence of ligand, or that binds ligand abnormally, might render the cell independent of growth factors for control of proliferation. The proto-oncogene *c-erb-B* corresponds with the epidermal growth factor receptor.

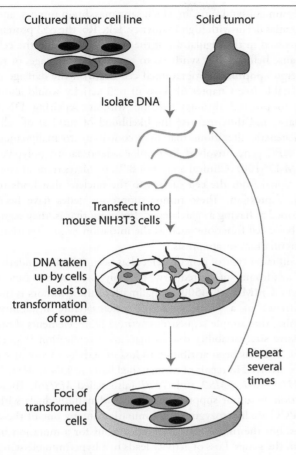

Figure 8.10 Identification of transforming genes by transfection of tumor DNA into mouse fibroblasts. DNA was isolated from tumor cell lines or from solid tumors. This was added to cultures of mouse NIH 3T3 fibroblasts, which grow indefinitely in culture but otherwise do not display a transformed phenotype. Some of the human DNA is taken up by the mouse cells and, in rare instances, results in transformation of the cells. These transformed cells had abnormal appearance, grew to high density, and could be cultured in soft agar (indicating lack of requirement for a solid surface on which to grow). The process was repeated for several iterations, using DNA from the transformed cells, effectively purifying the transforming genes from the rest of the human DNA. Analysis of the human DNA in the transformed cells revealed homology with known viral oncogenes.

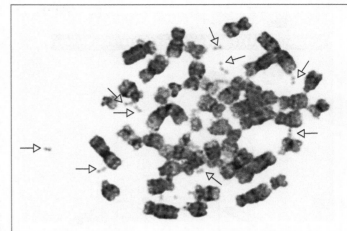

Figure 8.11 Double minute chromatin bodies (arrows) in tumor cell metaphase. (Courtesy of Dr. Andrew Carroll, University of Alabama at Birmingham.)

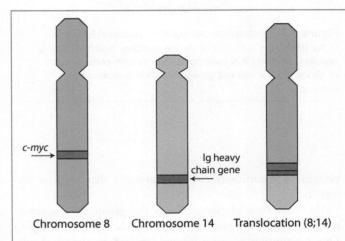

Figure 8.12 Translocation between chromosomes 8 and 14 in Burkitt lymphoma, juxtaposing the *c-myc* proto-oncogene into the immunoglobulin (Ig) heavy-chain locus. This alters the regulation of *c-myc* expression, contributing to the malignant phenotype. (Modified from Taub *et al.* 1982.)

The viral *v-erb-B* is a truncated form of this receptor with abnormal activity. Binding of a growth factor leads to dimerization of the receptor and activation of tyrosine kinase domains, which leads to phosphorylation of tyrosine residues on the receptor as well as other membrane proteins. Phosphorylation serves as an activating signal that leads the proteins to interact with others. Some of these other proteins also have tyrosine kinase activity and transmit an activation signal to target pro-

teins by phosphorylation. An example of such a downstream target is the *src* gene product.

The third class of membrane-associated proteins has the ability to phosphorylate serine or threonine residues. These include the product of the *raf* proto-oncogene. Another group consists of proteins that bind guanosine triphosphate (GTP), of which ras is the prototype. Ras is activated by signals transmitted from membrane receptors and, in turn, transmits a signal by modification of other proteins. Oncogenic *ras* mutations lead to overexpression of the activated form of the

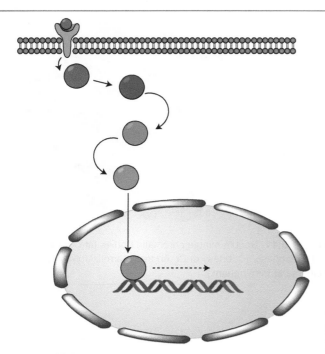

Figure 8.13 Prototypical cell-signaling pathway. A growth factor binds to a specific membrane receptor, which initiates a signaling cascade that culminates in activation of transcription of genes required for cell growth or differentiation in the nucleus.

protein or insensitivity to other proteins that regulate *ras* activity.

The final class of oncogenes is the group that controls transcription in the nucleus. These include *myc*, *jun*, and *fos*. Direct activation of these factors can lead to abnormal cell proliferation or differentiation in the absence of appropriate signals transmitted across the cell membrane and through the cytoplasm.

The mechanism of action of tumor suppressor genes is also coming to light. The Rb protein binds to and inhibits action of E2F proteins that are involved in control of transcription of proteins required to initiate DNA synthesis. Phosphorylation of Rb disinhibits E2F, leading to onset of the S phase. Loss of Rb therefore removes this control point, leading to rapid transit from G1 to S. Some tumor viruses effect the same outcome by producing proteins that bind to, and interfere with the ability of Rb to inhibit, E2F proteins. The *NF1* gene product, which is mutated in individuals with neurofibromatosis type 1 (NF1), is a GTPase-activating protein (GAP), which regulates ras activity by stimulating GTPase activity. Loss of the *NF1* gene product is believed to lead to unimpeded ras activity. The *TP53* gene is mutated in a wide variety of tumor types and is involved in a familial cancer syndrome,

Li–Fraumeni syndrome, in which sarcomas, brain tumors, and leukemias occur with high frequency. Like Rb, the p53 protein is involved in the regulation of the cell cycle, causing the cell to pause before DNA synthesis to repair DNA damage, or to undergo **apoptosis** (programmed cell death) if the damage is irreparable (see Chapter 6). Loss of p53 activity would allow cells to proceed through division without repairing DNA damage, and thus increase the likelihood of survival of cells with genetic alterations that may contribute to malignancy. The *APC* gene, involved in familial adenomatous polyposis (MIM 175100) (Clinical Snapshot 8.2), regulates transmission of a signal from the cell surface to the nucleus that leads to *c-myc* expression. These tumor suppressor genes have been described as having a "gatekeeper" function; that is, they regulate basic cell functions such as the initiation of proliferation, differentiation, or apoptosis.

A different type of genetic defect has been found to underlie the syndrome of hereditary nonpolyposis colon cancer (HNPCC) (MIM 114500). A hallmark of these tumors is the occurrence of a phenomenon of microsatellite instability, meaning that simple sequence repetitive DNA elements show excessive size variability due to inaccurate replication (Figure 8.15). This has been attributed to loss of activity of any of six genes involved in repair of mismatched bases in DNA: *MSH2*, *MLH1*, *PMS1*, *PMS2*, and *GTBP* (also called *MSH6*). These function as tumor suppressor genes, in that individuals with HNPCC are heterozygous for a mutation in any one of these genes, but the tumor cells are homozygous for a mutation in one of the genes. Loss of activity leads to a hypermutable state, in which mutations accumulate in other dominant or recessive oncogenes, leading to tumor progression. A similar mechanism underlies an increased risk of malignancy associated with DNA repair disorders (see Chapter 2). These are recessively inherited, and increased risk of malignancy is due to an accelerated rate of accumulation of mutations, some of which activate dominant oncogenes or inactivate tumor suppressor genes. The genes involved in HNPCC and DNA repair disorders have been referred to as caretaker genes.

A third class of genes that predispose to tumor formation is typified by *PTEN* and *SMAD4*. These genes are involved in juvenile polyposis (MIM 174900), in which benign polyps occur that have an increased risk of malignancy. The heterozygous mutation leads to abnormal proliferation of the stromal cells surrounding colonic epithelial cells. This is believed to result in an altered microenvironment and consequent aberrant cell growth, leading to malignant transformation. These genes have been described as functioning as "landscapers."

The products of oncogenes and tumor suppressor genes are part of a network of proteins that control cell growth. They represent steps in the pathway from the cell surface to the nucleus. A defect anywhere along the chain can render the cell incapable of responding to signals to stop dividing and differentiate or can trick the cell into a cycle of unstoppable proliferation.

👁 Clinical Snapshot 8.2   Hereditary Colon Cancer

Alice is a 40 year old who is referred for counseling following a recent diagnosis of colon cancer. She had presented with rectal bleeding and was found to have an adenocarcinoma of the rectum. A colonoscopy had then revealed multiple adenomatous polyps throughout the colon. Alice is an only child, but her mother had died of colon cancer at age 50. She has no further information about her family history.

Colorectal cancer is the second most common form of cancer in the United States. Although most cases occur sporadically, there are two major syndromes associated with autosomal dominant inheritance: familial adenomatous polyposis (FAP) and hereditary nonpolyposis colon cancer (HNPCC). Individuals with FAP develop multiple adenomatous polyps in the colon and rectum (Figure 8.14), as well as in the stomach and duodenum. Polyps may begin in childhood and continue throughout life, and cancer occurs in almost all affected individuals, most commonly in the third or fourth decades. Other manifestations include congenital hypertrophy of the retinal pigment epithelium, dental anomalies, and soft-tissue tumors. FAP is due to mutations in the tumor suppressor gene *APC*.

Individuals with HNPCC have about an 80% lifetime risk of colon cancer but do not develop adenomatous polyps. Women with HNPCC are also at risk of endometrial carcinoma. Other cancers associated with the disorder include small bowel carcinoma, urinary tract tumors, and glioblastoma. HNPCC is due to mutation in one of several DNA mismatch repair genes. These behave as tumor suppressors in that heterozygous mutation in the germline puts the individual at risk of loss of both alleles in the tumor, leading to defective DNA repair, an accumulation of mutations, and malignant change.

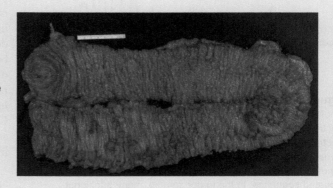

Figure 8.14 Multiple polyps of the colon in a patient with familial adenomatous polyposis. (Courtesy of Dr. Ernesto Drelichman, University of Alabama at Birmingham.)

Epigenetics and MicroRNAs in Cancer

In addition to inherited or acquired mutations in tumor suppressor genes and oncogenes, there is evidence that both epigenetic changes and changes in expression of microRNAs play a role in oncogenesis. We have already explored the role of epigenetic marking of DNA and histones as well as microRNAs in the regulation of gene expression. It should therefore come as no surprise that disruption of these processes can contribute to the dysregulation of cell growth that is at the basis of cancer initiation and progression.

Epigenetic changes appear to act in cancer through at least three distinct mechanisms. Firstly, cancer genomes tend to have a general hypomethylation of DNA, which becomes more pronounced as the tumor progresses toward more malignant behavior. This may result in expression of some genes that are normally not expressed, including imprinted genes. It may also predispose to chromosomal instability, leading to accumulation of mutations that drive progression of malignancy. The second epigenetic change is hypermethylation of the promoter regions of some tumor suppressor genes. This leads to reduced expression of these genes in the absence of mutation. Tumor-specific patterns of hypermethylation have been implicated in inactivation of genes such as *Rb*, mismatch repair genes, and

BRCA1, among others. The mechanisms of hypermethylation are not known. The third mechanism is hypermethylation of genes that encode microRNAs, leading to reduced expression of specific microRNAs and consequent aberrant gene regulation.

Aside from hypermethylation, other changes in microRNA expression have been implicated in cancer. Specific patterns of aberrant microRNA expression, including both over- and underexpression, may characterize particular tumor types, and can be used as a diagnostic or prognostic marker. Increased levels of a microRNA that interacts with a tumor suppressor could inactivate the tumor suppressor; reduced expression of a microRNA that normally regulates an oncogene could result in overexpression of the oncogene. The mechanisms of alteration of microRNA expression include, as noted in this chapter, not just aberrant methylation but also other mechanisms, such as chromosomal rearrangement at the site of a microRNA gene cluster as well as microRNA gene deletion or amplification.

The Molecular Basis of Oncogenesis

The transformation of a cell from normal to malignant comprises a series of genetic changes in oncogenes and tumor suppressor genes. In the familial cancer syndromes, and perhaps

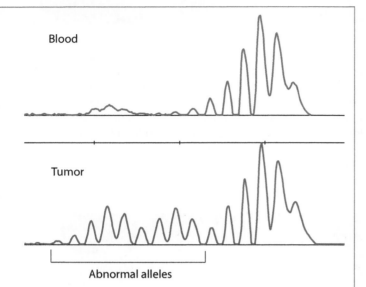

Blood

Tumor

Abnormal alleles

Figure 8.15 Microsatellite instability. A microsatellite repeat is amplified by PCR, and the length of amplified DNA analyzed by electrophoresis. The traces indicate band intensity along the electrophoresis gel. In blood DNA a set of bands is seen corresponding with two alleles of slightly different size. Multiple bands are seen due to inaccuracies of PCR amplification of the repeated sequence. In the tumor sample, many additional bands are seen due to instability of the repeat during DNA replication. (Courtesy of Dr. Ludwine Messiaen, University of Alabama at Birmingham.)

in sporadic cancers as well, loss of a tumor suppressor gene appears to be rate limiting: It is the change that sets into motion a cascade of events wherein genetic damage accumulates, leading to a complex set of abnormal properties. There can be a snowballing of genetic change. As the tumor cells accumulate genetic damage and cell division becomes more rapid and disordered, additional damage occurs. Other tumor suppressor genes may be mutated or lost, and oncogenes are activated. Novel genes may be created by translocation of two genes into one. The fusion proteins encoded by these new genes may confer new, abnormal properties to the cell. Some changes are deleterious and lead to cell death. If, however, a change occurs that causes the cell to grow faster or to be freed from dependence on a growth factor, that cell will have an advantage over others and may become the predominant cell type in the tumor. Tumor growth, then, is a process of natural selection. When the tumor finally is diagnosed, the tumor cells are highly evolved products of hundreds of generations of mutation and selection (Figure 8.16). Recent studies based on sequencing of tumor cell genomes are revealing the full complexity of genetic rearrangements in tumor cells (Hot Topic 8.1).

Knowledge of genetic changes in malignancy has significantly improved the approach to cancer diagnosis and management. In the leukemias, cytogenetic analysis has long been used for diagnostic purposes. The first tumor-specific chromosome change to be identified was the Philadelphia chromosome in chronic myelogenous leukemia. Although originally believed to be a deleted chromosome 22, this eventually was found to represent a translocation of chromosomes 9 and 22, juxtaposing the proto-oncogene *abl* to a gene called *bcr* to generate a novel fusion gene. Detection of the Philadelphia chromosome is used in the diagnosis of leukemia and in following response to treatment. The first appearance of Philadelphia chromosome–positive cells in the bone marrow of patients after treatment is often the first sign of relapse. Sensitive detection methods based on polymerase chain reaction (PCR) now provide early detection of such relapse, allowing treatment to be reinitiated before the tumor burden becomes substantial. The importance of the Philadelphia chromosome in developing a new treatment for chronic myelogenous leukemia will become apparent in the "New Treatments for Cancer" section of this chapter. Cytogenetic studies are also important in the assessment of acute myelogenous leukemias, helping to predict which are likely to respond to treatment and which are likely to relapse.

Diagnosis of cancer has been further refined using new approaches based on the analysis of patterns of gene expression. Tumor cells that look alike through the microscope may have very different clinical behavior and response to therapy. These differences may be reflected in expression of different sets of genes, which can now be analyzed using cDNA microarrays or next-generation sequencing of cDNA (RNA-seq) (Methods 8.1). Expression analysis is showing promise as a means of subclassifying tumors that may eventually guide choice of treatment and help determine prognosis.

Genetic testing can be used not only to diagnose and monitor cancer in affected persons but also to identify some individuals at risk of developing malignancy in the first place. This can be done for members of families with the syndromes listed in Table 8.1. Those who inherit a *TP53* mutation are at risk of developing sarcoma, brain tumor, or leukemia, characteristic of Li–Fraumeni syndrome. If the pathogenic mutation in the family is known, then any family member can be offered testing. This can lead to careful surveillance for tumor formation, and in some cases strategies for risk reduction, including treatment with certain medications or by surgery. We will explore this in greater detail in the second half of this book. The ability to offer genetic risk assessment also raises ethical issues, such as testing children for risk of cancer (Ethical Implications 8.1).

New Treatments for Cancer

Cancer is indeed a genetic disease, sometimes inherited but always showing somatically acquired genetic damage. The discovery of genes that underlie the transformation and progression of malignant cells is one of the great achievements in

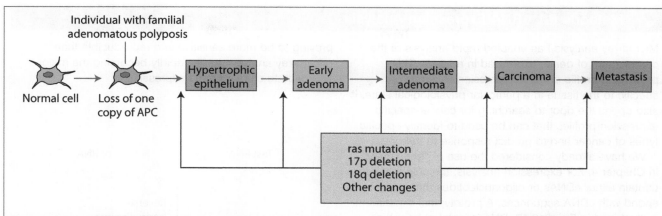

Figure 8.16 Multistep pathway from normal cell to metastatic colon carcinoma. The rate-limiting step is postulated to be loss of the *APC* gene on chromosome 5. Individuals with familial adenomatous polyposis (FAP) inherit the first mutation (*APC* gene) and need to acquire only a second mutation. Other individuals need to acquire both mutations in the same cell lineage. This leads to a hypertrophic epithelium. Additional genetic damage is then accumulated, including loss of sequences on chromosomes 17p and 18q as well as other changes. These can occur in any order but lead to progressively more abnormal cells including, eventually, cells capable of metastasis. (Source: Fearon and Vogelstein 1990.)

(!) Hot Topic 8.1   Cancer Genome Sequencing

There is a long history of analysis of tumor specimens using cytogenetics, which has revealed many tumor-specific chromosomal rearrangements. Molecular testing has similarly identified mutations in specific oncogenes or tumor suppressor genes. Cytogenetic studies are limited, however, by low resolution, and molecular testing requires a targeted approach, looking at known candidate genes. The advent of massively parallel next-generation sequencing has offered the possibility of doing an unbiased search of the entire genome of cancer cells to catalog the total content of mutations. As for germline studies (see Chapter 4), there is a major challenge in characterizing the millions of variants that inevitably are found in any specimen. The Cancer Genome Anatomy Project (see Sources of Information 8.1) is now systematically characterizing the genomes of a wide variety of tumor types. One recent study of glioblastoma (Cancer Genome Atlas Research Network 2008), a lethal brain tumor, revealed frequent mutations in mismatch repair genes and the *NF1*, *TP53*, *Rb*, and *PTEN* tumor suppressor genes, and activation of the *EGFR* gene and genes involved in the PI3 kinase signaling pathway. Sequencing of an acute myeloid leukemia (AML) specimen (Mardis *et al.* 2009) revealed 12 gene-coding sequence mutations and multiple other mutations in other regions that are conserved in evolution or are known regulatory regions. Some of these appear to be incidental to the tumor, and are believed to have been harmless changes present in the progenitor cell that gave rise to the leukemia. Several of the mutations were found to reside in genes previously known to be mutated in AML, but two were novel and subsequently found to be mutated in other AML specimens. Another study (Ley *et al.* 2010) has revealed mutations of the DNMT3A gene, which encodes a methylase involved in epigenetic marking of DNA, in AML, suggesting that disruption of methylation may be an important mechanism in AML tumorigenesis.

---

biology during the 20th century. Cancer diagnosis has been revolutionized, yet therapy still depends on the use of surgery or nonspecific killing of dividing cells with toxic drugs or radiation.

There is hope that new knowledge of the genetic mechanisms that underlie cancer may lead to novel approaches. A step in this direction has already occurred through the develop-

ment of more precise means of genetic diagnosis. Early diagnosis of relapsing chronic myelogenous leukemia by detection of the Philadelphia chromosome is an example. Genetic markers have also been used to distinguish histologically similar tumors that may respond differently to different means of therapy. An example is the distinction of Ewing sarcoma from neuroblastoma. These are histologically similar, small-cell, soft-

✓ Methods 8.1 RNA Expression Analysis

Microarray analysis has enabled rapid analysis of the complement of genes expressed in a tissue. This provides a profile of gene expression that may be specific to the tissue in a particular physiological state. It also opens the door to searching for cancer-specific expression profiles that can be used to identify specific types of cancer and to predict response to therapy.

We have already considered the use of "gene chips" in Chapter 4. For expression analysis, the chip features contain either cDNAs or oligonucleotides that correspond with cDNA sequences. A prototypical experiment is illustrated in Figure 8.17. RNA is isolated from the tumor to be tested and labeled with a red fluorochrome. RNA isolated from a reference sample, such as a nontumor cell, is labeled in green. Both RNA samples are then hybridized with the DNA in the chip. If a particular RNA is represented more in the tumor than in the reference sample, a feature will fluoresce in red; if the expression level is lower, it will appear green.

Thousands of cDNAs can be included on a single chip, providing a massive amount of data on the profile of genes expressed in the test sample. Various analysis systems have been devised to make sense of this vast dataset. One approach is to perform cluster analysis, grouping samples that have in common high or low levels of expression of particular genes. This approach has been used to separate tumors that look the same pathologically into groups that have different biological behavior or response to treatment.

Recently, next-generation DNA-sequencing technologies have been applied to expression analysis. RNA is isolated from the tumor and converted into cDNA. The population of cDNA molecules is then sequenced, and the number of times a particular sequence is identified in the mixture is an indication of the abundance of that transcript. This approach, referred to as RNA-seq, is proving to be more sensitive and reproducible than microarray analysis and is rapidly becoming the major approach to study of gene expression.

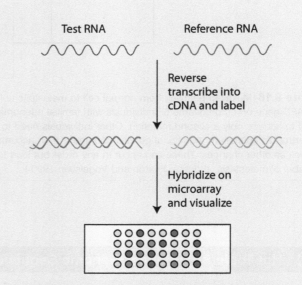

Figure 8.17 Microarray expression analysis. Thousands of different cDNAs are bound to a glass "chip," creating a grid with a different cDNA in each cell. RNA is isolated from a test and a control sample and made into two batches of cDNA. The test cDNA is labeled with a red fluorescent tag, and the control is labeled with a green tag. Equal amounts of both are hybridized with cDNA bound to the chip. If an RNA species is more abundant in the test sample, the cell will show red fluorescence, whereas if the RNA is more abundant in the control, the cell will show green fluorescence. Computer analysis of the patterns of red and green fluorescence can be used to establish a profile of differences in gene expression between the two tissues.

---

tissue tumors, yet they are treated differently. Although classic pathologic markers may not distinguish these tumors, Ewing sarcomas typically have an chromosome 11;22 translocation, whereas neuroblastomas are characterized by deletion of chromosome 1p.

Advances in therapy, though, are at a more primitive stage. Conventional modes of treatment are designed to kill all dividing cells. Side effects result from killing of nontumor cells, and treatment failures are due to failure to kill all tumor cells. Sometimes the tumor cells that survive develop drug resistance and may be more aggressive than their predecessors. Research in cancer therapy therefore is directed toward the development of agents that are more selective for tumor cells. Approaches include inhibition of tumor blood supply, taking advantage of cell surface markers that are unique to tumor cells, or developing means of altering the activity of genes involved in oncogenesis.

The latter has taken advantage of new knowledge of the molecular genetics of cancer. The same complexity of the system that regulates cell growth, which makes the cell vulnerable to genetic changes that lead to malignancy, also offers many possible sites of intervention. Drugs are being developed that interact either with oncogenes or with other cellular proteins that interact with oncogenes. A dramatic example is a drug developed to treat CML. The *bcr–abl* gene fusion encodes a novel hybrid protein, which has the kinase activity of abl, but is expressed in the cytoplasm rather than the nucleus, where abl is normally expressed. A small molecule was devel-

? Ethical Implications 8.1 Genetic Testing of Children

Should children be tested for risk of genetic disorders? It is common to offer genetic testing to children who display signs or symptoms of an inherited disorder. Achieving an accurate diagnosis can provide the basis for treatment and anticipatory guidance to the family as well as genetic counseling.

What about testing of children for adult-onset disorders? Should a child at risk be tested for disorders such as Huntington disease, breast and ovarian cancer, or colon cancer? The consensus in the genetic community is that testing should be offered only in instances where the child will directly benefit from the outcome of testing. This may be the case for familial adenomatous polyposis, since polyps begin in childhood. A child at risk will begin to have sigmoidoscopy at around 10 years of age. If the child is found to not have inherited an APC mutation, he or she can be spared from this uncomfort-

able procedure (at least until an age is reached where testing would be recommended regardless of family history). Familial medullary thyroid carcinoma, due to mutation of the *Ret* oncogene, can result in malignant thyroid tumors in children as young as 2 years old. Genetic testing of children at risk based on family history can be lifesaving, as those found to have the mutation should have thyroidectomy. Disorders such as Huntington disease or breast and ovarian cancer usually do not present in childhood. For such disorders, genetic testing is not recommended. Rather, it is suggested that testing be deferred until the child is old enough to understand the implications of testing and make an informed decision. The rationale is that the child will not immediately benefit from the results of testing, yet would be vulnerable to risks such as discrimination or stigmatization.

oped that binds to the ATP binding site of this fusion protein, preventing binding of ATP to the site and thereby inhibiting the kinase activity (Figure 8.18). This drug, called imatinib mesylate, has produced dramatic remissions of CML, which are largely refractory to conventional chemotherapy. The drug has also been used with success in some other tumors with mutation of oncogenes that have kinase activity. Imatinib mesylate does not cure the tumors, which develop resistance as mutations occur within the ATP binding site. Never-

theless, imatinib mesylate has a major role in treatment of CML and other cancers, along with either conventional or other mechanism-based therapies that may be used in combination.

Epigenetic and microRNA approaches are also being explored as possible avenues of therapy. Drugs that lead to demethylation of DNA or histone deacetylase inhibitors are in use for treatment of some forms of cancer. These drugs may work by restoring function of methylated genes such as

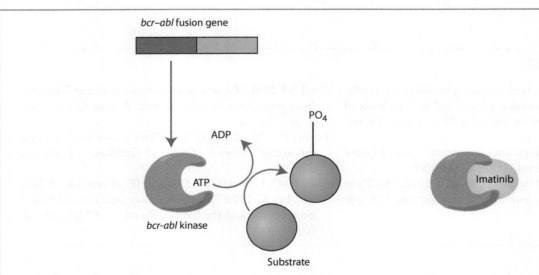

Figure 8.18 Mechanism of action of imatinib mesylate. The *bcr–abl* fusion gene encodes a fusion protein that binds ATP and phosphorylates other cytoplasmic proteins. Imatinib mesylate competitively binds the ATP binding site and thereby prevents the fusion protein from phosphorylating other proteins.

tumor suppressors, though they may also have the opposite effect of contributing to overall tumor hypomethylation. More targeted agents that reactivate specific hypermethylated genes are in development. Similarly, approaches to modulate micro-RNA expression are being investigated as potential therapeutic tools.

Knowledge of the genetic rearrangements associated with cancer can also assist with choice of treatment. Breast cancers that display amplification of the *Her-2* oncogene (human epidermal growth factor receptor 2) are sensitive to treatment with trastuzumab, an antibody that targets this oncogene. About 10% of individuals with non–small cell lung cancer respond to the kinase inhibitor gefinitib. Response can be predicted by finding mutations in the EGF receptor gene in the tumor cells.

Conclusion

A century of research has verified the hypothesis that genetic change is the major driver of initiation and progression of malignancy. This is producing major new approaches to prevention, diagnosis, and management. Individuals at risk on the basis of family history can be identified and offered programs of surveillance and prevention, a point we will explore further in the second half of this book. Genetic approaches are helping to supplement classical histology as a basis for diagnosing specific cancers and guiding choice of therapy. Ultimately, the greatest hope is the development of new treatments based on understanding the mechanisms of cancer.

REFERENCES

Cancer Genome Atlas Research Network 2008, "Comprehensive genomic characterization defines human glioblastoma genes and core pathways of glioblastoma", *Nature*, vol. 455:1061–8.

Knudson AG Jr 1971, "Mutation and cancer: statistical study of retinoblastoma", *Proceedings of the National Academy of Science of the USA*, vol. 68, pp. 820–3.

Fearon ER, Vogelstein B 1990, "A genetic model for colorectal tumorigenesis", *Cell*, vol. 61, pp. 759–67.

Ley TJ, *et al.* 2010, 'DNMT3A mutations in acute myeloid leukemia", *New England Journal of Medicine*, vol. 363, pp. 2424–33.

Malkin D, Li FP, Strong LC, *et al.* 1990, "Germline p53 mutations in a familial syndrome of breast cancer, sarcomas, and other neoplasms", *Science*, vol. 250, pp. 1233–8.

Mardis ER, *et al.* 2009, "Recurrent mutations found by sequencing an acute myeloid leukemia genome", *New England Journal of Medicine*, vol. 361, pp. 1058–66.

Taub R, Morton C, Lenoir G, *et al.* 1982, "Translocation of the c-myc gene into the immunoglobulin heavy chain locus in human Burkitt lymphoma and murine plasmacytoma cells", *Proceedings of the National Academy of Science of the USA*, vol. 79, pp. 7837–41.

Vogel F 1979, "Genetics of retinoblastoma", *Human Genetics*, vol. 52, pp. 1–54.

FURTHER READING

ACMG/ASHG 1995, "Genetic testing in children and adolescents, points to consider: ethical legal and psychosocial implications", *American Journal of Human Genetics*, vol. 57, pp. 1233–41.

Esteller M 2008, "Epigenetics in cancer", *New England Journal of Medicine*, vol. 358, pp. 1148–59.

Farazi TA, Spitzer JI, Morozov P, Tuschl T 2010, "MiRNAs in human cancer", *Journal of Pathology*, vol. 223, pp. 102–15.

Frank SA 2004, "Genetic predisposition to cancer – insights from population genetics", *Nature Reviews Genetics*, vol. 5, pp. 764–72.

Garber JE, Offit K 2005, "Hereditary cancer predisposition syndromes", *Journal of Clinical Oncology*, vol. 10, pp. 276–92.

Walter MJ, Graubert TA, Dipersio JF, Mardis ER, Wilson RK, Ley TJ 2009, "Next-generation sequencing of cancer genomes: back to the future", *Personalized Medicine*, vol. 6, pp. 1–15.

 Find interactive self-test questions and additional resources for this chapter at **www.korfgenetics.com**.

Self-Assessment

Review Questions

8.1   The nevoid basal cell carcinoma syndrome is characterized by the development of basal cell tumors in the skin, medulloblastoma of the cerebellum, and a number of congenital anomalies. It is transmitted as an autosomal dominant trait. The gene responsible for this disorder is linked to a locus on chromosome 9. Analysis of a polymorphic marker in the linked region in a tumor and nontumor sample from an affected individual reveals heterozygosity in the patient's blood cells but absence of one allele in the tumor. What does this imply about the mechanism of action of the responsible gene regarding tumor formation? If the disorder was inherited from the father of the patient referred to here, would you predict that the allele lost in the tumor would be the one inherited from the mother or father? Why might radiation therapy be a poor choice of treatment for cerebellar medulloblastomas in individuals with this syndrome?

8.2   Tumor suppressor gene mutations are often seen as constitutional mutations, but oncogene mutations generally occur sporadically. What would you expect to be the consequence of germline inheritance of an activating oncogene mutation?

8.3   Why is familial predisposition to cancer associated with an earlier age of onset of tumors than occurs sporadically?

8.4   What is a mechanism by which chromosome translocation can activate a proto-oncogene? Is it possible that a translation could inactivate a tumor suppressor gene?

8.5   What is the significance of microsatellite instability when found in a colon carcinoma?

Part Two

Genetics and Genomics in Medical Practice

CHAPTER 9
Chromosome Translocation

Introduction

Chromosomal analysis may be thought of as the first true genetic test, introduced in 1959 when trisomy 21 was found to be the cause of Down syndrome. A set of chromosomal aneuploidy syndromes was quickly discovered, making chromosomal analysis a standard part of the evaluation of an infant with congenital anomalies. Prenatal diagnosis by amniocentesis was introduced in the early 1960s. The ensuing decades have seen a progressive refinement of the approach to cytogenetic analysis, permitting precise characterization of chromosomal abnormalities at the submicroscopic and molecular levels. In this chapter we will explore the application of cytogenetic testing to diagnosis of an infant with multiple congenital anomalies. We will see how detection of the chromosomal basis for the child's problems leads to the ability to provide recurrence risk counseling and prenatal diagnosis. A variety of different approaches to prenatal diagnosis have been introduced, and pregnancies are now screened for the risk of Down syndrome. We will also look at advances in molecular cytogenetics that are rapidly changing the approach to cytogenetic analysis.

Human Genetics and Genomics, Fourth Edition. Bruce R. Korf and Mira B. Irons.
© 2013 John Wiley & Sons, Ltd. Published 2013 by John Wiley & Sons, Ltd.

Key Points

- Congenital anomalies occur in approximately 3% of pregnancies and are due to a wide variety of both genetic and nongenetic causes. Some multiple congenital anomaly syndromes are due to chromosomal abnormalities.
- Prenatal diagnosis by amniocentesis is commonly offered to women, especially those over 35 years of age due to an increased risk of trisomy, especially trisomy 21. Biochemical screening is being used to screen pregnancies for risk of trisomy.
- Chromosomal imbalance in a child can occur as a result of segregation of a balanced translocation in a parent. This leads to a risk of recurrence of the chromosomal abnormality in future pregnancies.
- The two most common approaches to obtaining fetal cells for prenatal diagnosis are amniocentesis (performed between 16 and 18 weeks' gestation) and chorionic villus biopsy (performed between 10 and 12 weeks' gestation).
- Cytogenetic analysis of fetal specimens may reveal a mixture of cells with or without a chromosomal abnormality, referred to as mosaicism. This may be indicative of true fetal mosaicism, or may arise during culture of the fetal cells.
- Molecular cytogenetic analysis, including fluorescence in situ hybridization (FISH) and array comparative genomic hybridization, are now being used to provide molecular characterization of submicroscopic chromosomal anomalies. This form of cytogenetic testing is now recommended as the first tier of testing in individuals with intellectual disability or autism spectrum disorders.

Part I

Karen was born after a full-term pregnancy. There were no medical problems during the pregnancy, but there was concern toward the end of term because her mother, Deborah, was not gaining weight as fast as expected. No prenatal testing had been done, as Deborah was 27 years old and there is no known family history of genetic problems. Deborah did have a blood test done during the second trimester, which she understood was to check that the baby was "developing normally," and she was told only that everything was "fine." An ultrasound examination done in the eighth month, though, showed the fetus to be small for gestational age. At birth, Karen weighs 4 pounds, 10 ounces. She is noted to have a number of unusual features (Figure 9.1), including widely spaced eyes, a prominent nose, large ears, and bilateral iris colobomata. She is brought to the special care nursery where, on day 2 of life, she is found to have a heart murmur due to a ventricular septal defect. Karen is examined by a geneticist, who suggests that she might have Wolf–Hirschhorn syndrome.

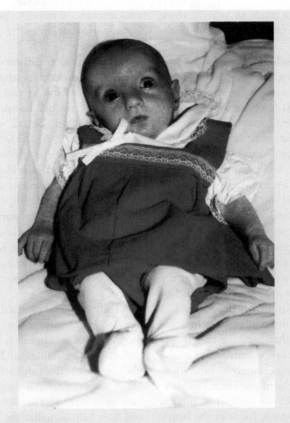

Figure 9.1 Child with Wolf–Hirschhorn syndrome.

Approximately 3% of all babies are born with a congenital anomaly. In most cases, these anomalies involve a single part of the body, for example, cleft lip or a heart defect. Usually the problems are compatible with survival and can be surgically repaired. The body is formed normally beyond the one area that is malformed. There are some infants, however, who have multiple congenital anomalies, indicative of a more generalized disruption of embryonic development. Some of the malformations may be obvious (e.g., facial or limb defects). Internal organs such as the brain, heart, and kidneys often are involved as well. Surgical treatment may be possible for specific malformations, but most defects of the central nervous system, which lead to neurologic problems and developmental impairment, cannot be corrected.

Multiple congenital anomalies can occur due to many causes, such as infections acquired in utero, exposure to toxic agents (teratogens), and genetic factors. Genetic problems include single-gene defects, chromosomal abnormalities, and multifactorial disorders.

Determining the etiology of multiple congenital anomalies can be challenging but is important both for care of the infant and for counseling of the family. Recognition of a pattern of anomalies can lead to the diagnosis of a syndrome – a constellation of distinctive features that is fairly consistent from individual to individual. Knowledge of features associated with a syndrome can alert the clinician to examine the child for internal anomalies that are not otherwise apparent. Some congenital infections can be treated with antibiotics to prevent further damage. The parents can be informed about future prospects for their child, both medically and developmentally. Finally, if a genetic disorder is identified, the family can be counseled about risks of recurrence.

Wolf–Hirschhorn syndrome consists of a set of multiple anomalies with a very distinctive facial appearance. The eyes are set widely apart, and the nose is prominent. A coloboma is a defect in the formation of the iris or retina. There is often a cleft lip and palate. Cardiac defects are common and may cause heart failure in the early days of life. Usually, the brain is severely malformed, resulting in profound developmental impairment. Wolf–Hirschhorn syndrome is due to a chromosomal anomaly, specifically deletion of material from the short arm of chromosome 4.

A chromosome deletion could have been detected by prenatal analysis, but there was no indication for such testing with this pregnancy. Amniocentesis is generally offered if the mother will be 35 years of age or older at the time of delivery, due to the increased frequency of nondisjunction with advanced maternal age. Although the risk of having a child with trisomy increases with maternal age, most pregnancies occur in younger women, and hence most births of children with trisomy occur to younger women. Efforts have been made to identify those at risk of carrying affected fetuses by means other than assessment of age.

Several approaches have been developed to provide early prenatal screening for Down syndrome. The first to be widely used involves biochemical testing of analytes in the mother's blood in the second trimester. Alpha-fetoprotein is a serum protein produced by the fetus. A small quantity is excreted through the urine into amniotic fluid, and some crosses the placenta into the maternal circulation. Congenital malformations that create defects in the fetal body wall lead to large increases in amniotic fluid and maternal serum alpha-fetoprotein levels. During the course of screening for such defects, it was noticed that low amniotic fluid levels tend to occur more often if the fetus has a chromosomal abnormality, particularly trisomy 21. It was later found that addition of two other measurements – unconjugated estriol and human chorionic gonadotropin (βhCG) – increased the sensitivity of the screen. Fetuses with Down syndrome are associated with low alpha-fetoprotein and estriol levels but a high βhCG level in maternal serum. Low values for the three substances indicate a risk of trisomy 18. It is estimated that applying this "triple test" will detect 70% of fetuses with Down syndrome at a false positive rate of 5%. Addition of another analyte, inhibin-A, increases sensitivity to around 80%. Use of ultrasound to identify physical features consistent with Down syndrome, such as shortened humerus or femur or echogenic focus in the heart, can increase sensitivity, but it is difficult to quantify this because of variation in the ultrasound approach used in different centers.

Although second-trimester screening is now routinely offered in most centers, approaches to first-trimester screening have been introduced and validated. The test involves measurement of nuchal translucency by ultrasound, as well as measurement of βhCG and pregnancy-associated plasma protein-A (PAPP-A) at 11–13 weeks. This provides a detection rate around 84% at a 5% false positive rate. Some centers combine first- and second-trimester screening, using a variety of approaches to calculate a final risk. Integrative testing provides a single risk figure based on the combined results of first- and second-trimester tests. Sequential testing involves first performing first-trimester screening and disclosure of results. If no prenatal test is done on the basis of these results, second-trimester screening is then done, with various approaches to risk assessment based on the first-trimester results.

A truly universal prenatal test for trisomy will require a risk-free and inexpensive means of fetal testing. Experiments are in progress with an approach based on analysis of fetal DNA in the maternal circulation. Some fetal DNA leaks across the placenta just as does alpha-fetoprotein. Genetic analysis of this DNA for the prenatal diagnosis of chromosomal abnormalities, such as Down syndrome, has recently been introduced and may help actualize the dream of a risk-free test.

Part II

Because Wolf–Hirschhorn syndrome is suspected, blood is sent to the laboratory for chromosomal analysis. Deborah and her husband Steven are told of the possible diagnosis. They are very anxious about Karen's future. They understand that the chromosomal analysis may take 2 weeks to be completed. Clinically, Karen is doing fairly well; her heart disease does not require treatment. She is being kept in the hospital mainly for nutritional support, until she gains some weight. Two weeks after Karen's blood sample is drawn, the laboratory reports that she does have a deletion involving material on the short arm of chromosome 4, with abnormal extra material attached to the end of 4 (Figure 9.2). Fluorescence in situ hybridization (FISH) studies are done, and reveal that the extra material is derived from chromosome 8. This confirms the clinical diagnosis of Wolf–Hirschhorn syndrome, though in addition she has partial trisomy for the short arm of chromosome 8. Deborah and Steven discuss the finding with Karen's pediatrician and with the geneticist who was asked to see her. They are told that Karen has no life-threatening problems but will likely have significant developmental impairment. They are not really surprised at this by now, having had several weeks to adjust to Karen's condition. After nearly 3 weeks in the hospital, Karen is now gaining weight, and she is ready to be taken home.

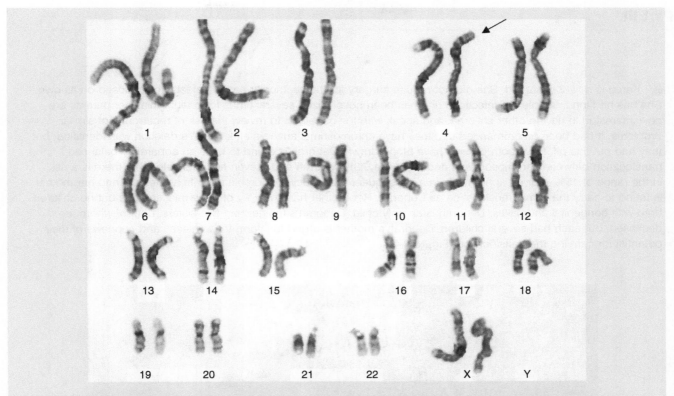

Figure 9.2 Karyotype showing evidence of deletion of the short arm of chromosome 4, with abnormal material present on 4p (arrow).

Wolf–Hirschhorn syndrome was described in the early days of clinical cytogenetics, before chromosome banding. It is associated with deletion of material from the tip of the short arm of chromosome 4. The congenital anomalies are thought to result from loss of multiple genes in the region. The paradigm of a complex set of developmental anomalies resulting from deletion of multiple contiguous genes has been invoked for many chromosomal deletion syndromes (see Chapter 6). Efforts have been made to map the extent of deletion with specific phenotypic features in affected individuals, but the specific genes that are responsible for various aspects of the phenotype are not known.

More refined methods of chromosomal analysis have revealed that some apparent deletions are actually the result of translocations between two or more chromosomes. Sometimes these

are visible with chromosome banding, but some require FISH to be detected. The translocation in this child involves loss of material from the short arm of chromosome 4 and gain of material from the short arm of chromosome 8. The phenotype would be expected to reflect genetic imbalance of both chromosomal regions. The fact that the child has features of Wolf–Hirschhorn syndrome suggests that the chromosome 4 deletion has the predominant effect, perhaps because a larger region of chromosome 4 was lost than was gained for chromosome 8.

Most likely, the unbalanced translocation was the result of segregation of a balanced translocation in one of the parents. Chromosomal analysis of both parents should be carried out, since if one carries a balanced rearrangement there is a risk of having additional children with chromosomal imbalance.

Part III

Karen is now 2 years old. She did not require surgery for the ventricular septal defect, which closed on its own. She has had innumerable ear infections and has been hospitalized several times for pneumonia. Her parents are now interested in having other children, and speak with the geneticist to review the risk of recurrence of similar problems. It had been recommended that they have chromosomal analysis after Karen's deletion was identified, but they had put this off. Now, both parents have blood drawn. Deborah is found to have an apparently balanced translocation between chromosomes 4 and 8 (Figure 9.3). Deborah and Steven are counseled that there is a risk – in the range of 15% – for an abnormality in a subsequent pregnancy. Deborah's parents are tested, and her mother is found to carry the same translocation as Deborah. Her mother has a history of three miscarriages but no children born with congenital anomalies. Deborah is an only child. Deborah's mother had two sisters, both of whom are deceased, but each had several children. Deborah's mother is urged to inform these nieces and nephews of their potential for carrying the translocation (Figure 9.4).

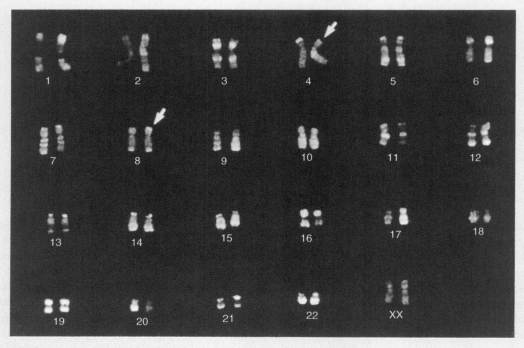

Figure 9.3 R-banded karyotype showing balanced translocation between chromosomes 4 and 8 (arrows). (Courtesy of Cytogenetics Laboratory, Brigham and Women's Hospital, Boston.)

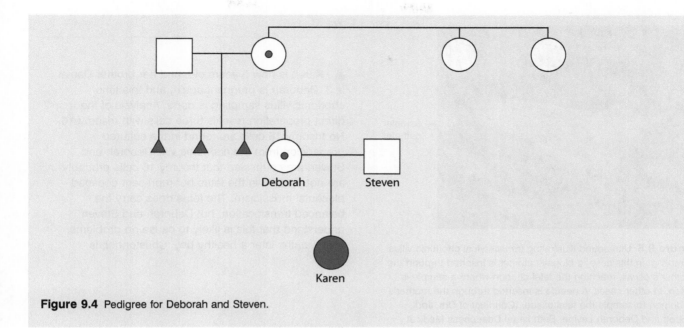

Figure 9.4 Pedigree for Deborah and Steven.

We have seen in Chapter 6 how meiotic segregation of a balanced translocation can give rise to gametes with gains or losses of chromosomal segments. Alternate segregation will produce either normal chromosomes, or gametes with the balanced translocation. The unbalanced products, however, will likely result in some perturbation of development. Often, the developmental effects are of sufficient magnitude that spontaneous abortion occurs. This is probably the fate of most chromosomally abnormal embryos, and may occur so early that the pregnancy goes unrecognized. Only the more subtle imbalances are likely to be compatible with development to later stages of pregnancy, or development to term. These subtle imbalances, however, may be of sufficient magnitude to produce major congenital anomalies.

The risk of production of unbalanced gametes is difficult to predict. It depends on many factors, including the size of the translocated segment. Also, the risk is often different depending on whether the mother or the father is the carrier, for unknown reasons. Recurrence risks are derived empirically, but in many cases a particular translocation is unique to a particular family, making it difficult to provide accurate risk assessment.

Finding a balanced translocation in an individual warrants counseling of other family members who may also be at risk. There may be a family history of congenital anomalies or, more commonly, of recurrent miscarriage. Chromosomal analysis should be offered to couples who have a history of recurrent miscarriage, especially first-trimester miscarriage, since most chromosomally abnormal embryos miscarry at this time in pregnancy.

Part IV

Deborah is now pregnant. Amniocentesis is done at 16 weeks and, 2 weeks later, a normal male karyotype is reported: 46,XY. Deborah and Steven are delighted when, 5 months later, a healthy baby boy is born.

For the prenatal diagnosis of genetic disorders, fetal tissue has to be obtained. There are two major ways of obtaining this tissue. At 10–12 weeks of gestation, a sample of the fetal placenta can be obtained with a biopsy catheter inserted either through the cervix or transabdominally – in either case, under ultrasonographic guidance (Figure 9.5). This is referred to as **chorionic villus sampling (CVS)**. The tissue can be used to isolate DNA or can be grown in culture. At 16–18 weeks of pregnancy, a sample of amniotic fluid can be withdrawn with a needle inserted transabdominally (**amniocentesis**) (Figure 9.6). This fluid contains fetal cells, mainly derived from skin and bladder (amniotic fluid is largely derived from fetal urine), that can be grown in culture.

Visualization of the chromosome structure requires access to dividing cells. Amniotic fluid cells must be grown in culture for several days, after which dividing cells are harvested and studied. Some cytotrophoblast cells obtained with chorionic villus tissue divide so rapidly that they can be harvested immediately for chromosomal analysis. Extra-embryonic mesoderm can also be obtained from this tissue and grown in culture.

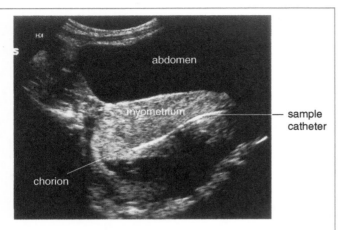

Figure 9.5 Ultrasound illustrating transcervical chorionic villus sampling. In this case, a biopsy catheter is inserted through the mother's cervix, reaching the fetal chorion where a sample is taken. In other cases, a needle is inserted through the mother's abdomen to sample the fetal tissue. (Courtesy of Drs. Jodi Abbott and Deborah Levine, Beth Israel Deaconess Medical Center, Boston.)

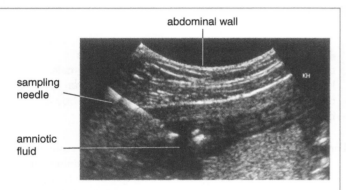

Figure 9.6 Ultrasound illustrating amniocentesis. A needle is inserted through the mother's abdomen into the amniotic cavity, where fluid is withdrawn for study. (Courtesy of Drs. Jodi Abbott and Deborah Levine, Beth Israel Deaconess Medical Center, Boston.)

When a parent is known to carry a balanced rearrangement, it is relatively simple to analyze fetal chromosomes to look for evidence of imbalance. FISH probes have been developed to permit rapid diagnosis of aneuploidy for the major chromosomes involved in live-born aneuploidy syndromes (13, 18, 21, and X). These probes bind to chromosome-specific DNA in uncultured interphase cells, permitting the presence of monosomy (for X) or trisomy to be detected rapidly. The approach does not detect structural rearrangements of chromosomes, or aneuploidy involving other chromosomes or chromosomal segments.

Part V

> Karen is now 5 years old, and her brother Daniel is 3. Deborah is pregnant again, and this time chorionic villus sampling is done. Analysis of the direct preparation reveals three cells with trisomy 16. No trisomy 16 cells are found in the cultured preparation from the chorionic villi. Deborah and Steven are counseled that trisomy 16 cells probably are not present in the fetus but represent confined placental mosaicism. The fetus does carry the balanced translocation, but Deborah and Steven understand that this is likely to cause no problems. Five months later a healthy boy, Christopher, is born.

When nondisjunction occurs during mitosis rather than meiosis, the result is chromosomal mosaicism. Detection of mosaicism by prenatal diagnosis can result in situations in which the phenotypic consequences are hard to predict. Not only is it difficult to know whether the fetus has physical abnormalities, but also the abnormal cells may not be derived from the embryo. Chorionic villus biopsy samples two cell types, neither of which is embryonic. Rapidly dividing cytotrophoblast cells are particularly prone to mitotic nondisjunction, and the mosaic chromosomal abnormalities often are not represented in the fetus. Cultured chorionic villus tissue is derived from extra-embryonic mesoderm. Amniotic fluid cells originate from fetal skin and bladder, as well as from the lining of the amnion. The latter, again, are not embryonic.

This has created a dilemma in genetic counseling for many families. Mosaicism noted in uncultured chorionic villus material should be confirmed with cultured material. Mosaicism that is confined to the cytotrophoblast is much less likely to be clinically significant. For amniotic fluid analysis, it is common to grow samples in multiple culture flasks or on coverslips in multiple culture dishes (Figure 9.7), permitting analysis of colonies derived from individual cells. Sometimes chromosomal mosaicism will arise by nondisjunction in culture. This is referred to as **pseudomosaicism**. If the chromosomal anomaly is not seen in multiple cultures, it is presumed to be pseudomosaic and probably is not clinically significant. On the other hand, if the abnormal cells occur in multiple cultures, true mosaicism is present. This is more likely to have phenotypic impact, although in some cases the proportion of affected cells may be low, and the exact phenotypic consequences may be difficult to predict. Many families who undergo prenatal diagnosis are not well prepared for the possibility of receiving results that are of uncertain clinical significance. This underscores the importance of genetic counseling as a component of the prenatal diagnosis process.

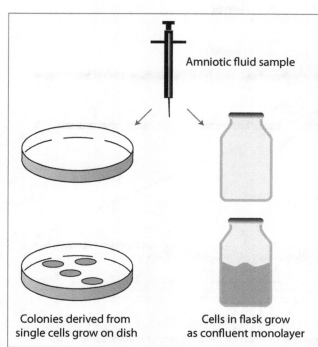

Amniotic fluid sample

Colonies derived from
single cells grow on dish

Cells in flask grow
as confluent monolayer

Figure 9.7 Amniotic fluid may be inoculated into culture dishes or flasks. In the dishes, single cells grow into discrete colonies. If cells are grown on cover glasses in dishes, they may be harvested in situ and directly examined with the microscope. In this way, cells within individual colonies may be directly examined. Cells that are inoculated into flasks grow as a confluent monolayer. These cells are enzymatically removed from the flask and harvested for chromosomal analysis.

Part VI

👤 Christopher is found to be healthy at birth with no abnormal physical findings noted, as expected, since he inherited Deborah's balanced translocation. At 4 years of age, he is referred to a geneticist because he has some developmental problems. Deborah tells the geneticist that early in life he had some feeding problems and poor weight gain, but that these resolved by the time that he was 2 years old. He is generally healthy, although he does have asthma and allergies. He had his tonsils removed for recurrent strep infections, and is followed by an orthopedist for flat feet that are treated with orthotics. His early motor milestones were somewhat delayed, but he walked independently at 15 months. From a motor standpoint, he is still "clumsy" and less coordinated than his siblings. His most significant developmental problem is a significant delay in expressive language (he can only say "momma"), although his receptive language is age appropriate.

On physical examination, he has a relatively big head for his size and some nonspecific facial features, including an unusual head shape with a broad, prominent forehead and prominent occiput, midface hypoplasia, unusual ears, a single transverse palmar crease on the right hand, broad large toes, and mild hypotonia. The geneticist sends a new cytogenetic test, a chromosome microarray, to look for an area of chromosome imbalance. Christopher is found to have a 6.6 megabase deletion of the long arm of chromosome 4 that involves the region of 4q13.3 to 4q21.21 (Figure 9.8). Blood is sent for chromosome analysis to determine if the deletion can be identified by standard cytogenetic methods. A focused analysis of chromosome 4 suggests the presence of a very subtle interstitial deletion (Figure 9.9). Christopher's parents are told that while there are no patients reported in the literature with his exact deletion, other patients with larger overlapping deletions have similar craniofacial features and developmental delays, so this deletion is most likely the cause of his problems.

(Continued)

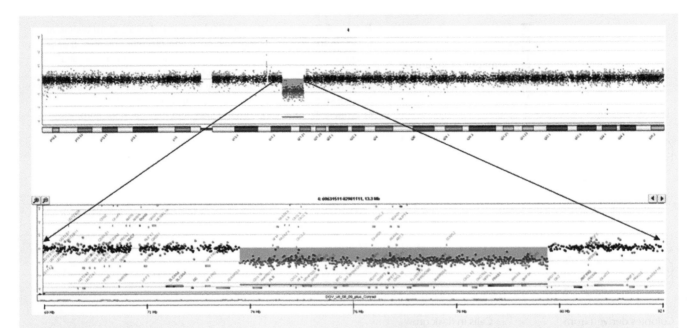

Figure 9.8 Chromosome microarray findings that illustrate the 6.6 megabase deletion on the long arm of chromosome 4. The figure at the top illustrates the "chromosome view" of the deletion, while the bottom figure illustrates a more detailed view of the deletion and the genes contained within the deleted segment. (Courtesy of Dr. Yiping Shen, DNA Diagnostic Laboratory, Children's Hospital Boston).

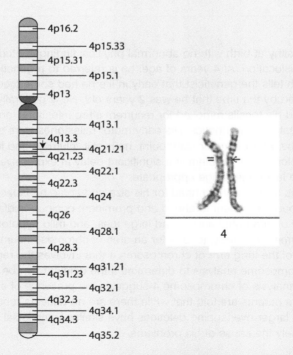

Figure 9.9 Illustration of the chromosome 4 deletion. The figure on the left illustrates the size and location of the deletion, which would contain one dark band, while the figure on the right illustrates the difficulty of identifying the deleted segment on a standard karyotype even with knowledge of the location of the breakpoints of the deletion. In the figure on the right, the arrow points to the deleted chromosome 4 on the right, while the two lines identify the location of the deletion on the nondeleted chromosome 4 on the left. (Figure on right courtesy of Dr. Allen Lamb and ARUP Laboratories, University of Utah.)

Chromosome microarray analysis, rather than a standard kary-otype test, has now become the first-tier test for the cytogenetic evaluation of children with developmental delay, intellectual disability, or autism spectrum disorders. This is due to the increased resolution of microarray technology, which allows for better detection of small deletions or duplications that cannot be "seen" by karyotype analysis, and results in a diagnostic yield that is up to 10–15% higher. While there are differences in how the currently available chromosome microarray tests have been developed, most of the microarrays in clinical use target areas of known clinically significant deletions or duplications, as well as other random areas of the genome, to look for chromosome imbalance. Analysis of these latter areas can result in the detection of copy number variants (CNVs) of either benign or unknown significance that can cause some counseling difficulties. Chromosome microarray analysis is increasingly becoming more useful in the evaluation of individuals with autism spectrum disorders where specific abnormalities have been identified more frequently (e.g., 16p11.2 deletion or 15q duplication), and for further evaluation of apparently balanced chromosome translocations, as it has been estimated that approximately 20% of these individuals have loss or gain of material that cannot be identified on a standard karyotype from a specimen obtained prenatally (chorionic villus or amniocentesis) or from blood obtained postnatally. However, since a chromosome microarray identifies areas of imbalance (gain or loss), it will not identify balanced translocations that can have genetic counseling implications. Therefore, a standard karyotype would still be the first-line test for individuals with recurrent pregnancy loss.

Clinical Cytogenetics

Chromosomal analysis was the first routine medical genetic test. In the early years of cytogenetics, several distinctive syndromes were discovered (see Chapter 6) that are due to changes in chromosome number. Several disorders due to large deletions or other rearrangements were described, but it was not until the advent of chromosome banding in the late 1960s that more subtle chromosome structural changes could be routinely detected. Over the years since then, the precision of chromosomal analysis has gradually improved, to the point now where molecular cytogenetic tools such as FISH and CGH arrays (see Chapter 6) permit detection of deletions or duplications with several thousand nucleotide resolution.

Standard chromosomal analysis includes a count of 20 or more metaphases to exclude mosaicism and banding, usually with Giemsa staining. Chromosomes are extended as much as possible to elicit fine structure and facilitate detection of small rearrangements. There is a wide range of indications for standard chromosomal analysis. It is performed to confirm a suspected diagnosis of a chromosomal aneuploidy syndrome such as Down syndrome, trisomy 13, Turner syndrome, or the like. In some cases, such as in a child with multiple, severe congenital anomalies, the analysis may be performed emergently. Since

the survival of children with trisomy 13 or 18 is very limited, it may be decided to withhold major surgical treatments if a diagnosis is confirmed.

Standard chromosomal analysis is the first-line genetic study performed for children with multiple congenital anomalies. The yield on chromosomal testing is low if there is only a single anomaly, such as isolated cleft palate, but increases if there are two or more anomalies or if the anomalies are accompanied by impaired cognitive development. High-resolution analysis may reveal very small rearrangements, such as small deletions, insertions, or duplications.

Another indication for standard chromosomal analysis is for couples who have experienced recurrent first-trimester miscarriages, or with a history of infertility. The goal is to search for a balanced rearrangement, such as translocation or inversion, that predisposes to the production of chromosomally unbalanced gametes. There are many other causes of recurrent miscarriage or infertility, so cytogenetic analysis is but one component of the evaluation. The yield on chromosomal analysis tends to be higher in couples who have had previous pregnancies that have come to term, since if one carries a balanced rearrangement it is expected that some normal gametes will be produced.

Molecular cytogenetics provides additional tools for special study. Individuals suspected of having a microdeletion syndrome can be tested using specific FISH probes. In most cases these microdeletions are overlooked with standard cytogenetic analysis. FISH can also be used with subtelomeric probes to search for small deletions in the subtelomeric region. The phenotype associated with these deletions is often a nondescript one, with developmental delay, intrauterine growth retardation, and sometimes a family history of similar problems or miscarriage.

FISH can also be helpful in the identification of chromosomes involved in rearrangements. Derivative chromosomes, that is, chromosomes that form as a result of segregation of a balanced rearrangement, can be difficult to identify with standard banding. Sometimes the constituent chromosomal segments can be identified by performing cytogenetic studies on both parents, looking for one with a balanced rearrangement. Otherwise, cocktails of chromosome-specific FISH probes can be used to paint specific chromosome regions, permitting identification of the abnormal material. Other techniques, such as comparative genomic hybridization or spectral karyotyping, can also be used. These require more complex technologies that are not always available within clinical laboratories. Moreover, there is limited clinical utility to identification of the exact origin of abnormal chromosomal segments, as it can be difficult to predict phenotype from this information.

CGH microarray analysis is becoming increasingly more utilized for clinical cytogenetics. It offers the advantage that deletions or duplications as small as just a few thousand bases can be detected without prior knowledge of the specific chromosomal region that is involved. It can therefore be used as a general screen for diagnosis of an individual with a disorder

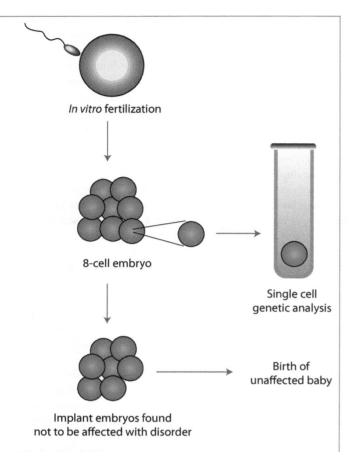

In vitro fertilization

8-cell embryo

Single cell
genetic analysis

Birth of
unaffected baby

Implant embryos found
not to be affected with disorder

Figure 9.10 Scheme of preimplantation diagnosis. Egg cells are obtained from the mother by insertion of a collecting catheter into the abdominal cavity, following hormone treatment to stimulate ovulation of multiple eggs. Fertilization of several egg cells is carried out in vitro. The embryos are brought to the eight-cell stage in vitro, and one or two cells from each embryo are biopsied using micromanipulation. DNA is extracted from the cells, and a sensitive assay, capable of detecting a single cell's DNA, is used to determine the genotypes of the biopsied cells. Only embryos found to be unaffected are implanted into the mother's uterus and brought to term.

that does not fit a specific syndrome. The major disadvantage to this approach is that it is insensitive to balanced rearrangement.

Any of these approaches can be used with prenatal samples obtained by chorionic villus biopsy or amniocentesis. In addition, blood can be obtained from the fetus by percutaneous umbilical blood sampling (PUBS). This is done after 18 weeks' gestation and is associated with a miscarriage rate as high as 2%. It is used to establish a diagnosis in cases where clinical suspicion of a chromosomal abnormality occurs too late for amniocentesis. This might be the case, for example, where abnormal ultrasound findings occur in the second trimester.

A new approach to prenatal testing involves **preimplantation diagnosis** (Figure 9.10). The most common approach is to perform testing on single blastomeres derived from an early embryo. Multiple oocytes are obtained by hormonal induction of ovulation and are harvested using a laparoscopic procedure. These are fertilized in vitro, and the embryos are allowed to divide to the eight-cell stage. A single blastomere is removed using a micropipette. This cell can be used for FISH studies to detect a chromosome rearrangement or trisomy for which the embryo is known to be at risk. DNA can also be isolated from the cell and tested for specific mutations known to be in the family. Embryos that are found not to have the genetic abnormality in question are then implanted into the mother's uterus and brought to term. (The loss of a single cell does not impair viability.) Preimplantation diagnosis offers testing at the earliest possible stage and is, in effect, a form of embryo selection. Most of the technology was developed as an approach to treatment of infertility, and diagnostic testing is often used for couples with a history of inability to become pregnant, sometimes because of a familial genetic disorder.

FURTHER READING

Bahado-Singh RO, Choi SJ, Cheng CC 2004, "First- and mid-trimester Down syndrome screening and detection", *Clinics in Perinatology*, vol. 31, pp. 677–94.

Bergemann AD, Cole F, Hirschhorn K 2005, "The etiology of Wolf–Hirschhorn syndrome", *Trends in Genetics*, vol. 21, pp. 188–95.

Brambati B, Tului L 2005, "Chorionic villus sampling and amniocentesis", *Current Opinion in Obstetrics and Gynecology*, vol. 17, pp. 197–201.

Eiben B, Glaubitz R 2005, "First-trimester screening: an overview", *Journal of Histochemistry and Cytochemistry*, vol. 53, pp. 281–3.

Kuliev A, Verlinsky Y 2005, "Preimplantation diagnosis: a realistic option for assisted reproduction and genetic prac-tice", *Current Opinion in Obstetrics and Gynecology*, vol. 17, pp. 179–83.

Lau TK, Leung TN 2005, "Genetic screening and diagno-sis", *Current Opinion in Obstetrics and Gynecology*, vol. 17, pp. 163–9.

Miller DT, Adam MP, Aradhya S, *et al.* 2010, "Consensus statement: chromosomal microarray is a first-tier clinical diagnostic test for individuals with developmental disabil-ities or congenital anomalies", *American Journal of Human Genetics*, vol. 86, pp. 749–64.

Reddy UM, Mennuti, MT 2006, "Incorporating first-trimester Down syndrome studies into prenatal screening", *Obstetrics and Gynecology*, vol. 107, pp. 167–73.

 Find interactive self-test questions and additional resources for this chapter at **www.korfgenetics.com**.

Self-Assessment

Review Questions

9.1 An amniocentesis is done because of advanced maternal age, and interphase FISH studies are done looking for evidence of trisomy 13, 18, and 21, as well as sex chromosome aneuploidy. Three signals are seen representing chromosome 21, indicating that the fetus will be affected with Down syndrome. Why is it important to still perform chromosomal analysis for counseling the couple?

9.2 A couple has a child with Down syndrome following a prenatal biochemical screen that did not indicate increased risk of Down syndrome in the pregnancy. They ask how the diagnosis could have been missed on the screen. What would you tell them?

9.3 A chromosomal analysis done on chorionic villus cells indicates trisomy 15, but follow-up amniocentesis shows normal chromosomes. Should the parents be reassured that the fetus will be normal, and that the initial result represents confined placental mosaicism? Are there other tests that should be done?

9.4 A child with multiple congenital anomalies has an apparently balanced translocation between chromosomes 2 and 11. Is it possible that the translocation is responsible for the child's problems? What would you do to further explore this possibility?

9.5 You are providing counseling to an adult with cleft palate and a history of congenital heart disease that was repaired as a child. He wants to know if there is risk of transmission of similar problems to the next generation. What kind of cytogenetic test would be appropriate in this setting, and if the result is positive, how would you counsel him?

CHAPTER 10
Molecular Diagnosis

Introduction

The diagnosis of genetic disorders has long been based on clinical assessment and use of various laboratory tests, including imaging; physiological tests; tests of blood, urine, or other body fluids; and biopsy of affected tissue. In some cases tests are expensive and can be invasive, even requiring hospitalization and surgery. Results are sometimes ambiguous, and it may require years before a definitive diagnosis can be achieved. Prenatal testing or testing in advance of symptoms for an individual at risk was impossible with such approaches. Molecular diagnosis can overcome these problems. If the gene for a genetic disorder is known and mutations can be detected, it can be possible to establish a diagnosis on the basis of testing DNA from any tissue, such as blood. In some cases, diagnosis can be definitive, rapid, and inexpensive, and can be established in advance of clinical symptoms or even prenatally. Molecular diagnosis has transformed the medical approach to genetic disorders, and is beginning to have an impact on medical decision making in the care of common disorders. In spite of its power, however, there are many pitfalls in the use of molecular diagnostic tests, both technical and ethical. In this chapter we will explore the use of a diagnostic test for one of the most common Mendelian disorders: neurofibromatosis type 1 (NF1). We will then look at some of the challenges faced in the development and interpretation of molecular tests.

Key Points

- Identification of the gene for a disorder permits diagnostic testing by direct mutation analysis.
- Some genetic disorders are associated with a wide range of allelic heterogeneity.
- Genetic testing may reveal variants of unknown significance that require special care in interpretation.
- Molecular genetic tests are often first developed in research laboratories, but clinical testing requires transfer of the test to a certified clinical laboratory.
- Genetic linkage analysis can be used to track a genetic trait through a family if the responsible gene is not known or mutations cannot be easily identified.
- Genetic tests can be evaluated in terms of analytic validity, clinical validity, and clinical utility.
- Genetic tests raise a number of potential ethical issues that should be considered in deciding to initiate testing.

Human Genetics and Genomics, Fourth Edition. Bruce R. Korf and Mira B. Irons.
© 2013 John Wiley & Sons, Ltd. Published 2013 by John Wiley & Sons, Ltd.

Part I

👤 Robert is a 10-month-old boy who has just seen his pediatrician, and his parents, Tim and Janet, are in a panic. They had noticed some brown spots on his skin beginning at about 4 months of age (Figure 10.1), and at first they assumed that these were harmless birthmarks. At first, just a few were noticeable, but over the past several months more have appeared to the point where they can't be ignored. Janet pointed these out to the pediatrician, who made note of the location of the spots in a diagram in the medical record. He then said that he would like to refer Robert to see a specialist. When Janet asked why, he mentioned a condition called "neurofibromatosis." He said that he didn't know that much about it, but that the condition could result in the formation of tumors. A referral was made to a medical geneticist, with the appointment set for 2 weeks later. Janet immediately went on the Internet to learn more, and did not like what she saw.

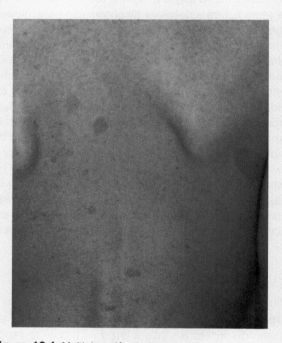

Figure 10.1 Multiple café-au-lait spots.

Café-au-lait macules are flat, tan or brown spots on the surface of the skin. The spots may be present at birth, but others tend to appear over the course of the first 1–2 years of life. They are present in both dark- and light-skinned individuals, and usually are easy to see in ordinary room light. Café-au-lait macules tend to tan, so it is not unusual to notice them in the summer months when a child is more likely to be exposed to the sun. Café-au-lait macules are common, with at least 10% of individuals in the general population having at least one spot, and some having two or three.

Individuals with neurofibromatosis type 1 (NF1) tend to have multiple café-au-lait macules, usually dozens or even hundreds. NF1 is one of three disorders classified as one of the "neurofibromatoses." The other two disorders are neurofibromatosis type 2 (NF2) and schwannomatosis. All three are characterized by the tendency to develop tumors of the nerve sheath, arising from Schwann cells. Individuals with NF1 develop neurofibromas, which are loosely packed accumulations of Schwann cells and other cells comprising the nerve sheath, as well as circulating cells called mast cells. Those with NF2 and schwannomatosis develop schwannomas, which are tumors composed entirely of Schwann cells. NF1 and NF2 include many features in addition to the characteristic tumors (Table 10.1). All three disorders are inherited as autosomal dominant traits, each due to mutation in a distinct gene. Only NF1 is associated with multiple café-au-lait macules as a presenting feature, though some individuals with NF2 also have several spots.

Table 10.1 Features of different forms of neurofibromatosis.

Disorder	Features	Gene	Frequency
NF1	Café-au-lait macules Skinfold freckles Neurofibromas Optic gliomas Lisch nodules Skeletal dysplasia Malignancy Learning disabilities	*NF1*: chromosome 17 Encodes neurofibromin: GTPase-activating protein	1:3000
NF2	Bilateral vestibular schwannomas Cranial and peripheral nerve schwannomas Meningiomas Ependymomas	*NF2*: chromosome 22 Encodes merlin – cytoskeletal protein	1:30000
Schwannomatosis	Schwannomas Pain	*SMARCB1*: chromosome 22 Encodes chromatin remodeling complex protein	~1:40000

Part II

👤 The 2 weeks between the visit to the pediatrician and the visit with the geneticist are an ordeal. Tim and Janet spend much of their time reading web pages on neurofibromatosis, some of which present very scary scenarios, showing people with deformities and tumors all over their bodies, and telling stories about children who have gone blind or even died. They have decided not to tell family members or friends, hoping that the diagnosis would turn out to be incorrect. They find it hard to believe that Robert could be affected with a condition as serious as NF1.

Finally the day comes for the visit with the medical geneticist, Dr. Scott. Dr. Scott first takes a medical history, which doesn't take long, as Robert has been healthy. She also takes a family history, which is similarly brief, as Robert is a first child, neither of his parents has similar skin spots, and there is no previous family history of neurofibromatosis. A physical exam is then done, revealing more than six café-au-lait spots, no skinfold freckles, and otherwise normal findings, except that Robert has a large head, in the 95th percentile for his age. Dr. Scott then explains that Robert has multiple café-au-lait spots, suggestive of the possibility of neurofibromatosis, though a definitive clinical diagnosis cannot be established with just this finding. She goes on to explain that children with neurofibromatosis eventually develop a second sign of the condition, permitting a definitive diagnosis. In the meantime, she says, there is no medication or other treatment, but Robert should be watched closely for development of possible complications, including having an eye doctor examine his eyes and follow-up in the genetics clinic once a year. She also says that a genetic test could be done that might permit a definite diagnosis to be made more quickly, but that the test would only determine if the diagnosis is indeed neurofibromatosis, and would not predict how severe the disorder might be. Tim and Janet have lived with uncertainty long enough, and ask that the test be done.

The diagnosis of neurofibromatosis is based on clinical features. Diagnostic criteria are used (Table 10.2), with the convention being that NF1 can be confidently diagnosed in any individual who fulfills at least two criteria. Many of the diagnostic features are age dependent, however, so it is often impossible to establish a clinical diagnosis in a young child. Most children present with multiple café-au-lait spots, defined as six or more spots measuring at least 5 mm prior to puberty or 15 mm after puberty. Freckles in the axillary or inguinal region are often the next sign to appear, but usually are not visible until 3–5 years of age. Neurofibromas may not be seen until puberty, though some children have small skin bumps that represent early neurofibromas. Also, a subset develops very large neurofibromas that cause major deformities or overgrowth; these are called plexiform neurofibromas. Lisch nodules are tan growths on the iris of the eye; they are commonly seen in adults with NF1

Table 10.2 Diagnostic criteria of NF1.

Feature	Comments
Café-au-lait macules	Six or more macules larger than 5 mm prepubertal or 15 mm postpubertal
Skinfold freckles	Axillary and inguinal
Neurofibromas	Two or more neurofibromas, or one or more plexiform neurofibroma
Lisch nodules	Melanocytic hamartomas on iris
Optic gliomas	Pilocytic astrocytomas of optic nerve or chiasm
Characteristic skeletal dysplasia	Long-bone dysplasia (usually tibial) or orbital dysplasia
Affected first-degree relative	Affected parent, child, or sibling

Note: An individual who fulfills two criteria can be diagnosed, but many of the features are age dependent.

Most, but not all, children who present with more than six café-au-lait spots at least 5 mm in size will go on to develop other signs of NF1. There is another condition, called Legius syndrome, which also leads to multiple café-au-lait spots, and may include skinfold freckles, hence fulfilling NF1 diagnostic criteria. Legius syndrome is associated with mutation of a gene that encodes a protein that operates in the same biological pathway as the *NF1* gene product (discussed in this chapter). Individuals with Legius syndrome do not seem to develop the various tumors associated with NF1, however, suggesting that it is a more benign condition. There are a variety of other rare conditions in which café-au-lait spots can also occur, though for the most part these are not difficult to distinguish from neurofibromatosis on clinical grounds.

There is no treatment for NF1 as yet, so management involves education of the patient and family and surveillance for treatable complications. In children, this involves regular follow-up visits looking for problems such as optic glioma, learning disabilities, growth of neurofibromas, and skeletal abnormalities. The process begins, however, with trying to establish an accurate diagnosis. Prior to the availability of genetic testing, this often meant waiting a year or more for an additional sign of NF1 to appear. Now, it is possible to identify the presence of an *NF1* mutation in upward of 95% of affected individuals using a blood sample. The advantages of doing the test include obtaining a definitive diagnosis, which may help mitigate parental anxiety, and, in the rare cases of Legius syndrome due to *SPRED1* mutation, indicating that the child is at low risk of development of tumors. An argument against testing is the relatively high cost (>US$1000), given that an *NF1* mutation is the most likely outcome, and finding the mutation would lead to a recommendation for clinical follow-up, which can be done with or without genetic testing. The genetic test, for the most part, does not predict severity of the disorder or specific complications (discussed in "Part III" of this chapter).

and do not affect vision, but are not reliably seen in young children. Optic gliomas are tumors of the optic nerve or chiasm that are seen in 15% of children with NF1. They are often asymptomatic, but they can impair vision or cause abnormal hormone secretion due to involvement of the hypothalamus. Characteristic skeletal dysplasia consists of bowing of a long bone, especially the tibia, which can result in fracture. There can also be a defect in the bones that comprise the orbit, often in association with plexiform neurofibroma in the region. Finally, given that NF1 is a dominantly inherited condition, having an affected first-degree relative (parent, child, or sibling) fulfills one diagnostic criterion.

Part III

Six weeks have passed since the visit to the genetics clinic, where a blood sample was taken, and Tim and Janet could not be more anxious as they wait for Dr. Scott to come into the room. Finally, she does, and they hear what they least expected: The genetic test results were inconclusive. Dr. Scott explains that the test is designed to look for a mutation in the *NF1* gene, and that 95% of individuals with NF1 will have a mutation in the gene. The problem is that not all changes in this gene have been definitively associated with neurofibromatosis. Most genetic changes associated with NF1 completely disrupt function of the gene. That is not what was found in Robert; instead, he had a "misspelling" in the gene that would cause the protein product of the *NF1* gene to be made incorrectly, but still to be made (Figure 10.2). Since there are some normal variations in the gene sequence, she explains, it is difficult to know if this particular one would cause neurofibromatosis or not. It is possible that the change is just a benign variant, but it is also possible that it would cause neurofibromatosis. The lab test results tended to lean toward this being clinically significant, but in order to further explore this, a sample is requested from Robert's parents for testing. Blood is therefore drawn from Tim and Janet, who leave the office both somewhat confused and frustrated by still more waiting.

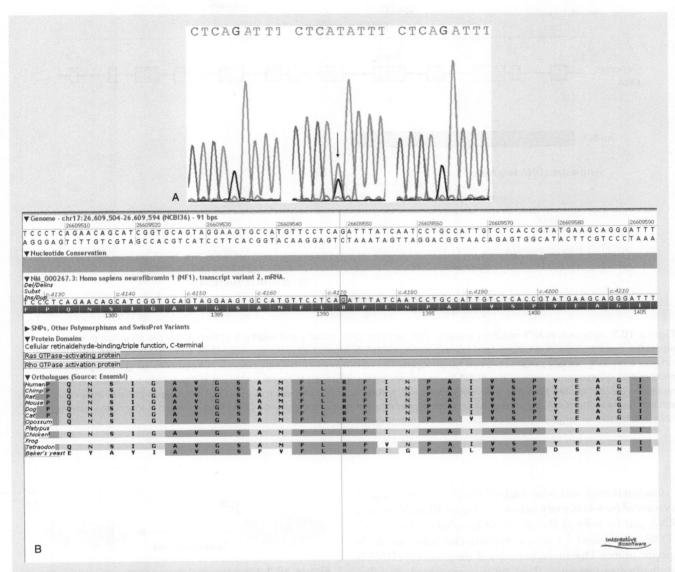

Figure 10.2 (A) DNA sequencing result from a region surrounding an *NF1* gene mutation. The mutation is indicated by the arrow, where two peaks are seen, one for G (black), which is the wild-type allele, and one for T (red), which is the mutation. Both are seen because the patient is heterozygous for the mutation. (B) Screen shot of a genome browser, showing the DNA and RNA nucleotide sequence and the amino acid encoded in the protein at this region in several species (*NF1* gene orthologues). At the site of the mutation, the wild-type sequence encodes an arginine (R), which is conserved across multiple species. The mutated codon (AGT) encodes a serine at this site.

The *NF1* gene spans over 300 kb and consists of 60 exons, encoding a 2818 amino acid protein referred to as neurofibromin. More than 1500 distinct mutations have been found, distributed throughout the gene and representing a variety of changes, including deletion of the entire gene; smaller intragenic rearrangements, deletions, or duplications; mutations in the coding sequence; and mutations within introns that affect splicing. Most of the mutations result in lack of gene expression through deletion, frameshift, stop codon, and so on, though a small proportion alter the amino acid sequence of the protein. Because of the great diversity of mutation types, no single approach to mutation analysis will detect the entire range of mutations. Sequencing of the entire coding region would detect mutations in exons, and extension of sequencing to the intron–exon borders would pick up many splicing mutations. However, mutations that reside deep within introns, and copy number changes such as deletions, would be missed by sequencing.

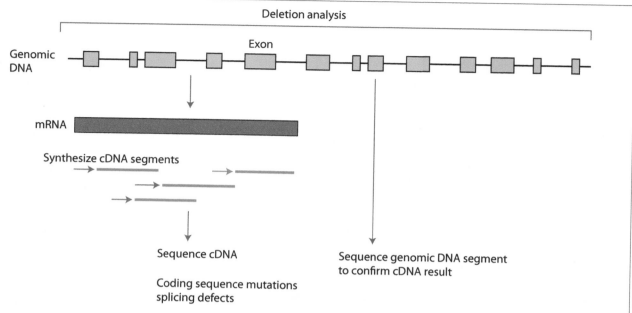

Figure 10.3 Approach to *NF1* mutation analysis. The genomic DNA (introns and exons) is shown at the top (diagram does not reflect the true intron–exon structure), and corresponding mRNA is shown below the genomic DNA. Both genomic DNA and RNA are isolated from cells, usually peripheral blood lymphocytes. The mRNA is used to synthesize cDNA fragments using *NF1* specific primers and reverse transcriptase. The cDNA fragments are then sequenced to reveal mutations in the coding sequence. Splicing mutations can be inferred from the cDNA sequence (e.g., finding an intron sequence in the cDNA or a skipped exon). Sequence variants found in the cDNA are verified by sequencing the relevant part of the genomic DNA. If no mutation is found, the genomic DNA is analyzed for large deletions or other genomic rearrangements.

Comprehensive mutation analysis therefore requires use of a variety of complementary techniques (Figure 10.3). Messenger RNA can be isolated (usually from lymphocytes) and *NF1* cDNA synthesized by reverse transcriptase using an *NF1*-specific primer. Due to the large size of the gene, the cDNA is synthesized in segments. These are then sequenced, revealing mutations in the coding region and also instances of aberrant splicing, such as exon skipping. The basis for the splicing mutations can then be determined by sequencing of the relevant region of genomic DNA. Deletions can be determined by demonstration of lack of heterozygosity for simple sequence repeat markers within the gene and confirmed by FISH or microarray analysis. Multiple ligation probe analysis (MLPA) can also be used; this is a variation of the PCR approach that detects deletions.

Interpretation of missense mutations in the *NF1* gene presents significant challenges. Neurofibromin functions as a GTPase-activating protein, stimulating the conversion of RAS–GTP to RAS–GDP, thereby terminating a cell growth signal (Figure 10.4). Although missense mutations have been demonstrated to interfere with this activity in some cases, there is no simple functional assay that can be performed on a clinical basis to validate new missense mutations. A pathogenic mutation would not be expected to be seen in unaffected

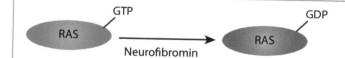

Figure 10.4 Neurofibromin stimulates the conversion of Ras–GTP to Ras–GDP. For details regarding the Ras signaling pathway, see Figure 8.13.

individuals, but rare benign variants might occur that have not been seen before in the general population. There are computer programs that can be used to predict whether a missense mutation might be expected to damage the function of a protein, but these do not prove pathogenicity. Finding that a variant occurs at an amino acid that is conserved in evolution is further evidence, but again is not conclusive. If the disorder affects multiple family members, it is possible to determine whether the mutation segregates with the disease phenotype in the family. If the parents of the affected individual are phenotypically unaffected, this would suggest that the affected individual represents a *de novo* mutation. This can be verified by testing both parents.

Part IV

👤 Tim and Janet return to see Dr. Scott after 2 weeks. They are told that neither one of them carries the genetic change that was found in Robert. Therefore, Robert's diagnosis of neurofibromatosis type 1 is confirmed. Tim and Janet are a little surprised to realize that having a definitive diagnosis was in some ways a relief after the weeks of uncertainty, though they are certainly not happy that Robert is affected with the disorder. Dr. Scott had previously discussed with Tim and Janet the natural history of neurofibromatosis, and the plans for follow-up, but she again spends time with them to review the plan now that a definite diagnosis is in hand.

The absence of the mutation in both parents indicates that it was indeed a *de novo* change in Robert, which together with the other evidence of evolutionary conservation and computer modeling strongly support its pathogenicity. The specific mutation does not, however, predict a specific phenotype. NF1 is a highly variable disorder, with differences in phenotypic expression occurring both within and between families. The only well-established genotype–phenotype correlations are the occurrence of a severe phenotype (with developmental impairment and large numbers of neurofibromas) in those with deletions of the entire gene and surrounding genes (1.4–1.5 million base pair deletions) and an exceptionally mild phenotype associated with a three-base (one amino acid) deletion in exon 17. There is some evidence that missense mutations may result in a large burden of internal neurofibromas with little skin involvement, but it is not clear whether any specific missense mutation is predictive of this mode of expression.

Part V

👤 Two years have passed, and Robert has been doing very well. He is growing and developing more or less normally, and has had his eyes checked each year without any worrisome findings. Then one day, Janet gets a call from her sister, Alice, who tells her that they have found café-au-lait spots on their daughter, Amy. Amy is just a year old and has been healthy, but has also been referred to a genetics clinic to explore the possibility of neurofibromatosis. This is a huge shock; after Robert's diagnosis, Tim and Janet had informed Alice, as well as Tim's two brothers, that Robert's condition was not inherited from either of them, and therefore that other family members were not at increased risk of having a child with neurofibromatosis. Amy's parents, indeed, have no signs of the condition. Amy is brought to see a medical geneticist, who arranges for genetic testing. An *NF1* mutation is found, and it is a different mutation from Robert's (Figure 10.5). Both sets of parents are told that this must be a rare coincidence; they find this hard to believe, but given that the mutations are different, no better explanation seems to be offered.

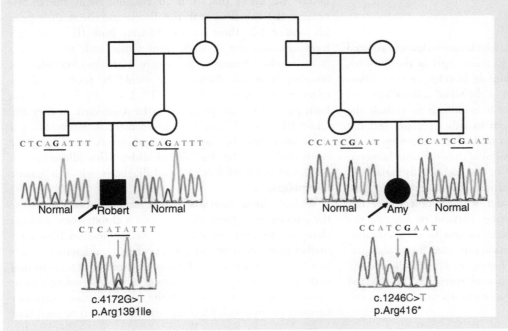

Figure 10.5 Sequencing results for Robert (left) and Amy (right), showing two *de novo* and distinct *NF1* mutations.

A stop mutation is highly likely to be pathogenic, and is clearly different from the missense mutation found in Robert. There is no known mechanism that could explain how two such different mutations might occur in the same family other than coincidence. The frequency of the *NF1* mutation has been estimated at around 1:10 000 per gamete per generation, making it one of the highest mutation rates known for a human genetic disorder. This indicates that there must be multiple mutated sperm or egg cells in every individual. Families have indeed been reported in which two relatives have the disorder due to independent *de novo* mutation.

Part VI

> Tim and Janet had always wanted to have two children, and feel that the time is right now to go forward and have a second child; Janet is now 6 weeks pregnant. They inquire about the possibility of prenatal testing to determine if the fetus has an *NF1* gene mutation. They understand that this is very unlikely, but they have already seen two very unlikely things happen in the family, and choose to go forward with amniocentesis in spite of the low risk. They have not entirely thought through what they would do if a mutation is found, and are expecting that none will be, yet wish further reassurance. An amniocentesis is performed at 16 weeks gestation; given the fact that two different mutations have been found in the family, the entire *NF1* gene sequence is determined in the amniocytes.

The penetrance of NF1 is 100%, which means that any affected individual would be expected to show signs of the disorder, such as café-au-lait macules, skinfold freckles, or neurofibromas. The absence of a mutation in the blood cells of Tim and Janet is further reassurance, but it is difficult to exclude the possibility of germline mosaicism in either parent. This has been documented in NF1, albeit rarely. Prenatal testing would definitively exclude the transmission of the mutation, however. Interest in prenatal testing for NF1 has been highly variable in different families. Some have expressed a desire not to have a child affected with the disorder, whereas others have not been interested in prenatal testing, particularly because the testing does not predict the severity or specific manifestations of the disorder. Some families have expressed interest in prenatal testing, even if the risk of having an affected child is low (as would be the case for unaffected parents of an affected child), mainly to obtain reassurance as early as possible in the pregnancy.

Part VII

> Tim and Janet are relieved to learn that no *NF1* mutation was found in the fetal DNA.

Molecular Diagnosis of Genetic Disorders

This case illustrates how molecular analysis can assist in the diagnosis of a genetic disorder. Molecular testing offers the advantages that it can be performed on any tissue source of DNA and does not require sampling of affected tissue. This means that diagnosis can be performed on blood or fetal samples (e.g., chorionic villus or amniotic fluid samples), obviating the need for invasive biopsy of tissues such as liver, kidney, muscle, brain, and so on, and also permitting prenatal diagnosis. It also can be done regardless of whether an individual is symptomatic, allowing for early diagnosis of individuals at risk of inheriting a genetic condition.

The first applications of molecular diagnosis involved linkage-based testing rather than mutation analysis. This was the case when genes involved in particular disorders had been mapped but not yet identified. Linkage is still used in instances where it is difficult to identify pathogenic mutations, either because the gene is unknown or because of the difficulty in finding mutations in large genes where a wide diversity of mutations may occur.

The basic strategy is shown in Figure 10.6. Here an individual (II-1) has an autosomal dominant disorder for which no laboratory diagnostic test exists. He is heterozygous for a marker gene closely linked to the disease gene that has two alleles, A and a. His partner is homozygous aa. In this family, we know that A is in coupling with the disease because II-1 inherited both the disease and the A allele from his mother, I-2. There are five children. Both III-1 and III-5 have inherited the A allele from father and, of course, a from mother. Because they received the marker allele in coupling with the disease, they would be predicted to be affected; and, indeed, they are. III-2 and III-4 got a from both parents and are predicted to be unaffected, as they are. Child III-3 would seem to be problematic, however. She got the a allele from her father and is therefore predicted to be unaffected, yet she has the disorder. This illustrates an important pitfall of linkage-based diagnosis, which is genetic recombination.

We have already seen how genetic recombination can change the association of particular alleles on a chromosome without changing the order of gene loci. Recombination between a marker gene and a disease gene can lead to a diagnostic error in a family linkage study. There are a number of ways to deal with this possibility. The likelihood of recombination can be estimated from knowledge of the recombination frequency between the two loci. Flanking markers can also be used (i.e.,

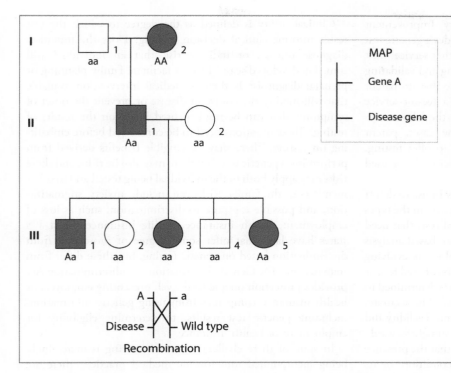

Figure 10.6 Linkage-based diagnosis in a family with an autosomal dominant disorder. Father II-1 is heterozygous for a closely linked marker with alleles A and a. A is in coupling with the disease gene in him, as he inherited both A and the disease allele from his mother, I-2. Children III-1 and III-5 inherit both A and the disease, and children III-2 and III-4 inherit both a and the nondisease allele. Child III-3 is a recombinant, as shown.

markers on either side of the disease gene) to identify recombinations when they occur.

There are a number of other limitations of the use of genetic linkage data for diagnostic purposes. Firstly, unlike most diagnostic tests, this approach requires study of a family, not just an individual. Relatives in two or more generations must be available and willing to participate in the study. Linkage studies have revealed a fairly high incidence of **misattributed parentage**. Most often this involves a situation in which the stated father of a child is not the biologic father (inferred from the fact that the child has an allele that could not have been inherited from the father). Often in such cases, a child's stated father is not aware that the biologic father of that child is a different person, setting up a sensitive and awkward situation in genetic counseling.

Secondly, linkage testing is not informative for all families. The parent who carries a mutant gene must be heterozygous for the linked marker or markers, and the alleles in this parent must be distinguishable from those of the partner. These criteria are more likely to be met if there are many markers available that are linked to a disease gene of interest. It also is helpful to have markers that are highly polymorphic, which means that there are multiple alleles at the locus and heterozygosity is common in the population.

Thirdly, and most important, is the issue of genetic heterogeneity. Because we are not directly determining the gene mutation, linkage-based testing relies on the assumption that the disease gene in the family is indeed linked to the marker gene. If diagnosis of the disease in the proband is incorrect, any inference of diagnosis based on linkage in another member of the family will also be incorrect. Even if the diagnosis in the proband is correct, however, genetic heterogeneity can provide misleading results. This would occur if there are many genes at different locations that can account for a given phenotype. If the wrong gene is tracked through the family, the results of linkage analysis will not indicate inheritance of the true disease-causing gene. Therefore, if genetic heterogeneity is known to exist, linkage studies must be used with great caution.

As more and more of the genes associated with medical disorders come to light, it is increasingly possible to offer genetic testing based on direct mutation analysis. This offers the significant advantage of being able to be performed on an affected individual, without the need for a family study in most cases. Direct mutation tests must be developed and validated for each gene. In some cases, such as sickle cell anemia, a single mutation accounts for virtually all affected individuals. In others, there may be a larger, but limited, repertoire of mutations known to be associated with disease, and in some there may be a great diversity of possible mutations, as is the case for the *NF1* gene.

Most genetic tests begin in a research laboratory where the gene is identified, but use of the test for clinical decision making involves validation and performance in a clinical diagnostic laboratory. In the United States, clinical laboratories are certified under the Clinical Laboratory Improvement Amendments (CLIA). A laboratory that provides a genetic test for diagnostic purposes and charges a fee for that service must be certified under CLIA. Aside from developing and validating a new test, the clinical laboratory must insure that no patent infringement occurs by offering testing on a fee-for-service basis. Many gene sequences are patented by the laboratories that first identified the sequence. In some cases, patent holders exercise rights to restrict the license to offer testing, and may force testing to be performed in specifically licensed laboratories.

There are a wide variety of technologies now in use to detect mutations. The specific approach depends, in part, on the types of mutations to be detected and the volume of tests that need to be done. Automated approaches to sequence-based analysis are increasingly being used, and the technology is evolving rapidly. In general, the analytical validity of DNA-based tests is very high; in other words, if a sequence variant is determined to be present or not present, that result is probably accurate, barring human error such as sample mixup. Clinical validity and clinical utility, on the other hand, may be less straightforward.

Clinical validity is defined as the likelihood that the presence of a sequence variant correctly diagnoses a condition, or its absence indicates that the condition will not occur. The clinical validity of tests such as an *NF1* mutation analysis is very high, although, as we have seen, variants of unknown significance may occur. Clinical validity may also be affected by instances of nonpenetrance, in which case presence of a mutation does not necessarily indicate the presence of disease.

Clinical utility is defined as the degree to which the test result informs clinical decision making. Does the mutation diagnose disease, or indicate risk that an individual will someday develop disease? Does it facilitate family planning or prenatal diagnosis? Is there a medical intervention available that will modify the course of disease or prevent the onset of symptoms that can be implemented based on the results of testing? These questions need to be considered before embarking on testing. There may be tangible benefits derived from performing a genetic test, but there may also be risks, and these risks may apply both to the individual being tested and to other members of the family. Risks can include anxiety, stigmatization, and possible exposure to discrimination, such as loss of employment, health insurance, or life insurance. Most US states have laws that offer some degree of protection from discrimination based on genetic testing, but these differ from state to state. The Genetic Information Nondiscrimination Act provides protection on a federal level, preventing employers or health insurance companies from using genetic information, including genetic test results, to determine eligibility for employment or health insurance.

In spite of these challenges, genetic testing is increasingly being incorporated into routine medical practice. There are many testing laboratories, both commercial and academic. An Internet database, available at www.genetests.org, can be used to identify a testing laboratory for any particular genetic disorder.

FURTHER READING

Neurofibromatosis

Boyd KP, Korf BR, Theos A 2009, "Neurofibromatosis type 1", *Journal of the American Academy of Dermatology*, vol. 61, pp. 1–14.

Ferner RE 2010, "The neurofibromatoses", *Practical Neurology*, vol. 10, pp. 82–93.

Molecular Diagnosis

Burke W 2009, "Clinical validity and clinical utility of genetic tests", *Current Protocols in Human Genetics*, vol. 9, p. 9.15.

Grosse SD, Kalman L, Khoury MJ 2010, "Evaluation of the validity and utility of genetic testing for rare diseases", *Advances in Experimental Medicine and Biology*, vol. 686, pp. 115–31.

Find interactive self-test questions and additional resources for this chapter at **www.korfgenetics.com**.

Self-Assessment

Review Questions

10.1 In the pedigree in Figure 10.7, a woman has had two brothers with Duchenne muscular dystrophy, an X-linked recessive trait. She is pregnant, and the fetus is found to be male. A linkage study is done, using two markers that flank the muscular dystrophy gene. The marker alleles are numbered in Figure 10.7. Based on the genotypes, what would you tell her is the risk that the fetus will have Duchenne muscular dystrophy?

10.2 A molecular diagnostic test reveals a single base change in a gene in an individual affected with an autosomal dominant disorder. The change causes an amino acid substitution in the protein. How would you judge whether this is a pathogenic change or a benign variant?

10.3 Some molecular diagnostic tests for large complex genes with multiple exons begin with sequencing of cDNA prepared from mRNA rather than genomic DNA. What is the advantage of this approach?

10.4 A 40-year-old man at risk of inheriting a Huntington disease allele is found to have 74 CAG repeats in his gene. Does this mean that he will definitely develop the disease?

10.5 You are counseling a family with Noonan syndrome. What is the mode of genetic transmission? What is the responsible gene? Is clinical genetic testing available?

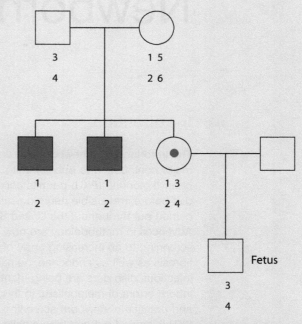

Figure 10.7 Pedigree and inheritance of Duchenne muscular dystrophy.

CHAPTER 11
Newborn Screening

Introduction

The introduction of newborn screening for inborn errors of metabolism was a major contribution to public health. Early detection of disorders such as phenylketonuria (PKU) permits children to be placed on a phenylalanine-free diet before irreversible neurological damage occurs. Newborn screening is carried out throughout the United States and in most of the developed world. Advances in methodology are now stimulating an expansion of newborn screening to an increasing array of disorders. Disorders such as cystic fibrosis as well as endocrine, hematologic, immunologic, neurologic, and infectious disorders are being identified in the newborn period, in addition to inborn errors of metabolism. In this chapter we will consider the principles and practice of newborn screening in depth. We will see how screening for PKU is carried out and how a child is managed after a positive screening test. We will look at general principles of inborn errors of metabolism, and consider various approaches to treatment. We will also look at how the expansion of disorders identified by newborn screening can identify the presence of more than one condition in a family as well as identify conditions that may have mild or benign clinical presentations.

Key Points

- Newborns can be screened for an increasing variety of conditions on the principle that early detection can lead to therapy that prevents severe, long-term medical problems. Technological advances are quickly expanding the scope of newborn screening.
- Children diagnosed with inborn errors of metabolism require lifelong care. An unexpected consequence of PKU is a risk of congenital anomalies in the child of an affected woman due to phenylalanine toxicity if the mother is not maintained on strict dietary control during pregnancy.
- There is a wide variety of pathophysiological mechanisms that underlie inborn errors of metabolism. These include defects in enzymes and coenzymes, with physiological consequences of product deficiency and/or substrate accumulation.
- A variety of approaches to the treatment of inborn errors of metabolism are in use or in development, including dietary management, coenzyme supplementation, removal of toxic metabolites, enzyme replacement, and gene therapy.

Human Genetics and Genomics, Fourth Edition. Bruce R. Korf and Mira B. Irons.
© 2013 John Wiley & Sons, Ltd. Published 2013 by John Wiley & Sons, Ltd.

Part I: December 1965

👤 Jocelyn is born after a full-term, uncomplicated pregnancy. Her birth weight is 3100 g, and she is a healthy and vigorous baby. She is being breast-fed and seems to be feeding well. A few drops of blood are taken from her heel on day 2 of life, just prior to her being discharged from the nursery with her mother (Figure 11.1); the blood is blotted onto a card and sent to the state laboratory. Her parents are told that this is a routine test done for all newborns, and so they put it out of their minds. They take Jocelyn home, and she continues to feed well and seems to be thriving. After 1 week, however, they receive a call from their pediatrician, who explains that an abnormal laboratory result has come back. At first Jocelyn's parents are mystified, unaware that any laboratory test had been done. The pediatrician then reminds them about the heel stick. He has arranged for the family to take Jocelyn to a special clinic at the nearby children's hospital.

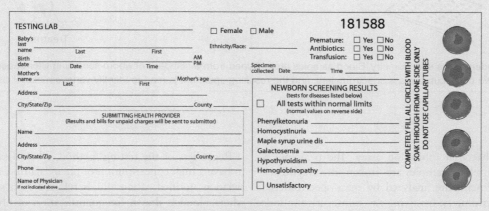

Figure 11.1 Spots of blood on filter paper card to be sent to a state laboratory.

The concept of the inborn error of metabolism was introduced in Chapter 3. These disorders are the consequence of mutation in genes that encode enzymes required for metabolism or catabolism of specific substances. Enzyme deficiency results in a buildup of substrate and/or deficiency of product, either or both of which can cause disease. Screening of newborns for several inborn errors of metabolism is standard throughout the United States and in most of the developed world. The rationale is that identification of infants with inborn errors can lead to institution of treatment prior to the onset of clinical signs of the disorder. This can prevent otherwise irreversible neurologic damage and other medical problems.

Screening generally is performed by obtaining a blood sample by heel stick just before the baby is discharged from the nursery. The specific disorders included in the testing panel vary from state to state in the United States. Screening began to be introduced in the 1960s, and disorders commonly included are PKU (MIM 261600); maple syrup urine disease, a disorder of branched-chain amino acid catabolism (MIM 248600); galactosemia, a disorder of galactose catabolism (MIM 230400); and homocystinuria (MIM 236200). In some areas, newborns also are screened for biotinidase deficiency, a lack of enzyme required to recycle the cofactor biotin (MIM 253260); sickle cell disease (MIM 603903); congenital

hypothyroidism; congenital adrenal hyperplasia (MIM 201910); and congenital toxoplasmosis. The criteria for screening for a particular disorder are as follows: (1) The disorder produces irreversible damage if untreated early in life; (2) treatment prevents the damage but only if begun in the newborn period, when the infant is asymptomatic; (3) the natural history of the disease is known; (4) a suitable screening test is available; (5) facilities for diagnosis and treatment are available.

The technology for newborn screening has recently undergone major changes. For decades, the mainstay of testing for PKU was a bacterial inhibition assay. Dried blood samples on disks of filter paper were placed onto an agar plate seeded with bacteria and with an analog of phenylalanine that inhibits bacterial growth. Phenylalanine in the blood sample would compete with the analog, permitting a halo of growth around the disk. The size of the halo was related to the concentration of phenylalanine in the sample. Similar assays were developed for many other metabolic disorders. The tests were simple, reliable, and inexpensive, but had to be performed separately for each disorder.

Recently, a new approach to newborn screening has been developed that uses mass spectrometry to detect abnormal levels of metabolites (Figure 11.2). This promises to allow diagnosis of a much larger number of metabolic disorders and

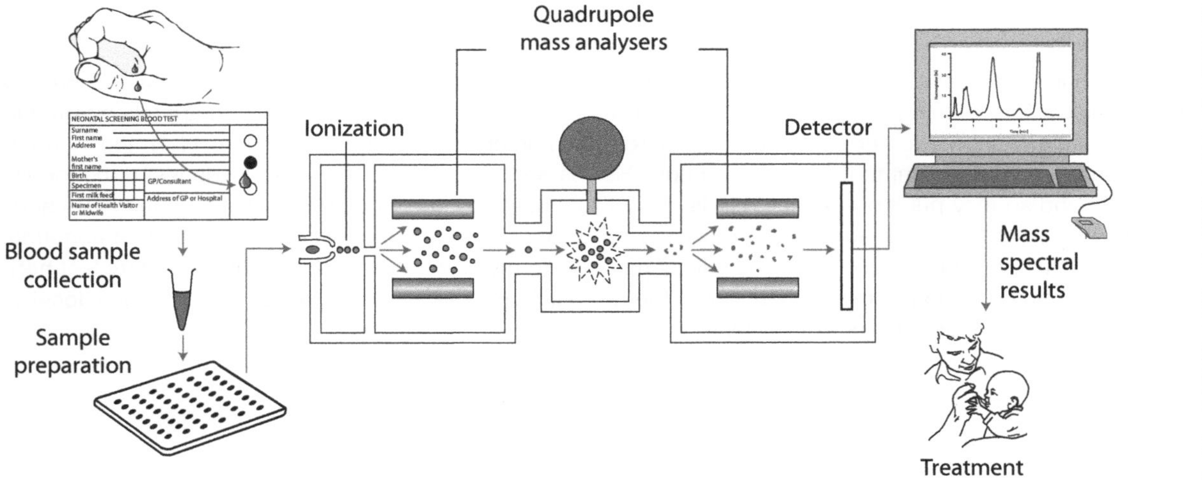

Figure 11.2 Tandem mass spectrometry. Blood samples are obtained from a standard newborn-screening filter paper. The blood is passed through two consecutive mass spectrometers, and the resulting spectrum is read to identify various metabolites in the blood.

has replaced the bacterial inhibition assay. The principle is that metabolites in blood samples are broken into fragments, and then the fragments are analyzed by mass spectrometry. Tandem mass spectrometry, involving two consecutive rounds of analysis, can be used to identify and quantify dozens of metabolites in a single analysis. Efforts are now underway to standardize the approach to newborn screening using tandem mass spectrometry. Some of the disorders that can be detected do not fit standard criteria for newborn screening, perhaps because the natural history is not well defined or there is no known treatment. Current efforts are focusing on a subset of disorders that are appropriate to include on a screening panel, with the hope that a similar set of tests will be accepted as standard across all regions of the United States and abroad.

Regardless of the testing method, when a sample is found to have a high concentration of phenylalanine, the baby's physician is notified. The child is referred to a specialty clinic, where blood is drawn for quantification of phenylalanine. A value greater than 20 mg/dL is indicative of classic PKU. Some newborns have phenylalanine values in an intermediate range (7–20 mg/dL), which is indicative of atypical or mild PKU. Either form of PKU is treated by reducing phenylalanine intake. Elevated levels of less than 7 mg/dL correspond with non-PKU benign hyperphenylalaninemia and require no treatment. Benign hyperphenylalaninemia mutations are missense mutations. PKU mutations also are usually missense mutations but might be mutations that lead to deficient production of protein (e.g., stop codons, splicing mutations, and deletions).

Part II: December 1965

The next day, Jocelyn is taken to the metabolism clinic. Her parents are told that the laboratory result indicates that Jocelyn probably has phenylketonuria. Jocelyn is examined, and the results are normal. Both blood and urine specimens are obtained. Jocelyn's parents are informed about PKU and, in particular, taught about the phenylalanine-free diet (Figure 11.3). Jocelyn will be fed with a special low-phenylalanine formula. Her parents are reassured that Jocelyn can be expected to achieve essentially normal cognitive development if this diet is adhered to. Nevertheless, they are in a state of shock, and are frightened. They spend considerable time talking with the clinic social worker and are introduced to other parents who have children with PKU. This somewhat reassures them. The next day, they get a call from the clinic nurse, telling them that Jocelyn's phenylalanine level was 25 mg/dL (the normal level being less than 2 mg/dL), confirming the diagnosis. Two weeks later, the urine pterin analysis is reported as normal, indicating that Jocelyn has classic PKU and not a cofactor deficiency in which the increased phenylalanine would be a secondary finding.

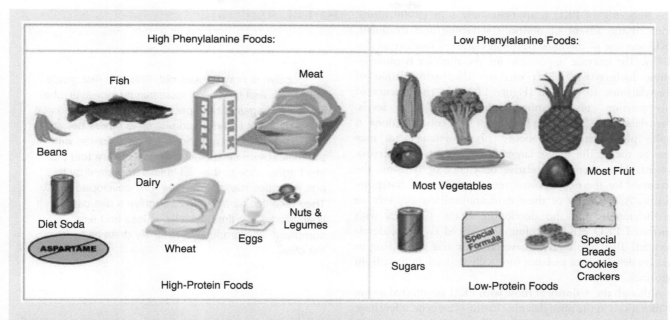

Figure 11.3 Example of foods permitted in a phenylalanine-restricted diet.

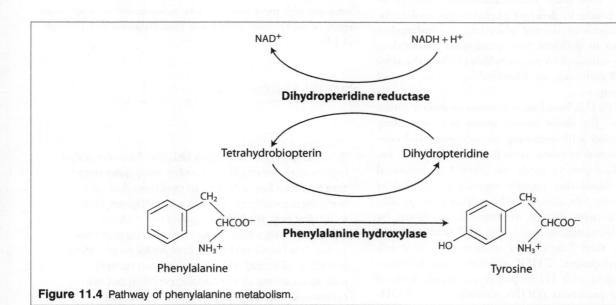

Figure 11.4 Pathway of phenylalanine metabolism.

The frequency of PKU is approximately 1 in 10 000 births. Prior to the advent of newborn screening and treatment, PKU was one of the most common causes of intellectual disability. The enzyme responsible for the disorder is phenylalanine hydroxylase, which catalyzes the hydroxylation of phenylalanine to tyrosine (Figure 11.4). In the absence of this reaction, phenylalanine builds up to high levels. Phenylalanine is believed to be toxic at high concentrations. A major phenylalanine metabolite, phenylpyruvic acid, may also be toxic. The major target for toxicity is the nervous system. Also, there is a relative deficiency of tyrosine, the precursor for the neurotransmitters dopamine and norepinephrine. A deficiency of these neurotransmitters is likely to be deleterious for the developing brain. Children with untreated PKU exhibit profoundly delayed cognitive development. They also tend to have fair hair and skin owing to relative deficiency of melanin (normally derived, in part, from tyrosine).

Although the majority of those with PKU are affected owing to mutations in the phenylalanine hydroxylase gene, a few have mutations in a different enzyme, dihydropteridine reductase (DHPR) (MIM 261630), or in the synthesis of biopterin. DHPR is involved in the reduction of H2 biopterin into H4 biopterin; H4 biopterin is a cofactor required for the hydroxylation of phenylalanine to tyrosine. It also is required for hydroxylation of tyrosine and tryptophan, which are critical in the synthesis of vital brain neurotransmitters. Absence of DHPR activity results in deficient phenylalanine hydroxylation in the presence of normal phenylalanine hydroxylase enzyme and also in deficient neurotransmitter production. Defects in the synthesis of biopterin, which produce the same effects as DHPR deficiency, are identified by a urine assay of biopterin and neopterin.

Treatment of PKU is based on restriction of dietary intake of phenylalanine. The major protein source is a preparation of individual amino acids excluding phenylalanine and containing supplemental tyrosine as well as carbohydrate, fat, and minerals. Low-protein foods are allowed in measured quantities, but foods that contain significant amounts of protein (e.g., meat, fish, cheese, and ice cream) are prohibited. Compliance with dietary treatment is monitored by testing blood phenylalanine levels. The goal is to maintain the level at less than 7 mg/dL, an amount considered safe for normal development. DHPR deficiency and biopterin synthesis are treated with H4 biopterin and supplements of neurotransmitter precursors (DOPA, carbidopa, and 5-OH-tryptophan), perhaps in conjunction with a low-phenylalanine diet.

The care of a child with PKU imposes many demands on a family to maintain compliance with the diet. It is best to provide care in a multidisciplinary clinic, where a physician, a nutritionist, a social worker, and (in some cases) other professionals might be involved. The family is likely to require considerable education and support.

Part III: April 1973

Jocelyn is now 7 years old. She is in first grade and doing well in school. Increasingly, however, she is rebelling against her special diet, mainly because it is not pleasant tasting, and she sees others her age eating tastier foods at school. After discussion with the metabolism clinic staff, her parents are told that strict adherence to the diet is less important by this age, because the brain is now fully developed. They take this as a sign that Jocelyn's diet can be liberalized. Over time, Jocelyn is less and less compliant, and gradually the family drifts away from the clinic.

The first few years of life are a critical time in terms of brain development. Compliance with the low-phenylalanine diet is especially important during this time. Formerly, it was considered safe to relax the diet later in childhood. The current view is that dietary relaxation during childhood or even in adolescence can lead to cognitive loss and emotional problems. Consequently, most centers now recommend at least some degree of compliance with a low-phenylalanine diet throughout life.

Part IV: March 1986

Jocelyn is now 20 years old. She has completed high school, although her grades were quite poor. She has also had a history of psychological and behavioral problems. Jocelyn has just given birth to a baby boy. His birth weight is only 2000 g, although he was born at term. He is microcephalic (small head size) and has a congenital heart defect (tetralogy of Fallot). His physicians are optimistic that they can repair the cardiac problem but are concerned that microcephaly predicts that his cognitive development will be delayed. His blood phenylalanine level is in the normal range at 2 weeks of life. He is being breast fed. There is no history of PKU in his father's family. Jocelyn is afraid and confused. She is not married and relies on her parents for emotional support.

There are many possible causes of the birth of a child with microcephaly and a congenital heart defect. In the child of a woman with PKU, however, by far the leading cause is a syndrome called maternal PKU. If the mother has not adhered to the low-phenylalanine diet, there will be high levels of phenylalanine in the fetal environment owing to the mother's defect, and the fetal phenylalanine hydroxylase activity will not be high enough to deal with this load. The consequence is an ironic outcome of treatment of a genetic disorder – toxicity in the next generation. In this case, the effects of high phenylalanine are particularly devastating. The fetus is exposed at a time when major organ systems, including the brain, are developing rapidly. It is common for these infants to have low birth weight, congenital heart disease, and inadequate brain development at the time of birth.

Part V: September 1988

👤 Jocelyn is pregnant again, by a different partner. Her son is now 2 ½ years old (Figure 11.5), and Jocelyn and the boy live with Jocelyn's parents. His heart defect has been surgically repaired, but he is severely developmentally impaired. He began walking only recently, and he is not yet talking. For this pregnancy, Jocelyn was counseled to start a phenylalanine-restricted diet prior to trying to conceive and to continue the diet throughout the pregnancy. Her compliance, which has been good, has been monitored by following blood phenylalanine levels. She is reassured that fetal damage from maternal PKU is very unlikely to occur in this pregnancy. She gives birth to a baby girl, Karen, who has a normal head circumference, weighs 8 pounds, and appears to have no other congenital or medical problems. She is discharged home at 2 days of age. Newborn screening reveals no abnormalities.

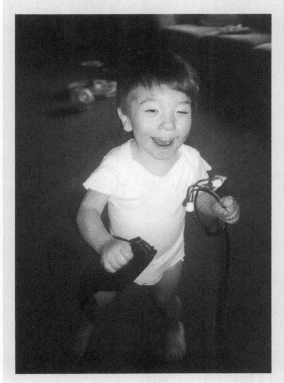

Figure 11.5 Child with dysmorphic facial features (broad nasal bridge and small nose) and microcephaly due to *in utero* effects of maternal phenylketonuria. (Courtesy of Dr. Harvey Levy, Children's Hospital, Boston.)

Maternal PKU is largely a preventable disease. The woman with PKU should be placed on a low-phenylalanine diet prior to the time of conception. The rationale for preconceptual treatment is that major events in organogenesis occur at a point very early in pregnancy when a woman may not realize that she is pregnant. Preconceptual treatment and continued close adherence to the diet throughout the pregnancy, however, have been shown to prevent the teratogenic effects of maternal PKU syndrome. Major efforts now are underway to identify women of childbearing age with PKU, educate them regarding the need to maintain the diet, and monitor them throughout pregnancy.

Part VI: April 2010

👤 Karen is now 21 years of age and has been healthy with no medical or developmental problems secondary to her mother's PKU during her life. She graduated from high school, completed training as a clinical assistant, and is working full-time at the children's hospital. She married last year and is currently pregnant with her first child. Her husband, Bill, is 23 years old, has no medical or developmental problems, and is of Northern European ancestry with no history of PKU or any other metabolic or genetic condition in his family. Karen's obstetrician discusses prenatal testing for PKU with her since she is a carrier for PKU, although Bill's carrier status is unknown. Karen declines prenatal testing, indicating that she is comfortable with testing the baby through newborn screening after delivery and treating the child if he or she is found to have PKU.

Karen delivers a 7 pound 8 ounce baby girl, Ellen, 2 days after her due date. The baby has no problems after birth and is discharged home on the second day of life. Prior to discharge, a heel stick blood specimen is taken for newborn screening, a test that now screens for over 30 conditions in addition to PKU, including other inborn errors of metabolism, cystic fibrosis, and several endocrine, hematologic, infectious, and immunologic conditions. Karen receives a call from her pediatrician several days later, asking her to bring in Ellen for further testing because she was identified as having elevated levels of octanoylcarnitine (C8) and decenoylcarnitine (C10:1), which can be seen in a condition called medium-chain acyl-CoA dehydrogenase (MCAD) deficiency (Figure 11.6). Further genetic testing reveals that she is homozygous for a single A985G missense mutation that confirms the diagnosis. She is referred for further evaluation and treatment to the metabolism clinic at the children's hospital, where additional metabolic testing confirms her diagnosis. Her parents are told that they should feed her at least every 4 hours and not allow her to go longer between feedings.

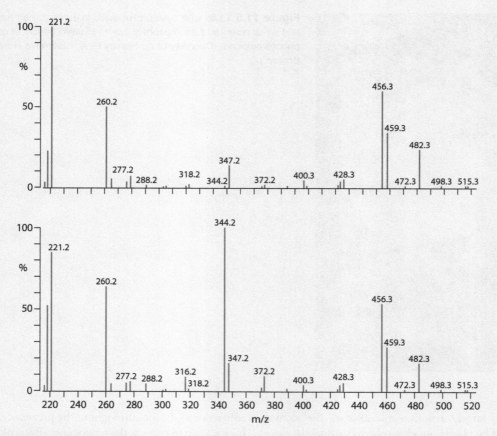

Figure 11.6 Mass spectrum of acylcarnitines following extraction of newborn-screening dried blood spot (DBS) and esterification with butanol. The peak at m/z 344.2 is C8 acylcarnitine (C8 AC), and the peak at MZ 347.2 is the internal standard, deuterated C8 acylcarnitine (^{2}H$_3$ C8 AC). Top: Normal newborn infant. Bottom: Infant with MCADD (DBS from day 2 of life). (Courtesy of New England Newborn Screening Program and Dr. Gerard Berry, Children's Hospital, Boston.)

Medium-chain acyl-CoA dehydrogenase deficiency (MCADD) (MIM 201450) is the most common of the fatty acid oxidation disorders and occurs with an estimated incidence of 1 in 10 000 births (see Figure 11.7). Approximately 60–80% of symptomatic patients are homozygous for a single A-to-G point mutation at position 985 of the MCAD gene, a missense mutation that originated in Northern Europe. Newborn screening for MCADD and the other fatty acid oxidation disorders became available with the introduction of tandem mass spectrometry in newborn-screening programs.

Mitochondrial fatty acid oxidation is very important for energy production, especially during fasting, when fatty acids provide 80% of required energy needs via ketone body synthesis in the liver and direct oxidation in other tissues. Long-chain fatty acids are important fuel sources for the heart and skeletal muscle. Fatty acids also provide energy for gluconeogenesis, and their oxidation spares glucose consumption.

Patients with fatty acid oxidation disorders generally present clinically during periods of fasting and/or acute illness that result in an increased metabolic rate and energy requirement. While patients with long-chain defects may present with cardiac and/or hepatic symptoms, those with MCADD generally have a more mild presentation. Unlike PKU, this condition does not require continuous treatment, but only at times of illness or metabolic stress. The majority of undiagnosed infants present with lethargy and hypoglycemia between 3 and 12 months of age (once the interval between feedings has lengthened, or nighttime feedings have been discontinued), or during an acute illness associated with decreased oral intake. Failure to recognize the signs and symptoms and institute glucose therapy promptly can result in coma and death. In fact, homozygosity for the A985G mutation has been associated with an increased incidence of sudden infant death (Wang *et al.* 2000). The ability to tolerate fasting improves with age and growth, so that episodes of hypoglycemia requiring therapy become less frequent, although many affected individuals will need to remember to avoid fasting and consume additional glucose calories during periods of illness or prolonged exercise or exertion.

While the majority of symptomatic individuals are homozygous for the A985G mutation, others are compound heterozygotes for another mutation in association with the A985G mutation. Genotype–phenotype correlations are less clear in these individuals, and some may be identified by newborn screening and have genotypes that are associated with a benign or mild clinical phenotype that may never have presented clinically, or presented later in life only during a significant illness or stress. This is particularly true in the case of newborn screening for MCADD where at least one family of

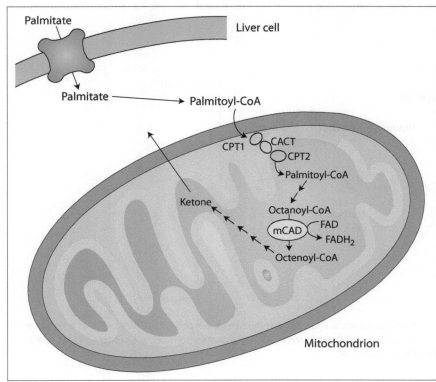

Figure 11.7 Mitochondrial fatty acid oxidation plays a critical role in hepatic synthesis of adenosine triphosphate (ATP) and ketones. A block in medium-chain acyl-CoA dehydrogenase (MCAD) enzyme activity results in an accumulation of medium-chain fatty acids esterified to coenzyme A and an impairment in energy production and ketone body formation.

four clinically asymptomatic individuals has been identified who were compound heterozygotes for the A985G and G842C mutations (Albers *et al.* 2001). This family may never have come to medical attention if it were not for newborn screening. It is unclear whether individuals with some of these more mild mutations may develop symptoms during periods of prolonged fasting, acute illness, or stress, so that lifelong vigilance is required.

Inborn Errors of Metabolism

Inborn errors of metabolism may result from mutations in enzymes or coenzymes, as is the case of PKU and MCADD, and may involve toxic buildup of substrate or product deficiency. There are, however, other pathophysiological mechanisms that apply to other biochemical genetic disorders. In addition, there are therapies that extend beyond dietary manipulation.

Another major cellular dysfunction associated with some metabolic disorders is the gradual accumulation of substances within the cell due to hereditary deficiency of enzymes required for their breakdown. This occurs in **lysosomal storage diseases**, in which one or another of the enzymes required to metabolize cell membrane components in the lysosome is missing. A hallmark of these disorders is the progressive buildup of membrane debris in the lysosome, leading to progressive loss of cell function. An example of a lysosomal storage disorder is Tay–Sachs disease (MIM 272800) (see Clinical Snapshot 7.2).

The defect underlying an inborn error need not reside in the gene for the enzyme or the coenzyme. Genetic defects may upset the mechanisms by which cellular proteins are targeted for specific organelles, leading to deficiencies of multiple enzymes. Such is the case for I-cell disease (mucolipodosis II) (MIM 252500), in which there is a failure in the trafficking of enzymes to the lysosome (Figure 11.8). Lysosomes become packed with undigested inclusions (hence the term "I-cells"). Lysosomal enzymes are glycoproteins that are targeted to lysosomes by binding mannose-6-phosphate residues to a receptor that transports the enzymes from the Golgi within vesicles. Children with I-cell disease have mutations that disrupt one of the enzymes required to phosphorylate mannose, resulting in the enzymes being secreted from the cell rather than incorporated into lysosomes. The disorder results in growth failure and severe neurological dysfunction, and is generally lethal.

Treatment of inborn errors of metabolism is aimed at reduction of the toxic substrate and/or replacement of missing product. This can be done, as we have seen, by dietary manipulation, but there are other approaches as well. One is to provide an alternative system to remove a toxic substrate. Deficiency of any of the enzymes in the urea cycle (Figure 11.9) can lead to buildup of ammonia, which is highly toxic. This can be removed emergently by dialysis, but chronic treatment involves administration of sodium phenylacetate and sodium benzoate, which complex with ammonia to form compounds able to be excreted safely in the urine.

Organ transplantation has been used to treat some metabolic disorders. Liver transplantation has been performed for some children with blocks in the urea cycle, for example. Advances in surgical technique and immunosuppression have vastly improved the safety and success of liver transplantation.

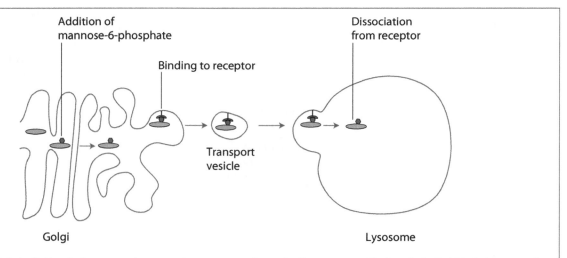

Figure 11.8 Protein trafficking to lysosome. Lysosomal enzymes are tagged with a mannose-6-phosphate that binds to a receptor within the Golgi. A vesicle pinches off from the Golgi and transports the enzyme to the lysosome. Within the lysosome, the enzyme dissociates from the receptor and the phosphate group is removed.

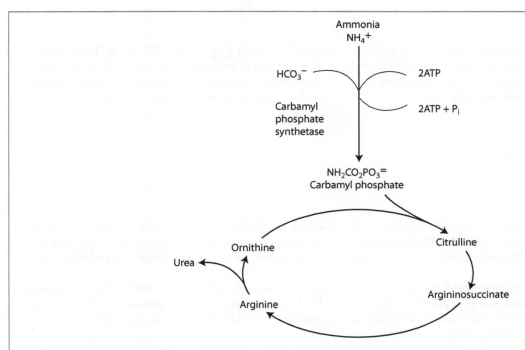

Figure 11.9 Major steps of the urea cycle. Ammonia is converted to carbamyl phosphate by the enzyme carbamyl phosphate synthetase, which reacts with ornithine to enter the urea cycle.

Likewise, bone marrow transplantation has been used to treat some lysosomal storage diseases. The rationale is that macrophages from transplanted bone marrow function as scavengers to engulf and digest membrane components that cannot be digested by the enzyme-deficient host cells. This has been tried with a set of disorders known as mucopolysaccharidoses. These disorders lead to buildup of proteoglycans (protein molecules with attached sugars) and are manifested clinically as progressive neurologic deterioration, growth failure, skeletal deformity, coarse facial features, and heart failure. Reduction in circulating mucopolysaccharide has been demonstrated in transplant recipients.

Because the pathogenesis of inborn errors of metabolism is based on deficiency of an enzyme, enzyme replacement would seem a reasonable therapeutic approach. Substantial progress toward enzyme replacement has been made in lysosomal storage diseases. The first to be treated in this way was Gaucher disease (MIM 230800), a disorder in which the enzyme glucocerebrosidase is absent. Macrophages become swollen with storage material and cause enlargement of the liver and spleen. In addition, the presence of engorged macrophages in bones leads to bone and joint pain. The missing enzyme can be purified in quantity from placenta, but initial efforts at treatment of patients by enzyme infusion were disappointing. It then was found that there are mannose receptors in the macrophage's cell membrane that are responsible for targeting mannose-containing substances for the lysosome. Chemical modification of purified glucocerebrosidase to expose mannose residues leads to efficient transport of the enzyme into the lysosomes of macrophages. Infusion of this modified enzyme, now produced by recombinant DNA methodology, has been demonstrated to be highly effective in reducing the size of the liver and spleen and reducing bone pain. A similar approach has been used more recently for treatment of other lysosomal disorders, including Fabry disease (MIM 301500); for some mucopolysaccaridoses; and recently for Pompe disease (MIM 232300), a disorder of glycogen metabolism.

The ultimate approach to treatment would be to replace the defective gene with an intact copy. Gene therapy protocols have also been tested on an experimental basis. These offer the possibility of replacing the defective gene, effecting a "cure" for the disorder. Most approaches are based on insertion of the gene encoding an enzyme into a virus, which then is used to infect cells, thereby inserting the gene into the cells. Major challenges include targeting the recombinant virus to the correct cells, obtaining physiologically appropriate levels of expression, and avoiding an immune response to the virus. Gene therapy is not yet in routine use for treatment of individuals with inborn errors of metabolism.

REFERENCES

Albers S, Levy HL, Irons M, Strauss AW, Marsden D 2001, "Compound heterozygozity in four asymptomatic siblings with medium-chain acyl-CoA dehydrogenase deficiency", *Journal of Inherited Metabolic Disorders*, vol. 24, pp. 417–18.

Wang SS, Fernhoff PM, Khoury MJ 2000, "Is the G985A allelic variant of medium-chain acyl-CoA dehydrogenase a risk factor for sudden infant death syndrome? A pooled analysis", *Pediatrics*, vol. 105, pp. 1175–6.

FURTHER READING

Kayler SG, Fahey MC 2003, "Metabolic disorders and mental retardation", *American Journal of Medical Genetics: Part C, Seminars in Medical Genetics*, vol. 117, pp. 31–41.

Levy HL 2003, "Historical background for the maternal PKU syndrome", *Pediatrics*, vol. 112, pp. 1516–18.

McCabe LL, McCabe ER 2004, "Genetic screening: carriers and affected individuals", *Annual Review of Genomics and Human Genetics*, vol. 5, pp. 57–69.

McCabe LL, Therrell BL Jr., McCabe ER 2002, "Newborn screening: rationale for a comprehensive, fully integrated public health system", *Molecular Genetics* and *Metabolism*, vol. 77, pp. 267–73.

National Institutes of Health 2000, "Phenylketonuria (PKU): screening and management", *NIH Consensus Statement*, Oct 16–18, vol. 17(3), pp. 1–33.

Find interactive self-test questions and additional resources for this chapter at **www.korfgenetics.com**.

Self-Assessment

Review Questions

11.1   Why are children with PKU not born with damage to the nervous system?

11.2   Why are children with lysosomal storage disorders usually not symptomatic at birth?

11.3   Enzyme replacement therapy for lysosomal storage disorders involves treatment with an enzyme preparation with exposed mannose-6-phosphate residues. Why is this modification necessary?

11.4   How does tandem mass spectrometry permit newborn screening for a larger number of disorders than previously used bacterial assays?

11.5   What are the general approaches used in the treatment of inborn errors of metabolism?

CHAPTER 12
Developmental Genetics

Introduction

We have introduced the concept of multiple congenital anomalies, and seen how the birth of an affected child can have a major impact on the entire family. Establishing a diagnosis for a child with congenital anomalies can be important for counseling of the family, regarding both future medical problems that may be anticipated and risk of recurrence in future offspring. Diagnosis has been historically based on clinical criteria, but advances in molecular genetics are rapidly revealing the genetic basis for congenital anomaly syndromes. This enables more precise diagnoses to be made, allows prenatal diagnosis to be offered, and in some cases predicts specific complications. It also reveals the underlying mechanisms of congenital anomalies, sheds light on normal development, and perhaps leads to future advances in prevention or treatment. In this chapter, we will consider the story of a child with multiple anomalies that include disparate systems. We will see how identification of the gene has improved the ability to provide diagnostic testing and counseling, and how the developmental mechanisms are coming to be understood. We will then look at the discipline of human dysmorphology, and glimpse some of the genetic systems that underlie human development.

Key Points

- The discipline of dysmorphology involves the use of clinical and laboratory approaches to establish the diagnosis underlying congenital anomalies.
- Establishing a diagnosis can provide a basis for counseling a family about the natural history and genetics of a disorder and may suggest specific approaches to management.
- Some congenital anomaly syndromes involve effects on widely varying organ systems. This may reflect the effects of disruption of multiple genes, or the possibility that a single gene participates in developmental processes common to various systems.
- Normal development is dependent on the activation or repression of genes under tight temporal and spatial control. Many of the genetic systems that underlie embryological development are coming to light.

Part I

👤 Jane's pregnancy has proceeded uneventfully right through the time of delivery. Jane and Albert are offered ultrasound examination during the pregnancy, and one is scheduled at 18 weeks, far enough along so that fetal growth and structure can be best evaluated. The ultrasonographer spends quite a bit of time taking all of the necessary measurements and views of the fetus. After the initial scans are taken, a fetal radiologist comes into the room and does further imaging. She tells Jane and Albert that the fetus is smaller than expected, and she is concerned that the heart and kidneys are not normally formed. She tells them that instead of two separate kidneys, it appears as though the fetus has a single horseshoe kidney, and that the heart appears to have an atrioventricular canal defect.

A genetic counselor comes into the room, talks to Jane and Albert more about the findings, and recommends that an amniocentesis be performed for fetal chromosome analysis since two major structural abnormalities are present. Although Jane and Albert would not terminate a pregnancy regardless of the outcome, they decide to proceed with the amniocentesis so that they have all of the information that they might need to make appropriate decisions regarding the remainder of the pregnancy. An amniocentesis is performed, and chromosome analysis reveals a normal 46, XX chromosome pattern. Additional fluorescence in situ hybridization (FISH) testing for a 22q11.2 deletion is negative (normal). Jane and Albert are referred for additional fetal imaging, specifically a fetal echocardiogram performed by a pediatric cardiologist at 20 weeks. The cardiologist tells them that the fetus has a large atrioventricular canal defect that will require surgical repair early in life. They decide to deliver at a large tertiary care center, rather than their local hospital, so that the baby can be cared for shortly after delivery by neonatologists and pediatric cardiologists. Labor begins spontaneously. It is obvious at the moment of birth that there are problems. The baby, a girl, is noted to have abnormal ears and an unusual face. Although she breathes spontaneously in the delivery room, it is immediately apparent that she is having respiratory distress. She is intubated in the delivery room and brought to the neonatal intensive care unit. Jane and Albert barely have time to see her and are confused and frightened.

It is common to offer ultrasound examination as a component of routine prenatal care. In addition to helping one recognize fetal malformations, ultrasonography provides accurate assess-ment of gestational age. Many couples find that having information about their baby's health prenatally helps them to plan, even if they do not choose termination of pregnancy in the event of fetal problems. The stressful environment of the delivery room is not a good place in which to first learn that a baby is in trouble. This baby apparently has multiple congenital anomalies, including abnormalities that were not identified by the prenatal ultrasound, as well as respiratory distress.

Chromosome analysis is typically performed when fetal anomalies are detected prenatally, as malformations are seen more frequently in the presence of a chromosome abnormality, such as Down syndrome (trisomy 21), trisomy 18, trisomy 13, or many partial-trisomy or partial-monosomy syndromes. Many of these chromosome abnormalities can be detected on a standard karyotype with high-resolution banding. Other "submicroscopic" chromosome changes may need additional testing by FISH or multiplex ligation-dependent probe amplification (MLPA) techniques, as they may not be detectable on a standard karyotype because of their small size. One example of the latter is the chromosome 22q11.2 deletion syndrome (see Clinical Snapshot 6.3). Since specific cardiac and renal abnormalities are seen in this condition, prenatal testing for this microdeletion by FISH or MLPA is indicated when cardiac malformations are seen prenatally.

Part II

👤 A geneticist is called to see the baby soon after her arrival at the medical center. She has been extubated, and although breathing on her own, is having some respiratory distress and feeding difficulty. On examination, she is small for gestational age and is noted to have several abnormal craniofacial findings, including a square face, a broad forehead, a small right eye, a prominent nasal bridge, tiny nasal openings, and short, wide, abnormally formed ears. Sloping shoulders are noted, and the geneticist also notices that the baby's face moves asymmetrically when she cries. The nurse tells her that a tube could not be passed down the nasal passages, indicating that they are smaller than normal. The cardiologists confirm the prenatal finding of an atrioventricular canal defect, and the baby is being closely monitored and treated for any possible cardiac problems that might occur prior to surgery.

The physical findings in this infant are indicative of a malformation syndrome that affects multiple organ systems. The clinical dysmorphologist tries to recognize patterns of abnormal development, with the goal of establishing an etiologic diagnosis. Major classes of anomalies are malformations, deformations, and disruptions. A malformation is the result of abnormal development of tissue. Developmental mechanisms

Figure 12.1 Diagram indicating association of tracheo-esophageal fistula, imperforate anus, vertebral defects, and radial defects. These malformations tend to occur together more often than might be expected due to chance. (Redrawn by permission from Quan and Smith 1973.)

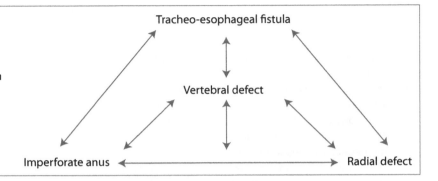

somehow are interfered with, and the tissue does not form properly. Deformation is defined as the distortion of a normally formed tissue by extrinsic pressure. An example is asymmetry of the skull due to pressure from a benign uterine tumor called a fibroid. Disruption is the damage of a normally formed tissue. For example, a tear in the amniotic cavity can trap a limb, amputating part of the extremity. Disruptions tend to be asymmetric, whereas malformations are more often (but not always) symmetric.

Various patterns of malformations are seen. Some comprise syndromes, such as Down syndrome. These are sets of congenital defects that are the consequence of some defined, ultimate cause. Down syndrome results from having an extra copy of chromosome 21. Syndromes can also result from exposure to teratogenic agents such as thalidomide. Whatever the cause – abnormality of one gene or a group of genes, or exposure to a teratogen – the outcome is perturbation of multiple developing systems in a reproducible way.

A second pattern of malformations is called a sequence. A sequence generally arises as the consequence of a single primary event, for example underdevelopment of the lower jaw in the Pierre–Robin sequence. Other anomalies that comprise the sequence are secondary effects of the primary malformation. In the Pierre–Robin sequence, the tongue is too large for the small mouth and interferes with closure of the palate, resulting in cleft palate. Here, cleft palate is not a primary malformation but a secondary consequence of underdevelopment of the jaw.

The third pattern is referred to as an association. It has been observed that particular sets of congenital anomalies tend to occur together more often than expected due to chance. These do not comprise syndromes; the causes are unknown, and many associations are etiologically heterogeneous. Indeed, the majority occur sporadically. One example is the VACTERL association, the major components of which are *v*ertebral anomalies, *a*nal atresia, *c*ardiac anomalies, *t*racheo-*e*sophageal fistula, *r*enal anomalies, and *l*imb defects (Figure 12.1). Various combinations of these features occur in different babies, reflecting the nonrandom association of these malformations. It is not known why these associations occur. They may reflect processes that have some molecular or morphologic event in common or processes that all occur at the same time in development.

The medical practice of dysmorphology is partly science and partly art. A dysmorphologist examines for both subtle and major anomalies, looking for recognizable patterns. Correctly establishing a diagnosis can help one to provide anticipatory guidance: What does the future hold? Is the child likely to have additional anomalies that are not obvious on cursory examination? It also permits accurate genetic counseling. Sometimes the recurrence risk will be high; at other times, the family may be surprised to learn that recurrence is unlikely.

Part III

Albert tells the care team that he and Jane have decided to name the baby Lisa. The geneticist suggests that Lisa be seen by an otolaryngologist to evaluate for choanal atresia and to evaluate the abnormally formed ears better, and by an ophthalmologist for further evaluation of the small eye. She also recommends that a hearing test be performed as well as further imaging of the ears by computed tomography (CT) scan and the brain by magnetic resonance imaging (MRI). Bilateral choanal atresia is confirmed by the otolaryngologist and by CT scan, which also reveals abnormalities of the temporal bones and inner ear bones (Figure 12.2). The ophthalmologist confirms that the right eye is abnormally formed, and CT scan also reveals colobomata of the optic nerves bilaterally, as well as pontine and inferior vermian hypoplasia (Figure 12.3). More detailed imaging of the brain will need to be performed by MRI, which will have to wait until the respiratory problems resolve.

👤 Lisa continues to have a problem breathing, which is felt to be due to her small nasal passages, and she requires tube feedings, as she is not able to feed comfortably by herself. Jane and Albert meet with the neonatologist later that evening, who explains that Lisa is sick but that no definite diagnosis has been made so far. The plan has been to provide maximum support as further information is collected. The other specialists have been called to see Lisa, but have not sent someone by yet.

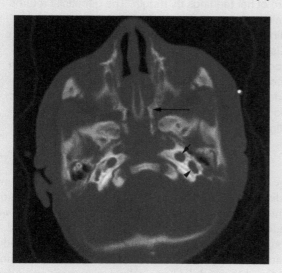

Figure 12.2 Temporal bone CT scan illustrating many features seen in CHARGE syndrome, including choanal atresia (long black arrow: lateral wall of the nasal cavity deviates medially and is opposed to the thickened vomer), abnormal cochlea (short black arrow: absence of internal cochlear structure and cochlear nerve canal), and hypoplasia of vestibule (black arrowhead: absence of semicircular canals). (Courtesy of Dr. Caroline Robson, Children's Hospital, Boston, and Harvard Medical School.)

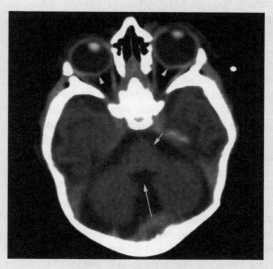

Figure 12.3 Brain CT scan illustrating pontine hypoplasia (short arrow) communication of the fourth ventricle with the retrocerebellar cerebrospinal fluid space due to inferior vermian hypoplasia (long arrow), in addition to small ocular colobomata (arrowheads). (Courtesy of Dr. Caroline Robson, Children's Hospital, Boston, and Harvard Medical School.)

The additional findings of choanal atresia and colobomata fit well with a rare condition called CHARGE syndrome (MIM 214800). This condition, first described in 1979, was initially called an association and is known by its acronym that stood for the physical abnormalities seen in the condition: *c*oloboma of the eye, *h*eart defects, choanal *a*tresia, *r*etarded growth and development, *g*enital hypoplasia, and *e*ar anomalies and deafness. CHARGE syndrome has an estimated prevalence of approximately 1 per 10 000–15 000 births (Figure 12.4).

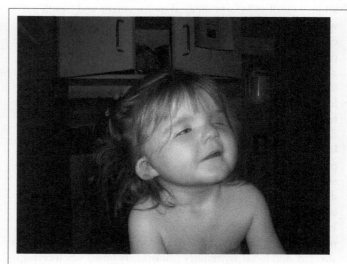

Figure 12.4 Picture of child with CHARGE syndrome that illustrates some of the craniofacial features of the condition, including a rectangular forehead, abnormally formed ears, and left microophthalmia. (Courtesy of Dr. Laurie Demmer, Tufts Medical School, Boston.)

Part IV

👤 Lisa is now almost 48 hours old. The geneticist meets with Jane and Albert and explains that Lisa has the clinical findings of CHARGE syndrome. It is explained that this disorder is characterized by a variable pattern of clinical and developmental problems, though not all of the associated problems are seen in every affected individual. They are told that many infants with CHARGE syndrome have respiratory and feeding problems in the newborn period, as Lisa has. She may require a feeding tube to supplement her feedings, and she may be smaller than other children her age. Recurrent infections, especially upper respiratory, are common. Since Lisa has colobomata of the optic nerves, they are told that she will likely have some visual problems, in addition to some degree of hearing loss due to the inner ear abnormalities noted on her CT scan. A family history is obtained, revealing no prior history of similar problems. This is Jane and Albert's first child. Jane had one previous miscarriage at 8 weeks of gestation. Jane and Albert are not related to one another. The geneticist tells Jane and Albert that the syndrome is usually sporadic, although recurrence in families has been reported in rare instances.

Knowing the medical and developmental problems that can be associated with the condition can help guide diagnostic evaluation, as well as inform medical management and health surveillance as this child grows older. The other abnormalities that can be seen in CHARGE syndrome include cleft lip and/or palate, esophageal atresia, limb anomalies, and vertebral anomalies resulting in scoliosis and kyphosis. Genital hypoplasia, including micropenis or cryptorchidism in boys and labial hypoplasia in girls, can be seen at birth. Hypothalamic dysfunction may also be present and result in abnormal pubertal development. Renal anomalies can cause vesicoureteral reflux, hydronephrosis, or recurrent urinary tract infections. The prognosis for central nervous system (CNS) function has been more difficult to predict. A small number of infants with this disorder have CNS malformations, including agenesis of the corpus callosum, cerebellar hypoplasia, or holoprosencephaly. Hypoplastic olfactory bulbs causing anosmia are seen in the majority of affected individuals. All cranial nerves can be affected, and facial asymmetry (more easily noted when crying) can be seen in up to 50% due to facial nerve palsy. Brainstem dysfunction leading to feeding and/or respiratory problems and abnormalities in thermal regulation have been reported. Intellectual disability is variable and can range from severe cognitive impairment to normal intelligence.

Part V

👤 Lisa continues to do well in the neonatal intensive care unit and is now breathing on her own and taking more of her feedings by mouth. The geneticist returns to talk to Jane and Albert about sending genetic testing to confirm the diagnosis of CHARGE syndrome in Lisa. The geneticist tells them that the gene responsible for CHARGE syndrome has recently been discovered, and confirmation of the diagnosis can be made in approximately 60–70% of affected individuals. Blood is drawn from Lisa and sent to a laboratory for testing.

The gene associated with CHARGE syndrome, *CHD7*, was first identified in 2004 using a microarray-based comparative genomic hybridization approach that identified a *de novo* microdeletion of 4.8 Mb on chromosome band 8q12.2. A previous patient with CHARGE syndrome had been found to have an apparently balanced translocation between chromosomes 6 and 8, which had originally drawn attention to these chromosomal regions. Further analysis of the genes within the deleted segment led researchers to the *CHD7* gene, which consists of 38 exons and codes for a protein made up of 2235 amino acids. Mutations of the *CHD7* gene in patients with CHARGE syndrome are spread across the coding regions and splice sites of the gene, and most are predicted to result in premature termination of translation of the protein, likely leading to haploinsufficiency. It is estimated that approximately 60–70% of individuals who meet diagnostic criteria for CHARGE syndrome have detectable mutations of the *CHD7* gene. Complete gene deletions, detectable by chromosome microarray analysis or MLPA, can be seen in additional patients.

CHARGE syndrome is an autosomal dominant condition that is usually sporadic, since most affected individuals represent new mutations. Recurrence risk is estimated at 2%, as both germline and somatic mosaicism have been identified in parents of affected children. Preimplantation genetic testing or prenatal diagnosis by means of chorionic villus sampling or amniocentesis is available for families with confirmed mutations of *CHD7*.

CHD7 encodes a chromodomain helicase DNA-binding protein and is part of the CHD family of proteins involved in chromatin remodeling and gene expression during early development. Analysis of *CHD7* expression patterns during early human development correlate well with the tissues affected in CHARGE syndrome (i.e., CNS, inner ear, and neural crest derivatives). It is believed that *CHD7* plays a critical role in chromatin remodeling, and its normal function is necessary for epigenetic control of target gene expression in mesenchymal cells derived from the cephalic neural crest.

Part VI

👤 Jane and Albert continue to visit Lisa in the neonatal intensive care unit, meet with all of the specialists involved in her care, and learn more about CHARGE syndrome. The geneticist tells them that a mutation of the CHD7 gene was identified in Lisa, confirming that she has CHARGE syndrome on a molecular basis. Although Jane and Albert have no signs of this condition, they are also tested to see if either of them carries the CHD7 mutation. Both have normal testing. Although it appears that Lisa has CHARGE syndrome on a de novo, or sporadic, basis, they are told that they have an approximately 2% risk of having another child with the same mutation in a future pregnancy, as germline mosaicism has been reported in this condition. Since Lisa's mutation has been identified, preimplantation genetic testing is available to them, as well as prenatal testing during the pregnancy. Prenatal testing could determine if a future fetus has inherited the CDH7 mutation, predicting how the child would be affected would not be possible due to the clinical variability associated with this condition. Lisa continues to do well, has her corrective heart surgery, and recovers well postoperatively. After one month, Jane and Albert take Lisa home.

This case illustrates a number of issues commonly encountered in genetic counseling. First, the problems are complex and usually are well outside the knowledge of lay individuals. The parents have never heard of the syndrome and may have little or no understanding of the principles of inheritance, let alone molecular genetics. Counseling is complicated further by the emotional trauma of having a sick child, for whom life-and-death decisions need to be made at the present time, in addition to new concerns regarding whether the couple is at increased risk of having another child with the same condition. This is especially important in conditions such as CHARGE syndrome, where very mild clinical manifestations, such as asymmetry of the ears (believed to be a variation of normal or a retinal coloboma noted only upon further examination), have been reported to be present in a parent found to have the same mutation as his or her child, giving the couple a 50% risk of having another affected child. It is often helpful to introduce a family to others who have firsthand experience with a genetic syndrome. Although specific manifestations and severity can differ from individual to individual, such contact provides at least a glimpse of what life may be like for a person with the disorder in question.

Inborn Errors of Development

Approximately 3% of all pregnancies end with the birth of a child with a birth defect. Usually, these are isolated defects, such as cleft lip or a neural tube defect; the child is otherwise healthy, although he or she may suffer serious consequences from the presence of the malformation. Many of these malformations occur sporadically and are believed to have a multifactorial etiology. Others are determined by single genes or chromosomal abnormalities. Aside from isolated malformations, some babies are born with a complex of multiple congenital anomalies.

Until recently, the molecular basis of syndromes of abnormal development was largely unknown. This vastly limited the tools available for diagnosis. The identification of genes involved in both normal and abnormal development is rapidly changing this picture. Normal development involves processes of cell replication, migration, and differentiation, tightly controlled in a spatial pattern and temporal sequence. Major developmental events are initiated through cell–cell signaling, with binding of a receptor leading to transduction of a signal to the cell nucleus to initiate a program of transcription of specific genes.

Some of the first genes involved in development to be discovered were initially studied in the fruit fly, *Drosophila*. Over the years, a curious set of *Drosophila* mutants had been identified. *Drosophila* species have the typical arthropod body plan of three segments – head, thorax, and abdomen. Rare mutants, referred to as homeotic mutants (the result of **homeotic genes**), have distinctive and often bizarre disruptions of body segmentation. The mutant Antennapedia, for example, has legs protruding from the head where antennae should be. Other mutants are characterized by segmentation defects (e.g., conversion of a legless abdominal segment into a thoracic segment with legs).

Many of the genes responsible for these phenotypes have been cloned. It has been found that they share a region of homology that has come to be called the **homeobox (Hox)**, which consists of approximately 60 amino acids (corresponding with 180 base pairs of DNA) that have DNA-binding properties. Other genes involved in the regulation of development share a different DNA-binding domain called the **paired box (Pax)**. The Pax box consists of 128 amino acids. In *Drosophila*, there are five Pax genes, most of which appear to be involved in body segmentation.

There are several groups of Hox genes in *Drosophila* that share sequence homology. One group, referred to as the homeotic complex (HOM-C), consists of eight genes. These genes are expressed in an anterior–posterior pattern in the *Drosophila* embryo, in a spatial order that is the same as their arrangement on the chromosome (Figure 12.5). The gene at the 3′ end of the complex is expressed in the head region, and loss of function of this gene causes disruption of development of head structures. Genes located in a 5′ direction are expressed in progressively more posterior segments. Areas of expression tend

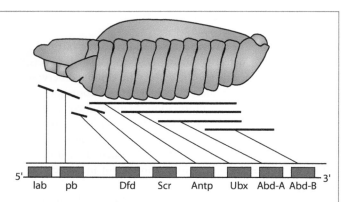

Figure 12.5 Domains of expression of genes of the HOM-C complex in *Drosophila*, with map of region shown at bottom. (Redrawn by permission from McGinnis and Krumlauf 1992.)

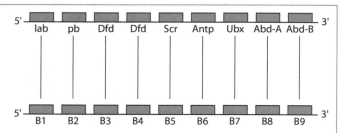

Figure 12.6 Genes of HOM-C complex in *Drosophila* (top), and homologous genes of Hox-2 cluster in mouse (bottom).

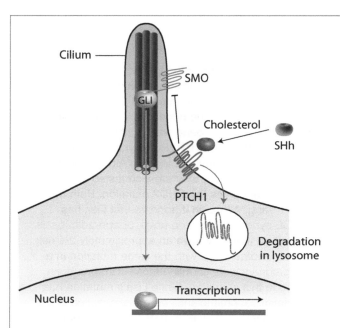

Figure 12.7 Diagram of sonic hedgehog signaling. The membrane receptor PTCH1 (Patched-1) inhibits SMO (smoothened), which is localized in the cilia. A sonic hedgehog ligand is activated by cholesterol and binds to PTCH1, which results in degradation of PTCH1 in the lysosome. This releases the inhibition of SMO, which then stimulates translocation of GLI to the nucleus, where it serves as a transcription factor for genes involved in cellular differentiation.

to overlap, however. The overlapping expression explains the transformation of one body segment into another in a homeotic mutant: When one Hox gene is not expressed in a segment, persistent expression of another leads to transformation of the segment. Pax genes also are expressed in specific segments in the *Drosophila* embryo. Both Hox and Pax proteins bind to DNA and activate the transcription of other genes. They are believed to act as switches that invoke tissue-specific developmental programs.

The discovery of Hox and Pax boxes prompted a search for homologous genes in higher eukaryotes, including humans. Using DNA probes for Hox or Pax boxes, regions of homology were indeed found. Moreover, mammalian Hox genes, like their *Drosophila* counterparts, are arranged in tandem arrays and are expressed in an anterior–posterior direction that mirrors their order on the chromosome (Figure 12.6). There are nine Pax genes in the human genome, seven of which also include Hox box sequences.

There are no known natural Hox mutants in the mouse, but study of Hox function has been accomplished by targeted disruption of these genes. A vector containing a mutant Hox gene has been introduced into mouse embryonic stem cells. The disrupted segment recombined with the wild-type gene and introduced the mutation into the mouse gene. The embryonic stem cells then were injected into mouse blastocysts, which in turn were implanted into a pseudopregnant uterus and brought to term. Breeding of these chimeric mice resulted in fully heterozygous animals. Mice with Hox mutations tend to have congenital anomalies in the body region where the mutant gene is expressed, indicating that the mammalian Hox genes, like their *Drosophila* counterparts, function to regulate the proper morphogenesis of different anterior–posterior regions of the embryo.

In contrast to Hox, three natural mouse Pax mutations have been identified. One is called undulated, the phenotype of which is skeletal deformities. It is due to a single base change in the Pax1 gene. The second mouse mutant is splotch, associated with Pax3 mutations. Splotch has arisen naturally several times, and different splotch alleles have been characterized. The third mouse mutant is referred to as smalleye, due to Pax6 mutations. The human homolog of this gene is responsible for the dominant-condition Waadenburg syndrome, which consists of deafness, widely spaced eyes, and a patch of white hair above the forehead.

Identification of the genes involved in development has revealed some unexpected connections between seemingly disparate conditions and has also challenged longstanding diagnostic classification schemes. For example, consider the gene *sonic hedgehog*. The pathway of *sonic hedgehog* action is shown in Figure 12.7. *Sonic hedgehog* mutations occur in some familial or sporadic cases of holoprosencephaly (MIM 142945), a major malformation of the CNS in which cleavage of the forebrain into two hemispheres fails partially or completely. Mutations in "patched," the sonic hedgehog receptor, are responsible for basal cell nevus syndrome (MIM 109400). This is an autosomal dominant disorder characterized by large head size, skeletal anomalies, and a predisposition to tumors, including benign basal cell nevi, basal cell carcinomas, and medulloblastomas. The developmental anomalies appear to be due to reduced gene dosage of patched (haploinsufficiency), whereas the tumors display loss of heterozygosity for patched, a classic tumor suppressor mechanism. Some sporadic basal cell carcinomas have been found to have smoothened mutations. Finally, the autosomal recessive Smith–Lemli–Optiz syndrome (MIM 270400) (cerebral dysgenesis, sometimes including holoprosencephaly, growth retardation, hypogenitalism, and limb anomalies) is due to a block in cholesterol metabolism. Cerebral anomalies in this disorder, and in fetuses exposed to drugs that inhibit cholesterol synthesis, may be due to aberrant *sonic hedgehog* signaling.

REFERENCES

McGinnis W, Krumlauf R 1992, "Homeobox genes and axial patterning", *Cell*, vol. 68, pp. 283–302.

Quan L, Smith DW 1973, "The VATER association – vertebral defects, anal atresia, t-e fistula with esophageal atresia, radial and renal dysplasia: a spectrum of associated defects", *Journal of Pediatrics*, vol. 82, p. 104.

FURTHER READING

Delahaye A, Sznajer Y, Lyonnet S, Elmaleh-Berges M, Delpierre I, Audollent S, Wiener-Vacher S, Mansbach AL, Amiel J, Baumann C, Bremond-Gignac D, Attie-Bitach T, Verloes A, Sanlaville D 2007, "Familial CHARGE syndrome because of CHD7 mutation: clinical intra- and interfamilial variability", *Clinical Genetics*, vol. 72, pp. 112–21.

Hunter AG 2002, "Medical genetics 2: the diagnostic approach to the child with dysmorphic signs", *Canadian Medicine Association Journal*, vol. 167, pp. 367–72.

Jongmans MCJ, Admiraal RJ, vander Donk KP, Vissers LELM, Baas AF, Kapusta L, van Hagen JM, Donnai D, de Ravel TJ, Veltman JA, Geurts van Kessel A, De Vries BBA, Brunner HG, Hoefsloot LH, van Ravenswaaij CMA 2006, "CHARGE syndrome; the phenotypic spectrum of mutations in the CHD7 gene", *Journal of Medical Genetics*, vol. 43, pp. 306–14.

Sanlaville D, Etchevers HC, Gonzales M, Martinovic J, Clement-Ziza M, Delezoide AL, Aubry MC, Pelet A, Chemouny S, Cruaud C, *et al.* 2006, "Phenotypic spectrum of CHARGE syndrome in fetuses with CHD7 truncating mutations correlates with expression during human development", *Journal of Medical Genetics*, vol. 43, pp. 211–17.

Veltman JA, Van Ravenswaaij-Arts CMA 2008, "CHD7 and the CHARGE syndrome", in CJ Epstein, RP Erickson, A Wynshaw-Boris (eds.), *Inborn errors of development*, Oxford University Press, London, pp. 995–1002.

Vissers LE, van Ravenswaaij CM, Admiraal R, Hurst JA, de Vries BB, Janssen IM, van der Vliet WA, Huys EH, de Jong PJ, Hamel BC, *et al.* 2004, "Mutations in a new member of the chromodomain gene family cause CHARGE syndrome", *Nature Genetics*, vol. 36, pp. 955–7.

Find interactive self-test questions and additional resources for this chapter at **www.korfgenetics.com**.

Self-Assessment

Review Questions

12.1 What is the difference between a disruption and a deformation? Would either one be the consequence of teratogen exposure *in utero*?

12.2 How did identification of the chromosome 22q11.2 deletion in the chromosome 22q11.2 deletion syndrome lead to new knowledge regarding the importance of the Tbx1 gene in cardiac development?

12.3 Molecular testing of the CHD7 gene will be abnormal and confirm the underlying molecular abnormality in approximately 60–70% of individuals with CHARGE syndrome. Does this eliminate the diagnosis of CHARGE syndrome in the other 30% of individuals with clinical findings consistent with this diagnosis?

12.4 A high proportion of dominantly inherited congenital anomaly syndromes are due to new mutations. Why is this the case?

12.5 What is the relationship between the orientation of Hox genes on the chromosome and their patterns of expression?

CHAPTER 13
Carrier Screening

Introduction

We have seen in Chapter 7 on population genetics that some genetic disorders occur at increased frequency in specific populations. The basis for this may reside in phenomena such as the founder effect or balanced polymorphism. The clinical importance is that ancestry may be a clue to the risk that an individual is a **carrier** for a recessive genetic disorder and that some couples may be at risk of having an affected child. There may not be a known family history of the disorder, so many couples learn of their risk only after the birth of an affected child. The principle of carrier screening is to identify such couples so that they can be counseled about their risk and the options available to deal with the risk. In this chapter, we will further explore the principles of carrier screening. We will look at how screening now is beginning to be performed on a wide scale, and how this compares with ancestry-based screening. We will also look at general principles of carrier-screening programs, and see some of the challenges faced in implementation.

Key Points

- Carrier screening involves testing of individuals for heterozygosity for genes that would produce significant disorders in the homozygous state. Couples found to be at risk if both partners are carriers can be offered counseling regarding their options to deal with the risk.
- An individual may be at increased risk of being a carrier for a particular genetic trait on the basis of ancestry. Many screening programs are targeted toward particular groups known to be at risk.
- Couples found to be at risk have many options, including prenatal diagnosis, adoption, use of an egg or sperm donor, or planning for the medical needs of an affected child.
- The decision to implement a carrier-screening program requires careful assessment of risks and benefits and provision of counseling, testing, and management resources. Carrier test results require careful interpretation and counseling of the couple.
- Genomic approaches are beginning to be applied to carrier screening, making it possible to significantly expand the scope of conditions for which screening is provided.

Part I

> 👤 Ruth and Ted were recently married and are now interested in starting a family. Both are of Ashkenazi Jewish ancestry and have known for a long time that genetic testing is recommended to determine their risk of having a child with a genetic disorder. Recently they read an article in a newsletter from their synagogue about testing for "Jewish genetic diseases." Ruth decides to discuss this with her gynecologist at her next visit, which is coming up soon.

The Ashkenazim are descended from Jews who settled in medieval times in the Rhine Valley of what is now Germany, and later expanded through migration into Eastern Europe. Although modern genetic analysis has shown admixture with non-Jewish Europeans, there are substantial blocks of preserved haplotypes shared among the Ashkenazim. This is indicative of a population bottleneck that is believed to have occurred in the 15th century, with subsequent major population expansion. This bottleneck has led to a founder effect in the Ashkenazi population that has in turn led to a number of recessive disorders that are seen at higher frequency in this group.

The first major carrier-screening program in the Ashkenazi population involved Tay–Sachs disease. We briefly discussed Tay–Sachs disease in Chapter 7. Prior to the onset of carrier screening, the frequency of Tay–Sachs disease in the Ashkenazim was approximately 1/3600. This equates to an allele frequency of 1/60 and a carrier frequency of 1/30. Tay–Sachs disease is divided into an acute infantile form, a juvenile form, and chronic and adult-onset forms. The acute infantile form begins in the first 3 months of life and progresses rapidly, with most children dying between 2 and 4 years of age. The juvenile form begins with neurological deterioration between 2 and 10 years of age and progresses during the early teen years, usually with death by about 15 years of age. In the chronic and adult-onset forms, neurological signs can be variable, and include motor dysfunction, muscle weakness and wasting, and, in some cases, cognitive deterioration and dementia. Tay–Sachs disease is a lysosomal storage disorder in which deficiency of the enzyme hexosaminidase A (HEXA) leads to accumulation of undigested GM_2 ganglioside in neurons. There is a correlation of degree of enzyme activity with the age of onset and rate of progression of the disease. The infantile form is associated with complete loss of enzyme activity, whereas the later onset forms tend to occur when enzyme activity is reduced to <15% but >5%.

Carrier testing was developed before the gene was discovered and is based on an assay of HEXA in plasma, or, in women who are pregnant or taking oral contraceptives, in peripheral blood leukocytes. There is clear differentiation of the enzyme activity in homozygous normal, heterozygous, and homozygous mutated individuals. The testing has high sensitivity and specificity and can also be done on cultured amniocytes, enabling prenatal diagnosis. The assay is typically done using an artificial substrate, and there are some alleles that lead to deficient ability to digest this substrate but normal activity on the natural substrate (and hence no disease). These "pseudodeficiency alleles" can be detected by DNA analysis, or by testing on a natural substrate in cultured cells.

Carrier screening in the Ashkenazi population was initiated in the early 1970s. The program has included public education, rigorous quality control of laboratory testing, and ready availability of genetic counseling. For ultraorthodox Jewish groups in which abortion is not acceptable but marriages are arranged, confidential screening has been used to avoid marriages between carriers. From 1971 through 1992, almost 1 million individuals had been tested and more than 36 000 carriers detected. Prenatal testing was done for more than 2400 pregnancies at risk. Prior to screening, approximately 60 new Tay–Sachs disease cases were identified around the world each year. Currently, the rate has fallen to 3–5 cases per year, comparable to the frequency in non-Jewish couples.

Since cloning of the gene for HEXA, more than 100 distinct mutations have been characterized. Testing of two mutations detects upward of 94% of Ashkenazi Jewish carriers. One is an insertion of the bases TATC into exon 11, which results in frameshift, found in 81% of carriers. The second is a mutation at the splice donor site of intron 12, which leads to abnormal splicing, found in 13% of carriers. Two percent of Jewish carriers have a glycine to serine change at codon 269, which leads to partial loss of enzyme activity. Because mutation analysis does not detect 100% of Ashkenazi Jewish carriers but enzyme analysis does, the biochemical test remains the "gold standard" for carrier detection.

The diversity of mutations in the Ashkenazi population is not what would be expected if only a founder effect accounted for the high frequency of the disorder in this group. It has been suggested, therefore, that there might also be a heterozygote advantage. Various hypotheses have been proposed, but none so far has been verified. Also population genetic studies have not revealed strong evidence for positive selection at the HEXA locus.

Part II

> 👤 The visit with the gynecologist, Dr. Sanger, goes well, with no problems seen that might interfere with starting a family. When Ruth asks about genetic testing, Dr. Sanger explains that this is easy to arrange. She could send a blood sample to a testing

laboratory that day, but recommends instead that both Ruth and Ted be seen together at a genetics clinic that has a program for providing testing for conditions seen in the Jewish population. She provides Ruth contact information for the clinic. That night, Ruth talks with Ted about the program, and the next day she calls for an appointment.

Tay–Sachs is one of several disorders for which carrier screening has been available since the 1970s. Another major example is screening for hemoglobinopathies. Hemoglobin, the oxygen-carrying molecule of the red blood cell (RBC), consists of two pairs of globin chains, each of which binds one heme molecule. The major form of hemoglobin in the adult, hemoglobin A, is a tetramer of two alpha-globin chains and two beta chains. There are other beta-like chains that can bind to the alpha chains and are expressed at different times in life. We discussed sickle cell anemia in Chapter 7, and have seen how relative resistance to malaria provided a selective advantage to heterozygous carriers of globin mutations, leading to their prevalence in parts of the world where malaria is endemic. Aside from sickle cell anemia, the other major hemoglobinopathy is thalassemia, defined as deficient production of either alpha or beta chains. Beta thalassemia is especially prevalent in the Mediterranean region, and is due to various mutations that impair beta-globin synthesis, including promoter mutations, stop mutations, frameshifts, and deletions. Alpha thalassemia usually occurs as a consequence of deletion of alpha-globin genes. Normally there are two duplicated alpha-globin genes in each copy of chromosome 16, so individuals usually have four gene copies. Loci exist with deletion of one or both genes from the chromosome. Deletion of all four genes is lethal *in utero*, resulting in hydrops fetalis, whereas deletion of two gene copies results in a clinically asymptomatic carrier state. Deletion of three of the four genes leads to clinical signs of alpha thalassemia. This phenotype, as well as hydrops fetalis, is most often seen in Southeast Asia, where the allele consisting of deletion of both gene copies is typically seen.

The high prevalence of thalassemia in some parts of the world has led to several organized population-screening programs, most notably on Sardinia and Cyprus (Figure 13.1). This has included public education and screening for carrier status, with prenatal diagnosis offered to carrier couples. The programs have vastly reduced the frequency of thalassemia in these populations, just as was the case for Tay-Sachs disease among the Askenazim. In other parts of the world, carrier screening has been offered on the basis of ancestry, with specific tests being offered to individuals with known descent from high-risk groups (Table 13.1).

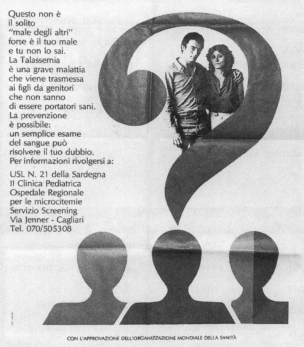

Figure 13.1 Poster publicizing the thalassemia-screening program in Sardinia. (Courtesy of Dr. Antonio Cao.)

Part III

Ruth and Ted meet with a genetic counselor, Deborah Stein, in the genetics clinic. Ruth and Ted had been told before the appointment that they should ask their parents about whether there is any family history of any genetic problem; they had been given a list of things to ask about. Deborah constructs a pedigree diagram for Ruth's and Ted's families, but does not turn up any specific conditions that would affect a pregnancy for Ruth and Ted. She then explains the rationale for genetic testing, and recommends that Ruth and Ted have testing for a set of 19 disorders. Blood is drawn from each of them, and a return appointment is arranged.

Both Tay–Sachs disease and hemoglobinopathies are amenable to screening using non-DNA-based tests – enzyme assay for Tay–Sachs and RBC studies and hemoglobin electrophoresis

Table 13.1 Major disorders subject to carrier screening in specific populations.

Population	Disorder	Test	Carrier frequency
Ashkenazi Jewish	Tay-Sachs disease	Enzyme/DNA	1/30
	Cystic fibrosis	DNA	1/29
	Familial dysautonomia	DNA	1/36
	Canavan disease	DNA	1/40
French Canadian	Tay-Sachs disease	DNA	1/70
Asian	Thalassemia	Hematologic	Population specific
Mediterranean	Thalassemia	Hematologic	Population specific
African	Sickle cell anemia	Hematologic	1/10
Northern European	Cystic fibrosis	DNA	1/25

Table 13.2 Comparison of testing outcomes using a 70% or 90% sensitive mutation screen.

| Outcome | 70% detection rate | | 90% detection rate | |
	Frequency	Risk of cystic fibrosis (CF) in offspring	Frequency	Risk of CF in offspring
N/N	0.9447	1/30 000	0.929	1/250 000
N/C	0.054	1/300	0.069	1/1000
C/C	0.00078	1/4	0.0013	1/4

N = normal result; and C = carrier result.

for hemoglobinopathies. This made it possible to offer screening before the advent of DNA testing. As the genes associated with various other autosomal recessive disorders were discovered, the ability to search for mutations at the molecular level opened new opportunities for carrier screening. In the Ashkenazi Jewish population, conditions such as Canavan disease and familial dysautonomia were gradually added to the list (see Table 13.1). Cystic fibrosis, which is described in Chapter 4, occurs with increased frequency in the Ashkenazi population, in addition to its high frequency in those of Northern European descent. After the *CFTR* gene was discovered, molecular-based carrier screening became a possibility.

The history of cystic fibrosis carrier screening illustrates both the potential power and challenges in launching a carrier-screening program. In 1997, a Consensus Development Conference held at the National Institutes of Health (NIH) recommended that cystic fibrosis testing be offered to individuals with a family history of the disorder and for all couples contemplating pregnancy or currently pregnant, but not to the general population. There was concern, however, that the medical community was not well prepared to offer testing and counseling on this large scale. A task force was set up to help establish the resources necessary to implement the NIH panel's

recommendations. After several years of discussion, in 2001 a joint committee of the American College of Medical Genetics and the American College of Obstetricians and Gynecologists issued joint recommendations that cystic fibrosis mutation screening be made available to all couples contemplating pregnancy. A standardized mutation panel was defined, consisting of the 25 mutations that occur at a frequency of at least 0.1% of all *CFTR* mutations in a US pan-ethnic panel. Explanatory brochures were created, along with informed consent documents.

The sensitivity of the screening test differs in different populations. No mutation screen detects 100% of possible *CFTR* mutations, and therefore lack of detection of a mutation does not guarantee that an individual is not a carrier. Even if both partners are not found to carry a cystic fibrosis mutation, they are still at risk of having a child affected with a mutation not included in the testing. The impact of this can be seen if one compares the outcomes of a test that detects 70% of mutations and one that detects 90% of mutations (Table 13.2). With either test, a finding that both partners are carriers leads to a one-in-four risk of cystic fibrosis in an offspring, and reliable prenatal testing is possible. Finding that neither partner is a carrier substantially reduces the risk of having an affected child, although that risk still is not zero. Couples need to be informed that this screening test does not detect all possible mutations and that some couples considered to be at very low risk may, rarely, still have an affected child. The most problematic scenario, however, is the middle one: One partner is found to be a carrier, and the other is not. This will be a common occurrence, happening in 5% or so of couples with a 70% sensitive screen and in more than 6% of couples with a 90% sensitive screen. In each case, the risk of having an affected child is increased over the population risk, as one partner is known to be a carrier and the other might still be a carrier for an undetected mutation. In such couples, mutation analysis will not identify cystic fibrosis in a fetus, as the second *CFTR* mutation is undetectable. Consequently, mutation screening has alerted the partners to their increased risk yet has offered nothing further in the way of prenatal diagnosis. The sensitivity of mutation screening, moreover, is highly variable among different ethnic groups. Only 30% of cystic fibrosis mutations in the Asian-American population are detected with most com-

monly used testing schemes, for example. In these populations the level of uncertainty provided by a negative test is even greater.

Aside from the complexities introduced by incomplete ascertainment of mutations, there are also counseling challenges due to genetic heterogeneity. It has become clear that not all *CFTR* mutations lead to the classical syndrome of cystic fibrosis. For example, some mutations lead to the pulmonary complications without the pancreatic insufficiency. An even milder phenotype associated with particular *CFTR* mutations has been identified in some males with infertility due to congenital bilateral absence of the vas deferens (CBAVD). Other syndromes associated with *CFTR* mutations include chronic pancreatitis or chronic sinusitis. The particular phenotype associated with a rare combination of two mutant alleles may be difficult to predict.

Further complication is introduced by the existence of a polymorphism within intron 8 of *CFTR*, in which individuals may have a run of 5, 7, or 9 thymidine bases (5T/7T/9T) (Figure 13.2). The 5T allele is associated with skipping of exon

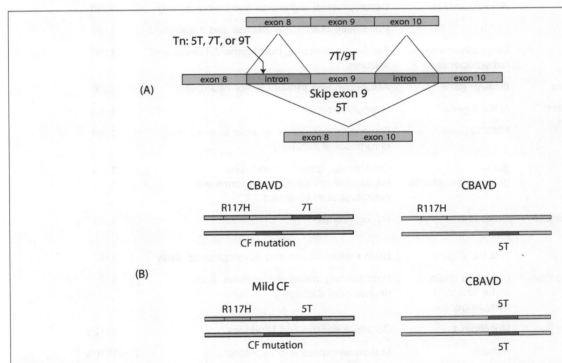

Figure 13.2 (A) Poly T polymorphism in intron 8 consists of three alleles, in which there can be 5T's, 7T's, or 9T's. The 9T allele is the most common and leads to normal splicing of the *CFTR* transcript. Normal splicing also occurs with the 7T allele, but exon 9 is skipped if the 5T allele is present. (B) Genotypes associated with CBAVD or mild cystic fibrosis (CF) associated with the poly T polymorphism and the R117H mutation. R117H acts as a mild CF mutation on the same chromosome with (also called "in cis with") a 7T allele, but has a greater phenotypic effect if in cis with a 5T allele. If there is a CF mutation on the opposite chromosome (also called "in trans with"), R117H in cis with 7T results in CBAVD but in cis with 5T results in mild CF. CBAVD may also occur with R117H in trans with a 5T allele, or with homozygosity for 5T. It is unknown whether the 5T chromosomes carry another, undetected CF mutation.

9 and reduced *CFTR* expression. The presence of the 5T allele may modify the expression of a mild *CFTR* allele on the same chromosome. Some males with CBAVD have been found to have a *CFTR* mutation on one chromosome and a 5T allele on the other; whether the chromosome with the 5T allele includes another undetected *CFTR* mutation is unknown. *CFTR* mutation status must therefore be interpreted in the context of other variants in the gene, at least in some cases, highlighting the importance of careful genetic counseling in reporting results to patients.

The founder effect in the Ashkenazi population has led to an increased frequency of many disorders aside from Tay–Sachs

disease. Since the advent of molecular genetic testing, the list of disorders offered for carrier screening has gradually been expanded. A current listing of 19 conditions for which screening is commonly offered is provided in Table 13.3. Some of these are much less common than Tay–Sachs disease, but the rationale for carrier testing is that specific mutations in the Ashkenazim can be detected reliably and the conditions have major medical effects in the homozygous state. Some, like Tay–Sachs or Canavan disease, are not treatable. Others, like cystic fibrosis or Gaucher disease, are amenable to some forms of treatment, though their medical burden may nonetheless be significant.

Table 13.3 Nineteen conditions included in the current Ashkenazi Jewish carrier-screening panel.

Condition	Enzyme or gene	Features	Ashkenazi carrier frequency
Bloom syndrome	Helicase	Sun-sensitive rash, growth deficiency, and risk of cancer	1:100
Canavan disease	Aspartoacylase	Developmental regression and macrocephaly	1:40
Cystic fibrosis	CFTR	Pulmonary obstructive disease and malabsorption	1:25
DLD deficiency	Dihydrolipamide dehydrogenease	Feeding intolerance, developmental delay, and seizures	1:96
Familial dysautonomia	IKBKAP gene	Autonomic and sensory motor neuropathy	1:30
Familial hyperinsulinism	ABCC8 gene	Hypoglycemia	1:66
Fanconi anemia C	FANCC gene	Congenital anomalies, aplastic anemia, and chromosome instability	1:89
Gaucher disease	Beta-glucosylceramidase	Osteopenia, bone fractures, and hepatosplenomegaly; some forms with neurological involvement	1:14
Glycogen storage disease 1a	Glucose-6-phosphatase	Hypoglycemia	1:41
Joubert syndrome	TMEM216 gene	Brain malformations and developmental delay	1:92
Maple syrup urine disease	Branched chain alpha keto acid dehydrogenase	Poor feeding, metabolic acidosis, and neurological damage	1:81
Mucolipidosis IV	Mucolipin-1	Cognitive decline and blindness	1:125
Nemaline myopathy	Nebulin	Muscle weakness and hypotonia	1:108
Niemann Pick A	Sphingomyelinase	Hepatosplenomegaly and developmental decline	1:90
Spinal muscular atrophy	SMN1 gene	Hypotonia and profound weakness	1:41
Tay Sachs disease	Hexosaminidase A	Developmental decline, seizures, and blindness	1:30
Usher syndrome IF	PDCH15 gene	Deafness and blindness	1:141
Usher syndrome III	CLRN1 gene	Deafness and blindness	1:107
Walker Warburg syndrome	Fukutin gene	Muscle, eye, and brain dysfunction	1:149

Part IV

🔒 Ted and Ruth return to the clinic, and are not particularly anxious about the results. They had been warned that they might well turn out to be positive for something, even perhaps more than one thing, but hopefully they would not both be positive for the same condition. Deborah provides each with a printout of their results, and proceeds to explain the findings. Indeed, both are positive, and unfortunately, one of the tests, for Tay–Sachs disease, is positive in both Ruth and Ted. Ruth was found to have the insertion mutation and Ted the splicing mutation, which would lead to infantile-onset Tay–Sachs disease in a homozygote. They are somewhat surprised, as no one in either family had ever been diagnosed with the disorder. Deborah reminds them that Tay–Sachs is a recessive disorder, so although there are undoubtedly other carriers in both of their families, there had not been an instance in either family of two partners who were carriers and had an affected child. She explains Tay–Sachs disease in detail, and the options available to the couple to deal with the 25% risk of having an affected child. Ruth and Ted are taking all this in, though they are a bit overwhelmed. They are then surprised to hear that they have not heard everything. Ted is also a carrier for Gaucher disease. This does not convey risk to a future pregnancy, since Ruth is not a carrier, but it could possibly have implications for Ted's own future health.

Carriers for hexosaminidase A mutations are clinically asymptomatic, so it is not surprising that Ted and Ruth have no clinical signs to predict their being carriers. Similarly, it is not rare for an individual to be a carrier for more than one disorder. Gaucher disease is due to deficiency of the enzyme beta-glucosylceramidase, responsible for conversion of glucosylceramide to glucose and ceramide (Figure 13.3). Like Tay–Sachs disease, Gaucher disease is divided into clinical subtypes based on residual enzyme activity. Type 1 presents with bone disease (osteopenia and sclerotic lesions that lead to pain and fracture), hepatosplenomegaly, anemia, thrombocytopenia, and leukopenia. There can be coagulation disorders and lung disease as well. Type 1 does not affect the central nervous system, but types 2 and 3 have prominent neurological features, including motor dysfunction, cognitive impairment, and seizures. Type 2 has onset before 2 years of age and rapidly leads to death in early childhood; type 3 has later onset and slower progression. Four mutations account for about 90% of carriers in the Ashkenazi population. One of these, designated N370S (substitution of serine for asparagine at codon 409), is the most common, and leads to type 1 disease regardless of the other mutant allele. The clinical presentation otherwise depends on the specific combination of alleles and, in turn, the residual enzyme activity.

Type 1 Gaucher disease is now a treatable disorder, thanks to enzyme replacement therapy. This is based on intravenous infusion of purified enzyme generated in a cell culture system using a recombinant DNA–based approach. The enzyme is chemically modified so that it has exposed mannose-6-phosphate residues that bind to cell membrane receptors and lead to endocytosis into phagocytic vacuoles. These fuse with lysosomes, delivering the enzyme to this compartment. Treatment

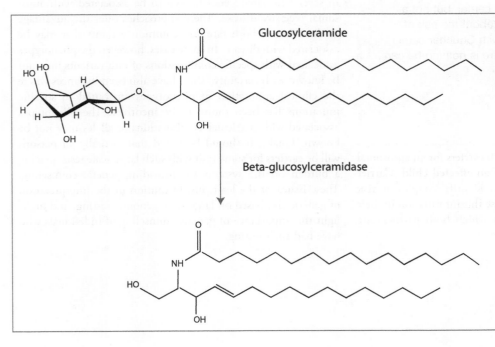

Figure 13.3 Beta-glucosylceramidase catalyzes the removal of glucose from glucosylceramide. Deficiency of this enzyme leads to Gaucher disease.

is highly successful at preventing or reversing the various pathophysiological processes, including bone disease, hepatosplenomegaly, and hematological disorders. Other therapeutic approaches are also available or in development, such as substrate reduction or chaperone therapies. Chaperones are chemicals that help to avoid misfolded proteins from being degraded, and instead help guide them to be processed in the endoplasmic reticulum and through the Golgi apparatus.

Features of Parkinson disease have been observed in individuals with type 1 Gaucher disease and in carriers. Parkinson disease is characterized by a movement disorder, including tremor and stiff, slow movements (bradykinesia), and sometimes by dementia. Although there are rare single-gene inherited causes, Parkinson disease most often occurs sporadically as a multifactorial trait. Studies have shown an increased odds ratio of Parkinson disease among affected patients and, to a lesser extent, among carriers. This may shed light on the underlying mechanisms of Parkinson disease, and suggests that carriers are at increased risk, but currently there is no preventative strategy to reduce this risk.

Part V

> 👥 Ruth is now 18 weeks pregnant. The pregnancy has gone well, and an amniocentesis was done at 16 weeks. She is back at the obstetrician's office, and she and Ted meet with another genetic counselor, who reports that the fetus is not affected with Tay–Sachs disease, though she is a carrier. Ruth and Ted are greatly relieved. They had told their parents and immediate family about the carrier test, and Ruth's sister had been tested and also was positive. Ted's brother is also a Gaucher carrier, but not a Tay–Sachs carrier. He has read about the risk of Parkinson disease associated with Gaucher carrier status, but has decided that there is nothing he can do about that.

Carrier Screening

Most couples learn that they are both carriers for an autosomal recessive disorder after the birth of an affected child. Carrier screening offers an opportunity to identify couples at risk before this time, allowing them to use this information in their planning. Options for a couple in which both partners are carriers include the following:

- Choosing not to have children
- Artificial insemination or egg donation
- Prenatal diagnosis and termination of an affected pregnancy
- Prenatal diagnosis and planning for care of an affected child
- No prenatal testing

Carrier-screening programs have been in existence for more than 40 years, and historically have focused on detection of carriers for disorders known to be found at increased frequency based on ancestry. We have seen the power of this approach in the Ashkenazi Jewish population, as well as in individuals at increased risk of carrying globin gene mutations. The advent of DNA-based testing, and more recently the ability to perform high-throughput analysis of large numbers of mutations, is rapidly changing the approach to carrier screening. There is an increasing trend toward universal screening panels that are not focused on detection of limited numbers of mutations in specific ancestry-based groups. In part, this reflects the fact that the incremental costs of screening for large numbers of mutations in any individual are very low. The practice also reflects the fact that not all individuals are aware of their complete ancestry. Finally, the low cost of simultaneously screening large panels of mutations makes it possible to include disorders that are rare, on the assumption that the few couples who are at risk would prefer to know about this risk prior to the birth of an affected child.

Large pan-ethnic carrier test panels can be done using multiplex SNP detection systems such as microarrays. Tests of this kind have begun to be offered commercially, in some cases with marketing direct to consumers. One study has explored the possibility of using next-generation sequencing as an approach to carrier detection, using an exon-capture approach applied to several hundred genes known to be associated with autosomal recessive disease. These approaches offer the advantage of detection of both rare and common variants that may be associated with disease. In some cases, however, the phenotypes associated with specific combinations of rare variants may not be known with certainty. There have also been instances where the clinical annotation of phenotypes attributed to specific mutations has been found to be incorrect. The phenotypes associated with particular combinations of alleles may not be known. Finally, it should be noted that virtually all persons will be carriers for some trait with such large-scale tests, placing a burden on the systems for providing genetic counseling. These issues, at the least, justify caution in the interpretation of genetic risk based on large-scale genomic testing, and highlight the importance of genetic counseling of individuals who have had such testing.

FURTHER READING

Atzmon G, Hao L, Pe'er I, *et al.* 2010, "Abraham's children in the genome era: major Jewish diaspora populations comprise distinct genetic clusters with shared Middle Eastern ancestry", *American Journal of Human Genetics*, vol. 86, pp. 850–9.

Bray SM, Mulle JG, Dodd AF, *et al.* 2010, "Signatures of founder effects, admixture, and selection in the Ashkenazi Jewish population", *Proceedings of the National Academy of Sciences of the USA*, vol. 107 (16), pp. 222–16, 227.

Cao, A 2002, "Carrier screening and genetic counseling in beta-thalassemia", *International Journal of Hematology*, vol. 76 (Suppl. 2), pp. 105–13.

Goker-Alpan O, Schiffmann R, LaMarca ME, *et al.* 2004, "Parkinsonisn among Gaucher disease carriers", *Journal of Medical Genetics*, vol. 41, pp. 937–40.

Scott SA, Edelmann L, Liu L, *et al.* 2010, "Experience with carrier screening and prenatal diagnosis for sixteen Ashkenazi Jewish genetic diseases", *Human Mutations*, vol. 31, pp. 1240–50.

Watson MS, Cutting GR, Desnick RJ, *et al.* 2004, "Cystic fibrosis population carrier screening: 2004 revision of American College of Medical Genetics mutation panel", *Genetics in Medicine*, vol. 6, pp. 387–91.

 Find interactive self-test questions and additional resources for this chapter at **www.korfgenetics.com**.

Review Questions

13.1   A couple request screening for globin disorders. One partner is of African descent, and one of Mediterranean descent. Are they at increased risk of having a child with a globin disorder?

13.2   Why are some carrier screens done by using biochemical testing (e.g., Tay-Sachs disease), and others by DNA testing?

13.3   Why is it important to consider ancestry in interpretation of a carrier screen for a disorder with allelic heterogeneity such as cystic fibrosis?

13.4   One of the pitfalls in carrier screening by testing for specific DNA mutations is that a negative test does not exclude carrier status, since an individual may still carry a mutation that was not included in the screening panel. Aside from cost, why is complete sequencing of a gene not an ideal solution to this problem?

13.5   Is there any point in offering carrier screening to couples who would not terminate an affected pregnancy?

CHAPTER 14
Genetic Risk Assessment

Introduction

One of the major promises of the Human Genome Project is the prospect of understanding the genetic basis of common disorders. This offers the possibility of genetic testing to identify individuals at risk with the hope of providing approaches to reducing that risk or providing treatments to improve outcome. There are many challenges faced in implementation of this approach, however. Common disorders result from a complex interaction of multiple genetic and nongenetic factors. Genetic testing may in some cases suggest an increased risk, but is not predictive of the actual risk of disease. There can also be ethical, legal, and social pitfalls, including concerns about stigmatization or discrimination resulting from a positive test in a healthy individual. We will consider these issues in this chapter, focusing on a relatively new development – the advent of direct-to-consumer genomic tests. We will explore the basis for this testing and the clinical utility of test results. We will also look at the ethical and regulatory issues raised by this approach, and consider what this may be telling us about the future of genetic testing in the management of common disorders.

Key Points

- Genome-wide association studies have revealed single-nucleotide polymorphisms (SNPs) in which specific alleles are associated with risk of various common disorders.
- Genotyping of individuals for specific SNPs can be used to estimate risk of disease, though the tests are not diagnostic.
- Direct-to-consumer genome-wide genetic tests are available and provide information on risk of disease, carrier status for some recessive disorders, some pharmacogenetic traits, and information about some other common nonmedical phenotypes.
- Genetic tests for disease risk should be evaluated in terms of analytical validity, clinical validity, and clinical utility, as is the case for other genetic tests.
- A distinction can be made between predictive tests, which identify whether an individual has inherited a gene mutation that may eventually lead to a genetic disorder, and predispositional tests, in which an individual may be found to be at increased or decreased risk of a multifactorial disorder.

Human Genetics and Genomics, Fourth Edition. Bruce R. Korf and Mira B. Irons.
© 2013 John Wiley & Sons, Ltd. Published 2013 by John Wiley & Sons, Ltd.

Part I

👤 Neal has just returned from a dinner party with a group of close friends, and he is intrigued by one part of the conversation. One of his friends was talking about having recently sent his spit for genetic testing, and has received an extensive report about what he described as his "genetic profile." He learned about his risk of heart disease and diabetes, and said that he has begun a diet to lose weight inspired in part by the results of the testing. Neal is surprised to learn that this wasn't arranged by his friend's physician – anyone could do it just by logging into a site on the Internet. The next morning Neal does a search and finds the site to which his friend had referred. After exploring the website and reading some background material, he decides to go ahead, pleasantly surprised that the cost is just a few hundred dollars. He creates a user name and password, types in his credit card information, and hits "Enter."

Most common medical conditions, for example coronary artery disease, diabetes, and hypertension, are multifactorial in etiology. We explored the theory of multifactorial inheritance in Chapter 5, and introduced the idea of the case-control study for identification of single-nucleotide polymorphisms associated with multifactorial conditions. The goal of this work is in part to identify genetic factors that can be used to predict risk of disease, but also it is intended to reveal genes that contribute to disease in the hope of elucidating pathogenetic mechanisms.

The concept of direct-to-consumer marketing of genetic testing has generated some controversy. The tests are not marketed as medical tests, and come with disclaimers that results are not intended to be used for medical decision making. It is, of course, impossible for the companies that offer the tests to control how individuals will use the results. The tests are conducted in laboratories that are certified as clinical laboratories. In the United States, this means they are certified under the Clinical Laboratories Improvement Amendments (CLIA), which address general laboratory practice but do not specifically address issues in genetic testing.

Those who support the direct-to-consumer model argue that the genetic information belongs to the individual, and therefore the medical profession does not have a right or obligation to stand in the way of individual access to personal genetic information. Some argue that the educational information provided by the companies is as good as or better than what most medical practitioners would be able to explain to patients. Some of the companies offer access to genetic counseling as part of the cost of testing, whereas others do not, though they

may recommend that an individual seek genetic counseling to better understand the results of testing.

Those who are opposed to the direct-to-consumer model argue that, regardless of company disclaimers, some people will use the results to make medical decisions without the benefit of professional medical advice. They argue that most of the tests have not been validated to demonstrate either clinical validity or clinical utility, and that consumers will not understand the limitations of the tests or the significance of the results. There is some concern that individuals will embark on unproven or unwise lifestyle changes or medical regimens, ignore commonsense advice such as maintaining an ideal weight, or embark on expensive follow-up tests that increase the costs of medical care.

Both the risks and benefits of direct-to-consumer genetic testing currently remain the subject of debate. Governmental regulation of testing is also under consideration. Tests vary widely in terms of the quality of information provided and claims of utility. Some, for example, purport to predict longevity, athletic ability, or the nutritional value of specific foods. At least for now, there are a wide variety of tests available on a direct-to-consumer basis, with little consumer guidance to assist in deciding of whether or where to obtain testing.

Part II

👤 A few days later, Neal receives a package in the mail from the testing company. It contains a plastic "test tube" labeled with a bar code, a funnel-like cap, a plastic bag, and a mailer. He reads the instructions – actually reads them a few times – and then begins the process. First he logs onto the website to connect the code number of the collection kit with his account. Then he begins to provide his DNA sample. This involves spitting into the tube through a funnel until his saliva reaches a line on the tube. Though not really difficult, it requires more effort than he expects to generate that much saliva. It takes about 4 minutes, after which he closes the cover, which breaks a seal and releases a preservative into the tube. He then replaces the funnel with a cap provided in the kit and shakes the tube to mix the contents. The tube is then put into the plastic bag, which in turn goes in a mailing box. He drops this in a mailbox and is done.

The specific technologies used by the various direct-to-consumer companies differ from company to company, but for the most part involve rapid and low-cost testing of hundreds of thousands of SNPs. Many of these involve use of microarrays (see Chapter 4), in which specific oligonucleotides are attached to a substrate, such as a glass "chip" or a silica bead.

Oligonucleotides are included that represent the sequence of different alleles of a particular polymorphism. Detection systems determine which oligonucleotides hybridize with DNA from a specific sample, which determines the individual genotype for a given SNP (Figure 14.1). These assays can be run simultaneously on hundreds of thousands of SNPs and require very small quantities of DNA for testing; hence the DNA present in saliva, derived mostly from epithelial cells in the mouth, provides a sufficient sample for testing.

Part III

After sending in his saliva, Neal had moved on to thinking about other things, so he is almost surprised when he receives an email telling him that his genetic results are ready. That evening, he logs onto the site. There is a lot of information, but he figures that the place to start is with his risk of disease. His highest risk is that of prostate cancer. He clicks on the link to that risk and finds that his lifetime chance of getting prostate cancer, given his ancestry (European), is about 24 per 100, compared with a population risk of about 18 per hundred. Looking down the list of other conditions (Table 14.1), he notices age-related macular degeneration, where his risk is about 10% compared to a population risk of 6.5%. He is not aware of anyone in his family who has been affected with either condition. Most of the conditions for which he was found to be at increased risk are things he has never heard of, and, for the most part, his risks are between 1.2 and 1.5 times the average. There is just one exception: His risk of Parkinson disease is more than three times elevated, and this condition did affect his paternal grandfather. Looking more carefully at the information provided, he learns a lot about Parkinson disease that he didn't know. One thing he does not learn, though, is what he can do to reduce his elevated risk. Aside from knowing the early signs, there does not seem to be much that can be done. There are also quite a few conditions for which his risk is lower than the population risk, things like type 1 diabetes. His risk of migraines is said to be lower than average, which interests him because he has had a number of migraines (or at least that's what he thinks they are). His risk for a large number of conditions is about the same as the population risk. Things on this list include obesity (he is not obese, though he has gradually put on about 20 pounds in the last 20 years) and coronary artery disease. That is one thing he had thought he might be at increased risk for, since his father had needed a coronary bypass procedure done (though he eventually died of cancer).

Table 14.1 Some examples of Neal's disease risk compared with population risk of these conditions based on his genetic testing.

Condition	Neal's risk	Population risk	Neal's risk compared to population risk
Parkinson disease	4.8%	1.6%	3
Age-related macular degeneration	10%	6.5%	1.5
Prostate cancer	24%	18%	1.3
Melanoma	3.3%	2.9%	1.16
Type 2 diabetes	27.8%	25.7%	1.08
Obesity	65.9%	63.9%	1.03
Gallstones	6.2%	7.0%	0.88
Coronary heart disease	39.7%	46.8%	0.85
Rheumatoid arthritis	1.3%	2.4%	0.6
Celiac disease	0.05%	0.12%	0.44
Type 1 diabetes	0.2%	1.0%	0.24

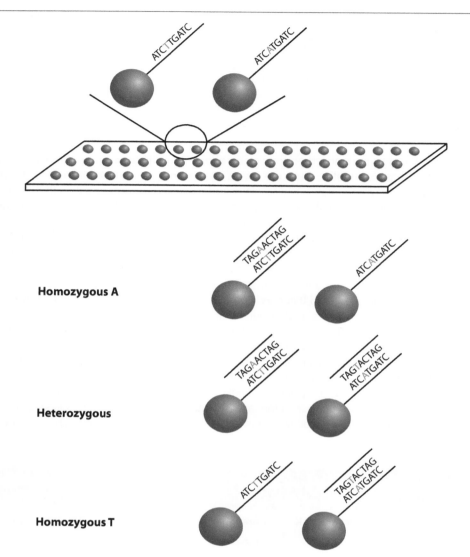

Figure 14.1 Detection of a single-nucleotide polymorphism using bead array. The polymorphism in this case is the presence of an A or a T in the sequence: TAG(A/T)ACTAG. An oligonucleotide with the sequence TAGAACTAG or TAGTACTAG is attached to a silica bead and attached to a solid substrate in a microarray. Fragmented DNA from a patient sample is then hybridized with the array. If the patient is homozygous for the A allele, the sample will hybridize with the bead containing the T; if the patient is homozygous for the T allele, the sample will hybridize with the bead containing the A; if the patient is heterozygous, hybridization will occur with both beads. Whenever hybridization does occur, a signal is emitted from that bead, allowing it to be detected. The various beads in the array have attached oligonucleotides that detect various alleles at different loci. Hybridization of the patient DNA to the array allows simultaneous genotyping for hundreds of thousands of loci.

We have seen in Chapter 5 how case-control studies can be used to calculate the odds ratio of disease in individuals who carry a specific SNP allele compared with those who do not. The odds ratio can be used to estimate the risk of disease in an individual who carries a particular SNP over a lifetime, or in a particular time interval. This is based on estimates of disease risk in the general population. An odds ratio of 1.3 would result in a lifetime disease risk of approximately 24% if the population risk is 18% (i.e., 18% × 1.3 = 24%).

There are several caveats to this approach, which can be explained in the context of the analytical validity–clinical validity–clinical utility paradigm that was introduced in Chapter 10. In this case, analytical validity refers to whether the specific SNP genotypes are determined correctly by the assay. Quality control studies indicate a very high analytical validity for modern SNP genotyping assays. It is always possible, of course, that human error could occur, such as sample mix-up. This could happen in the laboratory, or, for a direct-to-consumer test, could happen at the point of sample collection if multiple individuals (say, family members) are being tested at the same time. Also, a test that has 99.99% accuracy may still result in some erroneous genotypes if 1 000 000 simultaneous assays are done (around 100 errors in one million tests).

Clinical validity refers to how well a genetic result predicts risk of disease. There are several limitations on the clinical validity of risk assessment through SNP analysis. First, the odds ratio of disease is determined from one or more case-control studies done in specific patient samples. There is always a risk of error in these studies; some have been replicated numerous times, whereas others may result from a single study. The studies may have been done on populations of different ancestry from the particular person being tested, so it may be uncertain whether the odds ratio in the study applies to a person whose ancestors come from a different population. Disease risk is often calculated based on the results of multiple SNPs, and the particular set of SNPs, and the standards of evidence that lead to the inclusion of a particular SNP, may differ from company to company. In one published study, five individuals had testing done at three different direct-to-consumer companies; in some cases, significantly different disease risks were calculated. These were not based on erroneous SNP genotypes, but rather on different approaches used to calculate disease risk from the genetic data. It is also important to realize that disease risk is influenced by many factors other than genetic ones, and that only a proportion of the genetic contribution to a particular disease may be accounted for by a specific combination of SNPs.

Clinical utility refers to whether the genetic information is useful in guiding management. There are, at present, few common disorders for which specific risk modification regimens are available. For many conditions, for example obesity, diabetes, or cardiovascular disease, those at increased risk are advised to watch their weight and exercise more. These recommendations are commonly provided to, and often not heeded

by, individuals regardless of the results of genetic tests. There is no evidence to date that genetic test results provide additional motivation to follow these suggestions. There is also some concern that individuals found to have genotypes that indicate reduced risk might decide that they are immune to risk factors such as obesity, not realizing that the genetic results constitute only part of the picture in determining individual risk of disease.

Part IV

> 👤 After spending a good while reviewing his disease risks, Neal finds no great surprises and not much he can do to change his risks. He explores other areas as well. He finds a list of medications, none of which he is taking or has even heard of, where he is said to be more or less sensitive than the general population. One that does interest him is that he was found to be a slow metabolizer of caffeine – is that why he would be up all night if he had a cup of coffee after dinner, whereas his wife never seems to be bothered by this? He sees a lot of information about traits that do not seem to be important medically. The test correctly predicts his eye color as brown and his ability to smell a noxious odor in his urine after eating asparagus (he never knew that could be genetic or that some people could not detect this odor). There is also a list of conditions for which he might be a carrier. He was found to carry one cystic fibrosis allele, which surprises him, since no one in his family had ever been diagnosed with this condition.

The absorption, metabolism, excretion, and activity of various chemical substances, including medications, are, to an extent, influenced by specific genes. We will explore this in detail in Chapter 16. Caffeine is metabolized by the enzyme P450 1A2 (Figure 14.2). Individuals with different SNP genotypes in the CYP1A2 gene that encodes this enzyme differ in their rate of metabolism, and therefore may experience different effects of caffeine ingestion.

In principle, SNP testing for pharmacogenetic polymorphisms can be helpful in guiding choice of medication or customizing dosing for particular individuals to avoid side effects and maximize benefit. Testing for particular pharmacogenetic polymorphisms at the time when a drug needs to be prescribed may not be practical, however, since the result may not be available in time to initiate treatment. There would be an advantage, therefore, to having been tested in advance for a large number of possible pharmacogenetic SNPs and then referring to these when a therapeutic decision is being made. Given the very low cost of any individual SNP test in a

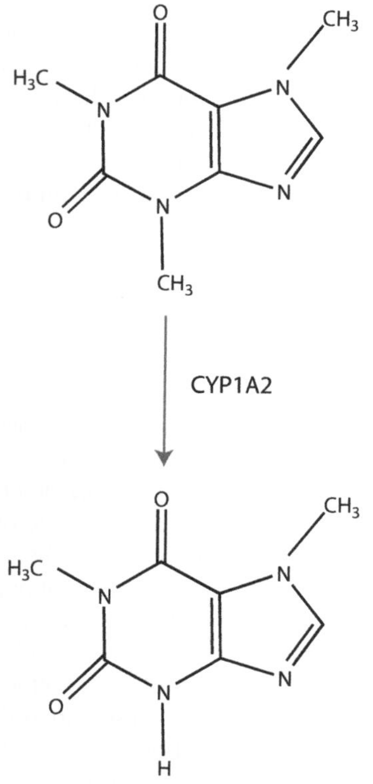

Figure 14.2 Metabolism of caffeine by CYP1A2.

microarray-based assay, there is essentially no incremental cost of testing these SNPs. The main limitations in their use are, firstly, that many physicians will not know how to interpret the information, and secondly, that there is no guarantee that the information will be available to a physician at the time a drug is prescribed. A result that is buried in a patient's record in a physician's office will be of little use if it is not readily visible at the time a drug is prescribed, and will be completely useless if a patient is treated by a different physician working at a different location.

Some direct-to-consumer tests include SNPs that are associated with autosomal recessive disorders, and therefore can be used to identify heterozygous carriers. We explored the notion of carrier testing in detail in Chapter 13. In some cases, the direct-to-consumer testing may show that an individual is a carrier for a condition for which testing had not been previously done. Given the high analytical validity of the testing, the result is likely to be correct, though it would be important to verify the result in a clinical laboratory if it is to be used in future prenatal testing. It should also be realized that the testing may not be designed to detect all of the mutations that may be seen in carriers, some of which will be missed on a SNP assay (such as deletions or duplications). Remember also

that Tay-Sachs screening is best done by enzyme assay rather than genotyping, since some carriers are missed by genotype-based testing.

Direct-to-consumer genetic tests may detect traits that are of no medical significance, but might be a subject of individual curiosity. Prediction of hair or eye color will obviously not surprise anyone, unless the prediction is wrong! Some people detect a noxious odor in their urine after eating asparagus, attributed to detection of a metabolite called methanethiol, which is under genetic control. Some of the SNPs associated with such traits have been discovered because of individuals who have participated in direct-to-consumer tests and self-identified their traits on surveys. The detection of these traits has been referred to as recreational genomics, though in fact it may demonstrate the power of the concept of direct-to-consumer genomic research and may also represent an opportunity to teach people about the influence of genetic factors on human characteristics, including risk of disease.

Part V

👤 One more thing catches Neal's eye as he continues to explore his genetic information. When he clicks onto a few disease areas, he finds that he has to read a warning message and click again that he really wants to open the page to see the information. This is fairly intimidating to him – does it mean that something really serious has been found? He does this for breast cancer – his maternal aunt had died of breast cancer, so he thought he might have inherited a risk factor – but is glad to learn that he did not test positive for breast cancer risk. One of these tests, though, is for risk of Alzheimer disease. On one hand, no one in his family had ever been diagnosed as far as he is aware. On the other hand, he knows that this is a common condition, and from what he knows about it he is more afraid of this than most anything else on the list of possible disease risks. He also knows that there is nothing he can do to reduce his risk of Alzheimer disease even if he does carry one of the genetic markers. After thinking about this for a few days, he finally decides to see his result; he is then relieved to see that his risk of Alzheimer disease is actually lower than that of the general population.

Most of the disease risks revealed by direct-to-consumer genetic tests reveal modest increases or decreases of risk, so test results are thought to be unlikely to result in major anxiety, but there are exceptions. There are well-defined gene mutations that result in substantial increase in risk of cancer, such as breast, ovarian, or colon cancer. We will consider examples of these in Chapter 15. Direct-to-consumer tests generally are not as comprehensive as targeted tests for these genes, but in some cases can reveal mutations that do substantially increase risk. In a clinical setting these tests are done with accompanying pre- and posttest genetic counseling, but this may not be the case in a direct-to-consumer test.

Testing for risk of Alzheimer disease poses issues that highlight some of the controversies surrounding direct-to-consumer genetic tests. Alzheimer disease is a form of progressive dementia that is common in the general population. It has long been recognized that a specific allele of the APOE gene is associated with increased odds of developing Alzheimer disease. ApoE is a lipoprotein that carries cholesterol. The gene includes three common variants referred to as ε2, ε3, and ε4, which can be distinguished by SNP testing. In individuals of European ancestry, ε4 heterozygotes may have twice the odds of developing Alzheimer disease, and homozygotes an 11-fold increase in odds. The effects of genotypes in other populations may be less well known. The means by which the ApoE genotype influences risk of Alzheimer disease is not known, and there are no known approaches to risk reduction for those found to be at increased risk. Because of this, ApoE testing has been widely viewed as not having clinical utility as a screening test (though it may be useful in the diagnostic evaluation of a person who is showing signs of dementia). Moreover, it has been feared that individuals found to be at significantly increased risk without having an option to reduce that risk might experience major adverse effects, including psychological distress, difficulty with relationships, or financial problems such as risk to employment or insurability. One study has challenged the notion of psychological harm resulting from knowledge of the ApoE genotype. Individuals at risk based on family history were offered testing and randomized to groups who were provided their genetic risk results or not provided those results. The study did not reveal evidence of psychological harm to those who were found to be at increased risk and were informed of this result. The decision to include ApoE on a direct-to-consumer test underscores the controversies surrounding whether potentially emotionally charged test results should be provided without accompanying professional medical interpretation and support.

Genetic Screening for Disease Risk

The ability to test for risk of disease in an asymptomatic individual is often cited as a major promise for the application of genetics in medical practice. The principle is that those determined as being at risk can be offered intervention either to prevent disease or to avoid serious complications. Genetic testing offers the advantages that it can be done at any time in life, is noninvasive, and does not depend on access to diseased tissue. Pitfalls are that tests may be of limited predictive value and clinical utility.

It is important to distinguish presymptomatic and predispositional tests. **Presymptomatic tests** apply to disorders that display age-dependent but complete penetrance, such as Huntington disease. An individual who tests positive will eventually develop the disorder if he or she lives long enough. The test is essentially deterministic of disease risk, though it may not predict time of onset or severity. A predispositional test can be used to estimate risk of disease but does not insure that an individual will or will not manifest the disorder. **Predispositional tests** apply to multifactorial traits, where multiple genes and/or environmental factors contribute to disease.

The clinical utility of presymptomatic or predispositional testing includes the possibility of informing family planning or enabling strategies to reduce risk or institute treatment. Presymptomatic tests for disorders that are transmitted as single-gene traits, often dominant traits, can be helpful for reproductive decision making. An individual who is at risk of inheriting the trait is also at risk of transmitting it. If the disorder displays age-dependent penetrance, however, the individual may not know if he or she has inherited the gene mutation until after reproductive age. This means that the trait may be passed onto offspring before the parent knows that he or she is affected. Genetic testing permits identification of the gene mutation prior to onset of symptoms, informing the decision-making process about having children and even prenatal testing.

Risk reduction or treatment strategies are based on the idea that either the disorder can be avoided altogether, or the occurrence of complications forestalled, by taking action on the basis of test results. In some cases, for example in testing for the risk of cancer, this may take the form of surveillance. Surveillance can be offered to anyone at risk, of course, but those known to be at risk on the basis of a genetic test might be more vigilant. In contrast, those found not to be at risk may not require close follow-up. This will be the case, of course, only if the family mutation is known and the individual has tested negative for the mutation. If the family mutation is not known, a negative test is harder to interpret, since there is always the possibility that a mutation is present but cannot be detected by the particular test employed.

Other forms of risk reduction include preventative surgery (often used by those at risk of cancer), modification of diet or habits such as cigarette smoking, or use of medication. There may be a compelling reason to pursue such strategies in those found to be at high risk, where the efficacy of risk reduction is well established. In some cases, though, there may be only a modest increase in risk on the basis of testing, and evidence of a benefit for risk reduction may be less clear.

There are potential risks of genetic testing to determine liability toward disease. Those who test positive may experience anxiety or stigmatization, or may be at risk for loss of insurance or employment. Those who test negative may erroneously assume that they can engage in self-destructive behaviors such as smoking, or forget that everyone is at risk of diseases such as cancer or heart disease and thus may not comply with routine screening recommendations.

The degree to which genetic predispositional testing will be incorporated into standard medical practice is not yet clear. This may depend on the evidence for clinical utility as well as the costs of testing, and costs of additional medical tests or interventions that may be done based on the outcomes of genetic tests. Whether direct-to-consumer testing will increase in use, whether it will become subject to government regulation, or whether it will give way to medically supervised testing also are unknown. The rapidly decreasing costs of whole-genome sequencing may also change the paradigm of medical application of genetics, since at some point it could become routine to sequence an individual's entire genome and make the results available to the individual and/or health providers. It is likely that the issue of predispositional testing will continue to be an area of intense debate and experimentation with various models as the technology of genotyping evolves and as the role of genetic factors in health and disease continues to be elucidated.

FURTHER READING

Bloss CS, Schork NJ, Topol EJ 2011, "Effect of direct-to-consumer genomewide profiling to assess disease risk", *New England Journal of Medicine*, vol. 364, pp. 524–34.

Eriksson N, Macpherson JM, Tung JY, *et al.* 2010, "Web-based, participant-driven studies yield novel genetic associations for common traits", *PLoS Genetics*, vol. 6, e10000993.

Green RC, Roberts JS, Cupples, LA, *et al.* 2009, "Disclosure of APOE genotype for risk of Alzheimer's disease", *New England Journal of Medicine*, vol. 361, pp. 245–54.

Khoury MJ, McBride CM, Schully SD, *et al.* 2009, "The scientific foundation for personal genomics: recommendations from a National Institutes of Health-Centers for Disease Control and Prevention multidisciplinary workshop", *Genetics in Medicine*, vol. 11, pp. 559–67.

Ng PC, Murray SS, Levy S, Venter JC 2009, "An agenda for personalized medicine", *Nature*, vol. 4611, pp. 724–6.

Find interactive self-test questions and additional resources for this chapter at **www.korfgenetics.com**.

Self-Assessment

Review Questions

14.1   What is the rationale for presymptomatic diagnosis of Huntington disease?

14.2   What is the difference between presymptomatic genetic testing and predispositional genetic testing?

14.3   What is the potential utility of presymptomatic testing for family planning?

14.4   An individual has a predispositional test that reveals he has an odds ratio of 2.5 of developing the disease. What does this mean?

14.5   How might predispositional testing render an individual vulnerable to stigmatization or discrimination?

CHAPTER 15

Genetic Testing for Risk of Cancer

Introduction

We have already seen that cancer is fundamentally a genetic disease. Although most of the genetic changes are acquired in somatic cells, some individuals inherit a predisposition. This may be based on mutation of one copy of a tumor suppressor gene or having a DNA repair defect. Risk of cancer in such individuals can be markedly increased, raising the possibility of genetic testing to identify such individuals in the hope of instituting preventative measures or surveillance to insure early diagnosis. An increasing number of cancer predisposition syndromes are being identified. In this chapter, we will consider one example associated with increased risk of breast and ovarian cancer. We will see how genetic testing can be used to identify people at risk based on family history, and the various options available to modify that risk. We will also explore some of the complexities faced in deciding to be tested, in interpreting test results, and in deciding on a course of action after a positive result.

Key Points

- Genetic predisposition to cancer is recognized by a pattern of familial transmission, as well as characteristics such as early age of onset and multifocality.
- A number of cancer predisposition syndromes have been identified, and some of these are subject to genetic testing.
- A positive genetic test result for cancer predisposition can be helpful in planning a program of surveillance or institution of medical or surgical approaches to risk reduction. It can also provide a basis for genetic counseling of family members.
- Like all predispositional tests, cancer genetic test results must be interpreted with caution, since not all individuals will develop cancer, and there are both risks and benefits to being tested.

Human Genetics and Genomics, Fourth Edition. Bruce R. Korf and Mira B. Irons.
© 2013 John Wiley & Sons, Ltd. Published 2013 by John Wiley & Sons, Ltd.

Part I

👤 The phone rings Tuesday at dinnertime, and Elaine almost decides not to get up to answer it. But she does, and her husband Jim sees her face fall and tears come to her eyes. It is Elaine's father, telling her that her mother had a mammogram today and a very suspicious mass was found. Elaine's mother is 55 years old and has been in good health. Her father explains that it was a "routine" mammogram, though in fact her mother had been worried about a lump in her breast. Actually, she has had lumps before – her breasts have been described as "cystic." Her physician had recommended that she have a mammogram annually, though in fact it has been more like 3 years since the last study. In any case, her mother is scheduled for a biopsy of the lesion later this week.

Breast cancer affects about one in eight women in North America. Many come to attention because of a breast mass, often noted by the woman herself. There are many possible causes of breast masses other than cancer. One common cause is fibrocystic disease, in which there are multiple, benign, fluid-filled cysts within the breasts. These can be readily diagnosed by ultrasound; brown bloodless fluid may be aspirated, which can relieve symptoms of pressure. The use of self-examination and mammography as screening tools has led to earlier diagnosis of breast cancer and improved prognosis. Although the issue remains controversial, mammography is now commonly recommended on an annual basis for women 40 years of age and older. Findings such as microcalcifications or densities (Figure 15.1) are followed up by biopsy.

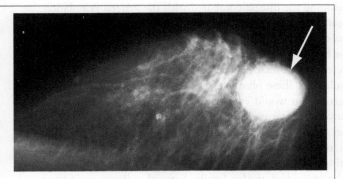

Figure 15.1 Mammogram showing breast carcinoma (arrow). (Courtesy of Dr. Wanda Bernreuter, University of Alabama at Birmingham.)

Part II

👤 Elaine goes to see her mother the next day, and stays with her during the coming week. The biopsy is done, and reveals an invasive ductal carcinoma (Figure 15.2). It is recommended that the mass be excised and that a sentinel lymph node biopsy be done. The possibility of modified radical mastectomy is also offered, although it is pointed out that there is no evidence that this will improve the outcome. Elaine's mother is very anxious to avoid this extensive surgery and elects to have the "lumpectomy." The surgery is performed, and the lymph nodes are found to be positive for tumor. The family is informed that the tumor is at stage IIA, since the tumor is less than 5 cm in diameter and there is evidence for lymph node metastases. The doctor points out that this is associated with a favorable prognosis of more than 80% 5-year survival.

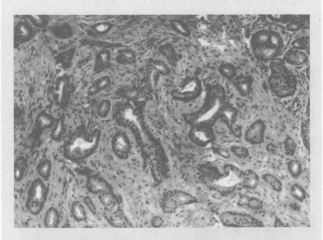

Figure 15.2 Photomicrograph showing infiltrating ductal carcinoma of the breast (hematoxylin and eosin stain). (Courtesy of Dr. Amy Adams, University of Alabama at Birmingham.)

Breast cancers are derived from epithelial cells, and are therefore classified as carcinomas. The most common pathology is referred to as invasive ductal carcinoma. In the past it was common to treat women with breast cancer by removal of the affected breast and dissection of surrounding lymph nodes. The radical mastectomy involves removal of the pectoralis major and minor muscles and axillary lymph nodes. This approach is rarely used today. The modified radical mastectomy leaves the pectoralis major in place. More recently, breast-conserving surgery, followed by radiation therapy of the involved region, has been shown to have similar efficacy to mastectomy for many tumors. Breast cancer staging is based on the size of the tumor, the degree of involvement of lymph nodes, and the presence of metastases to more distant sites. Smaller tumors, with less nodal invasion and no distant metastases, are associated with a more favorable prognosis.

Part III

👤 Elaine's mother, and, indeed, the whole family, is relieved to hear this relatively favorable prognosis. They are advised that she should have radiation treatments following the surgery, which are initiated. At a follow-up visit a few weeks later, they are informed that the tumor was negative for estrogen receptors and negative for HER-2/neu amplification (Figure 15.3). They are told that the HER-2/neu result is good news: It puts her in a more favorable prognostic category. The lack of estrogen receptors means that she will not benefit from treatment with tamoxifen; instead, they recommend a course of systemic chemotherapy.

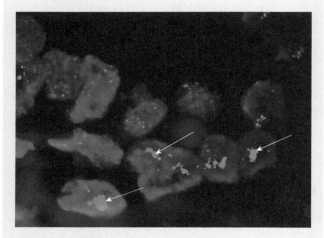

Figure 15.3 In situ hybridization showing amplification of the Her-2/neu gene (pink staining). (Courtesy of Dr. Andrew Carroll, University of Alabama at Birmingham.)

The approach to therapy depends on a number of variables, including the stage of the tumor, whether the woman is pre- or postmenopausal, and the results of genetic studies done on the tumor cells. Tumors that express estrogen or progesterone receptors tend to respond to treatment with hormone antagonists and are associated with a more favorable rate of long-term survival. Tamoxifen is an estrogen antagonist that has been shown to be effective in preventing recurrence of breast cancer

in women whose tumors are estrogen receptor positive. The drug is associated with side effects such as hot flashes and vaginal dryness, but is overall well tolerated. HER-2/neu is an oncogene that is amplified in some breast cancers. The gene encodes a membrane tyrosine kinase growth factor receptor. Overexpression of this gene, usually a result of gene amplification, is associated with poor prognosis. Given that Elaine's mother's tumor is estrogen receptor negative and that she has evidence of spread to the lymph nodes, it is recommended that she be treated with chemotherapy.

Part IV

👤 About 6 months have gone by since the initial diagnosis, and Elaine's mother is doing well. She has tolerated the chemotherapy reasonably well, although the treatment has, at times, been grueling. For Elaine, one effect of this experience has been to increase the degree to which she is interested in having regular breast examinations. She examines herself at least monthly, and has scheduled a visit with her gynecologist. It is while she is in the waiting room that she reads an article about the genetics of breast cancer. The article alarms her: Her mother's sister died of ovarian cancer at age 55 and her grandmother's sister was said to have died of breast cancer, although that was many years ago and details are not available. Elaine discusses this with her gynecologist. Based on this family history, he offers to refer her to speak with a cancer geneticist.

It has been clear for a long time that genetics contributes to risk of breast cancer. First-degree relatives of individuals with breast cancer face a 2–3 times increased risk of themselves developing the disease compared with the general population. Moreover, some families demonstrate transmission of breast cancer in an autosomal dominant fashion. Other members of these families may have ovarian cancer, and, in some, males are affected with breast cancer, a rare occurrence in the general population. These observations prompted a search for a gene or genes that would explain this risk, and culminated in the discovery of two genes that predispose to breast cancer. The genes are referred to as *BRCA1* and *BRCA2*. There are, in addition, other genes that predispose to breast cancer (Table 15.1). Testing may be offered for these based on clinical indications in the individual and/or family. Since the discovery of these genes, and the ensuing possibility of genetic testing, clinics have been set up to offer genetic counseling and testing for individuals thought to be at risk.

Part V

👤 It takes almost 2 months to get an appointment in the cancer genetics clinic, and it is necessary for Elaine to travel into the city – which she hates to do – for the appointment. She is given a form to fill out prior to the visit that requests detailed family history information. She speaks with her mother and father in an effort to fill in as much detail as she can, though they have only a relatively small amount of knowledge about other members of the family. Elaine is 24 years old, recently married, and has a 2-year-old daughter. Elaine has a sister, Carol, who is 28, and a brother, Michael, who is 30. Both Carol and Michael are healthy, and each has two children. Elaine's mother had a sister who died of ovarian cancer. She also has a brother who is 57 years old and has hypertension, but otherwise is well. Her mother's parents are both deceased: Her father died of a heart attack and her mother of an accident at age 48. They confirm that Elaine's grandmother was said to have had breast cancer, but they don't know much more than that. She died more than 40 years ago, so there is no prospect of getting additional records. At the counseling visit, Elaine relates all this to a genetic counselor. The counselor asks about her ethnic background, and Elaine answers that both her parents are of non-Jewish European descent.

Given the high frequency of breast cancer in the general population, it is not uncommon for an individual to have an affected relative. How much family history is enough to convey sufficient risk to suggest the possibility of a *BRCA1* or *BRCA2* mutation? The presence of multiple affected first- or second-degree relatives with any combination of breast or ovarian cancer at any age would suggest a genetic predisposition. Alternatively, if there are fewer affected relatives, young age of onset (<50 years) in an affected relative, the presence of a male relative with breast cancer, a relative with multiple primary cancers (bilateral breast cancer or breast and ovarian cancer),

and the presence of both breast and ovarian cancer in different first- or second-degree relatives would constitute risk factors. Ancestry can be important in risk assessment – there is a founder effect in the Ashkenazi Jewish (i.e., Jews descended from communities around Eastern Europe and Germany) population, for example, that increases the risk of specific *BRCA1* or *BRCA2* mutations. There are risk assessment computer programs that are used to determine the probability that an individual carries a *BRCA1* or *BRCA2* mutation. Of course, the occurrence of a known *BRCA* mutation in a relative constitutes a risk factor.

Table 15.1 List of genetic conditions, other than the *BRCA1* or *BRCA2* mutation, associated with predisposition to breast cancer. Breast cancer risk is dominantly inherited, except for the three listed as autosomal recessive.

Condition	Gene(s)	Clinical features
Li–Fraumeni syndrome	TP53	Multiple cancer types, including but not limited to sarcoma, breast, leukemia, glioma, and melanoma
Cowden syndrome	PTEN	Thyroid, breast, and endometrial cancer; macrocephaly; papillomatous papules; and tricholemmomas
Hereditary diffuse gastric cancer	CDH1	Diffuse gastric cancer and lobular breast cancer
CHEK2	CHEK2	Early-onset breast cancer
Ataxia telangiectasia	ATM	Carriers at increased risk of breast cancer
Lynch syndrome	Mismatch repair genes	Hereditary nonpolyposis colon cancer, and possible association with breast cancer
Peutz–Jeghers syndrome	STK11	Gastrointestinal polyps, mucocutaneous pigmentation, and breast cancer
Bloom syndrome	BLM	Autosomal recessive: Growth deficiency and risk of multiple types of cancer
Werner syndrome	WRN	Autosomal recessive: Premature aging and multiple cancers, including breast
Xeroderma pigmentosum	Nucleotide excision repair genes	Autosomal recessive: Sun sensitivity, neurological impairment, and multiple cancers, including skin and breast cancer

Part VI

👤 The visit with the genetic counselor goes on for over an hour. The counselor explains to Elaine about the genetics of breast cancer, and about the options available for genetic testing. She explains that testing is available for BRCA1 and BRCA2 mutations, although not all possible mutations are detected with current approaches to testing. She also reviews the potential risks and benefits of testing. Elaine has done considerable reading prior to the visit and has already decided that she would like to be tested. The counselor suggests that, given her non-Jewish background, she have complete sequencing of the BRCA1 and BRCA2 genes. She also suggests that Elaine's mother be tested first, to determine if she carries one of these mutations, prior to testing Elaine herself. Elaine agrees to discuss this with her mother and to get back in touch with the counselor by telephone.

The decision whether to undergo genetic testing for breast or ovarian cancer is a complicated one, and involves both technical and psychosocial issues. Both the *BRCA1* and *BRCA2* genes are large, and a wide variety of mutations have been found in affected individuals. Detection of all possible mutations is technically challenging and expensive, requiring complete sequence analysis of the coding region and intron–exon borders. A small proportion of mutations consist of gene rearrangements or deletions, which require additional testing. In the United States, *BRCA* testing is done by one laboratory – Myriad Genetics, Inc., which owns the patent on testing for mutations in these genes. In individuals of Ashkenazi Jewish background, testing may first be offered for two *BRCA1* mutations (187delAG, a two-base deletion at position 187, and 5385insC, a one-base insertion at nucleotide 5385) and one *BRCA2* mutation (6174delT) that are particularly common in this group. Searching for these mutations can be done at relatively low cost and might obviate the need for complete gene sequencing. In other populations, though, complete sequencing of the two genes is necessary. When possible, it is helpful to test an individual who is known to be affected with breast or ovarian cancer, since otherwise a negative test in an at-risk relative could indicate either that the individual did not inherit a mutation present in the family or that the risk of cancer in the family is not accounted for by a detectable *BRCA* gene mutation.

The risk–benefit analysis of testing for cancer risk is at least equally complex. There are proven approaches to risk reduction, but these may entail making major life decisions. The most extreme option, prophylactic mastectomy and oophorectomy, has proven benefit, but is a major and traumatic event.

Surveillance for cancer by physical examination, annual mammography and breast magnetic resonance imaging (MRI), transvaginal ultrasound, and serum testing for CA-125, a marker of ovarian cancer, may allow for earlier detection of cancer and improved rate of survival. Prophylactic administration of tamoxifen may be effective in reducing risk of breast cancer in *BRCA1* or *BRCA2* gene carriers. Many women will opt for testing in the hope of relief of anxiety about their risk, but, of course, they face a possibility of confirming their fears of being at risk of cancer. Also, some who test negative for a family mutation have experienced guilt at the fact that they have escaped a fate that affects others in the family, especially siblings. There has been much discussion about the stigmatization of cancer gene mutation carriers and tangible risks of discrimination, including denial of employment, health insurance, disability insurance, and life insurance. Legislation at the US federal level, in some US states, and in other countries addresses this by banning genetic discrimination. US federal law prohibits genetic information from being used to make employment decisions or to assess eligibility for health insurance, but it does not cover use of genetic information in determining eligibility for life insurance. Health insurance companies differ in their willingness to pay for genetic testing for cancer risk, though an increasing number in the United States are offering such coverage for individuals with established risk factors.

Part VII

👤 Elaine explains what she has learned to her mother and father, and asks her mother if she would be willing to undergo testing. Her mother gets very upset as the conversation progresses, and tearfully refuses to be tested. She has had enough of breast cancer, and is not interested in knowing whether she has passed a genetic risk of cancer on to her children. Elaine is disappointed and upset, but at some level understands her mother's reluctance. She calls the counselor back and explains that she would like to be tested, but that her mother has refused. The counselor arranges for Elaine to sign an informed consent document and for blood to be drawn for testing. It is arranged for Elaine to come back to the clinic in 2 weeks to hear the results. The time passes slowly, but finally Elaine and Jim come together to the clinic visit. Elaine is not surprised to hear that she has been found to carry a pathogenic mutation in BRCA1. She had already begun to think through what she would do if she tested positive, and has a long conversation with the counselor about her options.

The risk of cancer to a *BRCA1* or *BRCA2* mutation carrier is estimated from previous experience with carriers of similar mutations. In some cases the analysis is complicated by the fact that a mutation might be rare, so there is little experience with cancer risk in carriers. Direct sequence analysis also reveals some genetic variants that are of unknown significance, making it unclear whether they increase cancer risk at all. It is estimated that the *BRCA1* or *BRCA2* mutation conveys an 87% risk of breast cancer and a 44% risk of ovarian cancer in woman by age 70. The *BRCA1* mutation also conveys an increased risk of fallopian tube carcinoma, primary papillary serous carcinoma of the peritoneum, and prostate cancer in males. The *BRCA2* mutation is also associated with pancreatic cancer and breast cancer in males.

As noted in this chapter, there is no definitive treatment for mutation carriers that will eliminate the risk of cancer. The least that might be offered is surveillance, but studies indicate that prophylactic surgery can substantially reduce the risk of cancer. Bilateral mastectomy reduces the risk of breast cancer, though there is a possibility of cancer developing from small amounts of residual breast tissue. Mastectomy also does not address the risk of ovarian cancer. Salpingo-oophorectomy has been demonstrated to reduce the risk of both ovarian and breast cancers, and the benefit appears to apply if done after completion of childbearing.

Part VIII

Elaine and Jim are very concerned about her risk of cancer and feel that they must do everything in their power to avoid the possibility that she might develop cancer. They have one child, and feel that what is most important to them is protecting Elaine's ability to be there for her, and that they would be satisfied that their family is complete with one child. Elaine therefore opts to have a bilateral mastectomy. She inquires about also having salpingo-oophorectomy, and is advised that this is better done after menopause. Meanwhile, Elaine has spoken with Carol and Michael and discussed with them the possibility of their being tested. They both opt to be tested; Carol is negative, whereas Michael is positive. Michael has two daughters, and asks about whether they should be tested. Also, it has been increasingly difficult to keep Elaine's mother from realizing that several members of the family have been tested. The three children together decide to meet with their parents and break the news to their mother.

The news that an individual carries a breast cancer gene mutation has major implications for the family, as well as for the individual. In some cases, testing one person, such as a child, indirectly reveals mutation status in another, such as a parent. Carrier status is of greatest importance to women in the family, who are at risk for breast and ovarian cancer. Males, too, can

be at risk of cancer, mainly prostate cancer, and, principally for *BRCA2* carriers, breast cancer as well.

Genetic testing of children raises complex ethical issues. There is a long tradition of offering testing for certain disorders in children, such as muscular dystrophy. These studies are done to establish a diagnosis in a symptomatic child, and offer genetic counseling regarding recurrence risk and prenatal diagnosis for family members at risk of having a child with a devastating disorder. The situation is far different for cancer risk testing. Here, children are not symptomatic, and are not really at risk until they grow up. There is no intervention that would be offered to the child to reduce his or her risk. The consensus of opinion in the medical genetics community has been to test children only if they will benefit in the immediate future in terms of improved health care. Children at risk of inheriting a breast cancer mutation should be offered counseling at an appropriate age, when they can make their own informed decision about whether to be tested.

Part IX

Elaine has adjusted well following her surgery, and life is more or less back to "normal." She has become involved in a breast cancer advocacy group. Part of her role is talking with women who have been diagnosed or have been determined to carry a breast cancer susceptibility gene. She is also involved in fundraising efforts to support further research in the field.

The mechanism of action of the *BRCA1* and *BRCA2* gene products is not entirely known, but it appears that they are involved in the response of the cell to repair of DNA damage. Both genes act via a tumor suppressor mechanism, requiring homozygous mutation in tumor cells. There are multiple additional genes involved in the pathogenesis of breast cancer. In addition, there are genes that function as modifiers of risk of breast or ovarian cancer, as well as genes whose somatic mutation contributes to the progression of the cancers. It is hoped that further study of these genes will lead to better diagnostic tools as well as insights that may produce more effective therapies.

Familial Predisposition to Cancer

Cancer is a common disorder, affecting at least one in three individuals, so virtually everyone has a family history of cancer. There are, however, families in which the risk is transmitted as a single-gene trait with high penetrance. These families are characterized by autosomal dominant transmission of a tendency to develop cancer. The specific spectrum of cancers differs from family to family, but can be sorted into a number of familial cancer syndromes. Affected individuals within these families tend to develop their cancers at an earlier age than sporadically affected individuals, and may develop multiple, independent primary tumors.

As we have seen in Chapter 8, most instances of familial predisposition to cancer are the result of mutations in tumor suppressor genes. An at-risk individual inherits a germ line mutation and will develop cancer if the remaining nonmutated copy of the gene undergoes mutation in a susceptible tissue. The specific distribution of cancer types depends on the types of tissues in which the gene is normally expressed, and the specific role of the gene in that tissue. The major genes and syndromes are summarized in Table 8.1.

Identification of individuals at risk can be important from a number of points of view. In some cases, there may be specific treatments that can be provided to prevent cancer. For example, individuals who inherit a mutation in the RET oncogene are at high risk of developing medullary thyroid carcinoma, even in childhood. Prophylactic thyroidectomy in these individuals can be lifesaving. As with breast and ovarian cancer, surveillance programs can be instituted to insure early detection and treatment of cancer. Those at risk of colon cancer, for example, will be offered colonoscopy at a younger age than is routine in the general population. In some instances, the information may be used for family-planning purposes. This is especially true for conditions such as neurofibromatosis, where, in addition to a risk of malignancy, the syndrome causes major physical and developmental problems that may begin in childhood.

The approach to risk assessment begins with collecting family history information. Often, this is the indication for consideration of testing. As far as possible, the history should be documented to ensure that there is accurate information about types of cancers in affected relatives, age of onset, and so on. Information that is obtained secondhand is often inac-curate, and can lead to erroneous estimations of risks to relatives. Sometimes a physical examination will be warranted. This is typically the case in disorders such as neurofibromatosis, where specific signs and symptoms may be used to establish a diagnosis. In other disorders, however, such as breast and ovarian cancer syndrome, no physical signs will distinguish individuals at risk from others in the family.

How much family history of cancer does one need to have to warrant genetic testing? Cancer is common, and virtually everyone will have some family history of cancer. Specific criteria for testing have been developed for the various familial cancer syndromes. Ideally, genetic testing should first be performed on a member of the family known to be affected with cancer. The reason for this is that virtually all of the tests involve screening for mutations where not all possible mutations can be detected. Testing an affected individual maximizes the chance of finding a mutation if one is present, and provides the possibility of reliable testing for other family members at risk. The affected individual(s) may not be available for testing in some cases. If an unaffected individual is tested, a positive test will indicate that the person is at risk, but a negative test is harder to interpret. It may mean that the individual did not inherit the family mutation, that the family mutation could not be detected, or that there is no mutation in the family at all.

These complexities, as well as the ethical, legal, and social issues that were discussed in this chapter, warrant formal genetic counseling as part of the evaluation. Usually this involves at least two visits: an initial visit to gather information, make a decision about testing, and arrange for the testing, and a follow-up to report the results of testing. This paradigm is likely to be expanded to include other areas of risk assessment for inherited adult-onset disorders as the genes responsible for these conditions come to light.

FURTHER READING

American Society of Clinical Oncology 2003, "American Society of Clinical Oncology policy statement update: genetic testing for cancer susceptibility", *Journal of Clinical Oncology*, vol. 21, pp. 2397–406.

American Society of Human Genetics and American College of Medical Genetics 1995, "Points to consider: ethical, legal, and psychosocial implications of genetic testing in children and adolescents", *American Journal of Human Genetics*, vol. 57, pp. 1233–41.

Daly MB, Axilbund JE, Buys S, *et al.* 2010, "Genetic/familial high risk assessment: breast and ovarian", *Journal of the National Comprehensive Cancer Network*, vol. 8, pp. 562–94.

Kauff ND, Domchek SM, Friebel TM, *et al.* 2008, "Risk-reducing salpingo-oophorectomy for the prevention of BRCA1- and BRCA2-associated breast and gynecologic cancer: a multicenter, prospective study", *Journal of Clinical Oncology*, vol. 26, pp. 1331–7.

Prucka SK, McIlvried DE, Korf BR 2008, "Cancer risk assessment and the genetic counseling process: using hereditary breast and ovarian cancer as an example", *Medical Principles and Practice*, vol. 17, pp. 173–89.

Robson M, Offit, K 2007, "Management of an inherited predisposition to breast cancer", *New England Journal of Medicine*, vol. 357, pp. 154–62.

Find interactive self-test questions and additional resources for this chapter at **www.korfgenetics.com**.

Self-Assessment

Review Questions

15.1   A 50-year-old man presents with breast cancer. He has two teenage daughters. Is testing for a genetic cause of breast cancer indicated? If so, which gene or genes would be appropriate to test?

15.2   A 30-year-old woman requests counseling regarding her risk of breast and ovarian cancer. Her mother died of ovarian cancer, and her aunt currently has breast cancer. It is suggested that her aunt be tested before testing is done on her. What is the rationale for this recommendation?

15.3   A woman tests positive for a *BRCA1* mutation. She has two daughters, ages 5 and 7 years. When should the daughters be tested for the mutation?

15.4   A woman with a *BRCA2* mutation elects to have bilateral mastectomy and salpingo-oophorectomy. Does this guarantee that she will not get breast or ovarian cancer?

15.5   A woman with a family history of breast cancer is interested in testing, but expresses concern that being tested might result in her loss of health insurance. How would you counsel her regarding this risk?

CHAPTER 16
Pharmacogenetics

Introduction

A person's absorption, metabolism, distribution of, and reaction to, pharmacological agents are all under some degree of genetic control. It should therefore be no surprise that there are individual variations in how people respond to drugs. As the genes that underlie these responses come to light, it becomes possible to offer genetic tests that will predict adverse reactions, enable customization of dosing to insure optimal therapeutic levels, and tailor the choice of drug to individual needs. In this chapter we will explore the principles of **pharmacogenetics**, considering a specific case of adverse reaction to anesthetics called malignant hyperthermia. We will see how genetic studies are explaining the basis for this condition and how testing can be helpful to identify family members at risk. We will also glimpse the future of pharmacogenetics, which many predict will lead to an individualization of drug therapy.

Key Points

- Individual reaction to a drug can be influenced by genetic traits that affect absorption, biodistribution, excretion, and physiological effects.
- Genetic testing for specific polymorphisms involved in drug metabolism offers the possibility of avoidance of side effects and customization of treatment to the physiological needs of the individual.
- It is expected that pharmacogenetic testing will increasingly be used as a component of routine medical decision making.

Part I

👤 Eric was not looking forward to this day, though he was looking forward to not having frequent sore throats anymore. Finally, though, he is to have his tonsils taken out. At age 10, he is pretty well prepared for the surgery, but nevertheless frightened. His parents are with him right up to the point where he is taken to the operating room. The last thing he remembers is a nurse giving him some medication.

In the operating room, things are going smoothly. Eric is given a dose of succinylcholine to prevent coughing, and then an endotracheal tube is inserted. Anesthesia is halothane and nitrous oxide. The surgery begins, and the anesthesiologist settles into his routine of close monitoring. About 10 minutes into the operation, though, he begins to become concerned. The first sign is an increase in CO_2 levels monitored in Eric's exhaled air. Within minutes, Eric's heart rate increases to over 150 beats per minute and he begins to stiffen. Rate of ventilation is increased, but his pCO_2 remains elevated. Eric's temperature is also rising, now at 38°C. The anesthesiologist calls for the surgery to be stopped, and for additional help. He administers a dose of dantrolene and obtains a blood gas. Eric is found to have a mixed metabolic and respiratory acidosis. The halothane is stopped, and medications are administered to maintain anesthesia. Over the next half hour, the tachycardia resolves and Eric is transferred to the intensive care unit.

These signs and symptoms are typical for malignant hyperthermia. Malignant hyperthermia is a syndrome that occurs in rare, susceptible individuals who are exposed to one of several drugs (called "trigger agents") (Table 16.1). These drugs include depolarizing muscle relaxants such as succinylcholine and halogenated anesthetics such as halothane. Both are commonly used in general anesthesia. The muscle relaxant facilitates intubation, avoiding coughing and choking, and halothane is a widely used and generally safe anesthetic. Susceptible individuals are rare – one out of 15 000 children in Europe and the United States – but when they are exposed to a trigger agent, a life-threatening event may ensue.

The pathophysiology of malignant hyperthermia begins with a sudden and massive release of calcium from the sarcoplasmic reticulum into the muscle sarcoplasm. Normally, calcium release causes actin molecules to engage with myosin, leading to muscle contraction. The massive calcium release leads to sustained muscle contraction. There is a sudden increase in muscle metabolism, depleting ATP and leading to increased oxygen consumption. CO_2 production increases, leading to a respiratory acidosis, while the rise in muscle

Table 16.1 Trigger agents and safe agents for individuals susceptible to malignant hyperthermia.

Trigger agents
Depolarizing muscle relaxants (e.g., succinylcholine)
Halogenated anesthetics (e.g., halothane)
Safe agents
Nondeplorizing muscle relaxants (e.g., vecuronium)
Nitrous oxide
Intravenous anesthetics (e.g., ketamine and propofol)
Vasopressors (e.g., epinephrine and dopamine)
Other sedatives (e.g., opiates and benzodiazepines)
Source: Ali *et al.* (2003).

metabolism with depletion of oxygen causes an increase in lactic acid, leading to lactic acidosis. The increased CO_2 production is often the first sign of malignant hyperthermia. Heart rate increases to keep up with the increased oxygen demands. The acidosis is accompanied by increased blood potassium, which can lead to cardiac arrhythmia, and ventricular fibrillation or cardiac arrest may occur. The sustained muscle contraction and hypermetabolic state lead to increased body temperature, which may exceed 46°C and itself may be lethal.

Anesthesiologists are trained to recognize malignant hyperthermia and to react emergently. The anesthesia will be stopped immediately, substituting "safe" drugs that do not trigger malignant hyperthermia. Ventilatory rate is increased to remove CO_2. If necessary, anti-arrhythmia drugs are administered and acidosis may be corrected. The mainstay of treatment, however, is administration of dantrolene. Dantrolene works as a muscle relaxant, and specifically acts to inhibit calcium release in the muscle. It can be used to abort an attack, and can be lifesaving. The drug is continued for 24 to 48 hours, since repeat episodes are possible.

Part II

👤 Eric does not awaken until the next day, and he is surprised to find that he is connected to more tubes and lines than he has ever seen before. He expects his throat to be sore, which it is, but does not expect his whole body to be aching. His parents are at the bedside, and seem very relieved to see him awake. He asks what happened, and his mother begins to cry.

In fact, both his parents by now understand that Eric very nearly died. The night of the surgery, both the surgeon and the anesthesiologist spoke with them, and explained that Eric had experienced an episode of malignant hyperthermia. They were confused at first – they never expected to hear the word "malignant" following Eric's surgery. They were reassured to hear that Eric did not have cancer, but when the anesthesiologist explained what had happened they were not so reassured. But then they were relieved to hear that the episode had been effectively treated. Eric's body temperature, they were told, peaked at 39.5°C, requiring a cooling blanket, but his temperature did come down and it does not appear that any permanent damage was done. They were told that he will need to be kept on medication for several days. They also were asked if anything like this had ever happened to anyone else in the family.

Malignant hyperthermia was first described in 1960, in a study of an extended family in which multiple relatives of an affected individual were found to have elevated creatine phosphokinase (CPK) values. CPK is a muscle enzyme that leaks out of damaged muscle cells. The trait was found to segregate in the family as an autosomal dominant. Since then, it has become apparent that malignant hyperthermia is a classic dominant trait with incomplete penetrance. Although the trait is inherited as a dominant, the actual syndrome occurs only in indi-

viduals who are exposed to one of the trigger agents. Otherwise, an individual may go through life never experiencing an episode. Moreover, not all at-risk individuals have an episode even if exposed to a trigger agent. This makes it difficult to be sure whether a relative of a known affected has inherited the trait. Those who have the trait usually enjoy good health other than having a risk of the catastrophic event of malignant hyperthermia. Some may be at greater risk of heat stroke, and some have some degree of chronic muscle weakness. In some cases, individuals may have a myopathy referred to as central core disease, based on the appearance of muscle through the microscope (Figure 16.1). Most, however, have normal muscle function.

Part III

The answer to the question about family history is no, at least not to the knowledge of either of Eric's parents. Eric's subsequent hospital course is uneventful. His muscle aching takes weeks to fully resolve. His doctor had mentioned that a test he called CPK was very abnormal – as high as 30 000 the day of the surgery, and still 1000 a week later. Nevertheless, things went well, although Eric is upset to realize that he still has his tonsils. Arrangements are made to have them removed many months later. This time, a different anesthesia regimen is used without incident. Eric's parents are warned, though, that if Eric ever should need surgery in the future, his doctors should be informed about this event. Otherwise, though, both Eric and his family put the incident behind them.

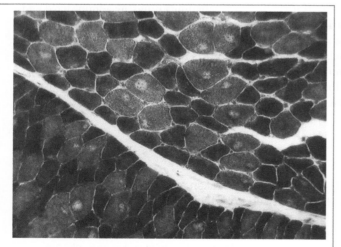

Figure 16.1 Photomicrograph of muscle showing central core disease. Pale areas within muscle cells are the pathological central cores. (Courtesy of Dr. Shin Oh, University of Alabama at Birmingham.)

If the patient survives the acute episode, complete recovery can occur. There can be a massive breakdown of muscle, which leads to a release of muscle protein, especially myoglobin, into the blood. Myoglobin can overload the kidney and lead to kidney failure in some instances. CPK also may leak out of the muscle, causing massive elevation in the blood. CPK itself is harmless, but is a marker of muscle breakdown. Individuals who have experienced an episode of malignant hyperthermia obviously need to avoid exposure to trigger agents in the future. This means that alternative "safe" agents must be used for surgical procedures. It is recommended to wear a bracelet warning of the risk, since it is possible that emergency surgery could be required at some point where the patient's prior medical history might not be available. The risk may apply to other family members as well, who should be advised to raise the issue if they should require surgery in the future.

Part IV

👤 Eric has never forgotten the incident, but over the next 15 years he does not require surgery again. He has told his doctors about the event, which has been noted in his medical record. Now, however, his mind is on his own son, Jonathan, who is 3 years old. Jonathan has a hernia, and Eric and his wife have just learned that he will require surgery. As the surgeon is explaining the procedure, it is Eric's wife, Jean, who brings up Eric's history. She thinks that she was told that this can run in families – could Jonathan be at risk? The surgeon requests additional information, and speaks with the anesthesiologist. They ask Eric for details about the episode. Of course, Eric doesn't remember much, and the hospital where the surgery was performed was closed years ago. Eric has no idea who the surgeon was. He calls his parents, though, who look through old papers, and they retrieve the information that Eric's episode was labeled "malignant hyperthermia." The anesthesiologist explains that they may need to use an alternative approach to anesthesia in Jonathan, to be on the safe side. He says that it is possible to do a test for malignant hyperthermia, but it will be difficult to do on a young child. He promises to look into testing more thoroughly, though, before the surgery is scheduled.

Testing for susceptibility to malignant hyperthermia is not easily done. The classical test involves biopsy of a relatively large sample of muscle, and test of the muscle for contraction on exposure to halothane and caffeine. The muscle must be tested within hours of biopsy, which means that the biopsy can be done only in a center that is properly equipped and experienced. There are only a few such centers anywhere in the world. As a result, testing is cumbersome and expensive. The test is 97–99% sensitive and about 90% specific. An at-risk individual may be treated as though affected, using safe anesthetics, rather than undergo the expense and inconvenience of biopsy. Moreover, it is difficult to remove a large enough sample of muscle from a child, making it unlikely that a young child will be tested.

Part V

👤 A few days later, Eric and Jean get a call from the anesthesiologist, who has spoken with a colleague in the genetics clinic. He says that genetic testing for

malignant hyperthermia may be possible, and arranges for Eric and Jean to be seen in the genetics clinic. They speak with a genetic counselor, who explains that genetic testing is available, though it does not always succeed in detecting the responsible mutation. It is arranged for a sample to be sent from Eric, with the understanding that Jonathan can be tested if Eric's test is positive.

Two genes have so far been discovered as being associated with malignant hyperthermia. The most common is designated *RYR1*; it is located on chromosome 19 and encodes a muscle cell membrane ion channel, referred to as the ryanodine receptor. The other gene is designated *CACAN1S*; it is located on chromosome 1 and encodes a protein called voltage-dependent L-type calcium channel, subunit alpha 1S. The *RYR1* mutation accounts for 70–80% of malignant hyperthermia, and the *CACAN1S* mutation for only about 1%. At least two other loci have been implicated by linkage, but the genes are not yet known.

The ryanodine receptor is so-called because it binds a toxic substance, ryanodine. It encodes a membrane protein that controls calcium release from the sarcoplasmic reticulum in muscle. Muscle contraction is initiated when acetylcholine is released from a motor nerve synapse at the muscle membrane. The depolarizing current is transmitted through membrane channels, T tubules, which make contact with the sarcoplasmic reticulum, a modified endoplasmic reticulum. The ryanodine receptor resides at the junction between the T tubules and sarcoplasmic reticulum (Figure 16.2) and triggers calcium release into the sarcoplasm upon depolarization of adjacent calcium channels, referred to as dihydropyridine receptors (DHPR). The increased calcium causes actin to engage with myosin, initiating muscle contraction.

The mutations responsible for malignant hyperthermia appear to lead to excessive calcium release, as a consequence of exposure to either succinylcholine, which elicits a large-scale membrane depolarization, or halothane, which interacts directly with the receptor. The two drugs acting together behave synergistically to trigger malignant hyperthermia episodes. Individuals who are not exposed to trigger agents may never have an episode. Most have normal muscle function, but some have a chronic myopathy, indicating some degree of calcium leakage without exposure to a trigger agent.

Part VI

👤 More than 2 months pass before the test results are available. Eric has been found to have a mutation at codon 2434, in which a leucine is substituted with proline. A cheek swab is taken from Jonathan. Four weeks later Eric and Jean learn that Jonathan did not inherit this mutation, which is a great relief. They are told, however, that other family members should be tested for the mutation. Eric speaks with his sister and brother, both of whom have children. His sister is found to have the same mutation, as does one of her children. Eric's brother does not have the mutation.

Molecular diagnosis of malignant hyperthermia poses many challenges. As has been noted, the *RYR1* gene is not the only one responsible for malignant hyperthermia. The *RYR1* gene includes 106 exons and encodes a protein of 5000 amino acids. Molecular testing is hampered by the complexity of scanning a large gene for mutations, and potential ambiguity in the interpretation of mutation data. A variety of different mutation types have been found in different affected individuals. Because of these challenges, mutation analysis is not used as the primary

diagnostic screen for malignant hyperthermia, in spite of the difficulties posed by the muscle contraction assay. Failure to find a mutation would not rule out the diagnosis, whereas false negative results cannot be tolerated in a potentially lethal disorder. Genetic testing can be useful in family counseling, however. If a known affected individual is tested and the mutation is found, testing can be offered to other relatives to determine whether they are at risk. Those found to be at risk would be managed with safe agents for anesthesia, whereas those who have not inherited the trait do not require such special treatment.

Pharmacogenetics and Pharmacogenomics

Malignant hyperthermia represents an example of a pharmacogenetic trait – a genetic trait in which expression of the phenotype requires exposure to a pharmacological agent. The effects of a drug in an individual are dependent on multiple variables: drug absorption, biochemical reactions that activate or inactivate the drug, distribution in the circulation, excretion, and interaction of the drug with its cellular target(s). Any of these variables can be subject to modification by genetic factors. The result is that the concentration of active drug can differ from person to person in spite of administration of the same dose, and the efficacy of the drug at any given serum concentration can likewise differ. These differences can include rare toxic reactions, such as is the case in malignant hyperthermia. Awareness of these inherited traits can be lifesaving, as we have seen, and can also avoid needless toxicity or, conversely, inadequate dosing in some individuals.

An important example of a drug metabolism pharmacogenetic trait involves the enzyme thiopurine methyltransferase (TPMT). TPMT is responsible for transfer of a methyl group to thiopurines, including the cancer chemotherapeutic agents 6-mercaptopurine and 6-thioguanine (Figure 16.3). Methylation of these drugs interferes with their ability to bind to DNA, and therefore inactivates the drug. Approximately one in 300 individuals is homozygous for a polymorphism that leads to deficient TPMT activity. These individuals fail to inactivate the drug, and therefore experience an exceptionally high level of activity from a standard dosage. 6-mercaptopurine is commonly used in the treatment of childhood leukemia. If drug dosage is not reduced in homozygous children, they may die from toxicity, since a standard dosage to them is, in effect, an overdose.

Another example is polymorphism of the gene CYP2D6, which encodes the enzyme debrisoquine hydroxylase, one of the P-450 family of hepatic oxidases. Oxidation by debrisoquine hydroxylase can modify a drug, either to an active or an inactive product (Figure 16.4). Common polymorphisms within the gene are associated with either excessive activity or diminished activity. Variants with decreased activity occur in 5–10% of whites in North America and 1–2% of African Americans. Gene duplications that result in rapid metabolism

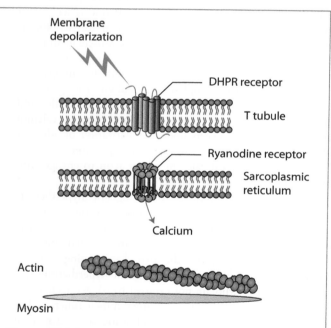

Figure 16.2 The ryanodine receptor resides in the sarcoplasmic reticulum membrane and is juxtaposed to the DHPR receptor in the T tubule, which is an invagination of the muscle cell membrane. Depolarization of the membrane results in opening of the ryanodine receptor, leading to entry of calcium into the cytoplasm. This, in turn, causes actin to interact with myosin, leading to muscle contraction. In individuals susceptible to malignant hyperthermia, mutation in the ryanodine receptor – or, more rarely, the DHPR receptor – leads to excessive calcium entry into the sarcoplasm.

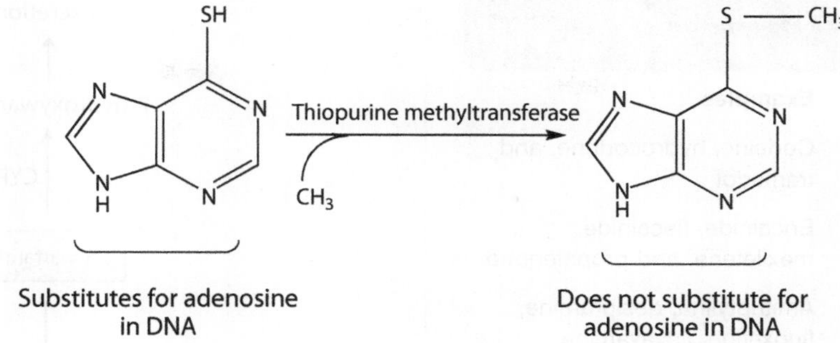

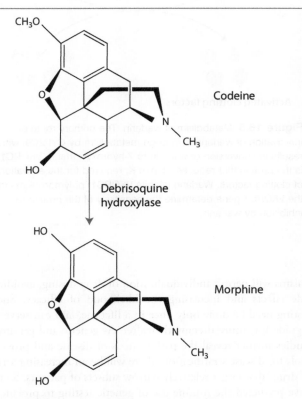

Figure 16.3 Thiopurine methyltransferase (TPMT) catalyzes methylation of 6-mercaptopurine and other sulfur-containing purines. The nonmethylated form is incorporated into DNA in the place of adenine, whereas the methylated form is not. In effect, then, TPMT inactivates the drug. An individual with low TPMT activity will accumulate a high concentration of the active drug, and be at greater risk of toxicity.

Figure 16.4 Conversion of codeine to morphine by debrisoquine hydroxylase. The pain-killing effects of codeine are dependent upon this reaction. Low debrisoquine hydroxylase activity will result in reduced efficacy, whereas high activity will cause excessive pharmacological effect.

occur in 5–10% of whites and 29% of Ethiopians. For a drug that is inactivated by debrisoquine hydroxylase, an individual with rapid metabolism will fail to achieve a therapeutic level and one with slow metabolism will accumulate the drug to the point of toxicity. For a drug that is activated by CYP2D6, rapid metabolism will lead to excessive activity, and slow metabolism to deficient activity. A list of drugs influenced by the polymorphism includes many in common use (Table 16.2).

Malignant hyperthermia is a prime example of a genetic variation that influences how a drug interacts with targets at the cellular level. Succinylcholine and halothane will induce malignant hyperthermia only in individuals with an at-risk genotype. Another example is a variant in a gene that encodes a sodium channel, *SCN5A*. The variant is present in 13% of African Americans, and places an individual at risk of cardiac arrhythmia when he or she is exposed to any of a number of commonly used medications, including some antibiotics.

The case of warfarin, a drug used to prevent blood clotting, illustrates both the potential power of pharmacogenetics and the challenges in implementation. Warfarin is the most common drug used to treat or prevent blood clotting. It is used, for example, to treat individuals with deep vein thrombosis, to prevent embolization of a blood clot to the pulmonary artery, where it might obstruct blood flow to the lungs (life-threatening pulmonary embolus). It is critical to get the dose of warfarin just right – too little risks blood clotting, whereas too much can lead to fatal hemorrhage. This is done by trial-and-error dosing – administering a standard dosage and monitoring the degree of impairment of blood clotting through a blood test. Two pharmacogenetic polymorphisms have been found to be important in determining the effects of the drug. One, *CYP2C9*, is involved in inactivating the drug, whereas the other, *VKORC1*, is involved in determining the sensitivity of the target protein (Figure 16.5). Testing polymorphisms in

Table 16.2 Examples of drugs metabolized by debrisoquine hydroxylase.

Drug class	Examples
Analgesics	Codeine, hydrocodone, and tramadol
Anti-arrhythmics	Encainide, flecainide, mexiletene, and propafenone
Antidepressants	Amitriptyline, desipramine, fluoxetine, fluvaxamine, imipramine, nortriptyline, and paroxetine
Antihistamines	Chlorpheniramine, diphenhydramine, and promethazine
Antipsychotics	Haloperidol, perphenazine, and thiridazine
Beta blockers	Carvedilol, metoprolol, propranolol, and timolol
Cough suppressants	Dextromethorphan

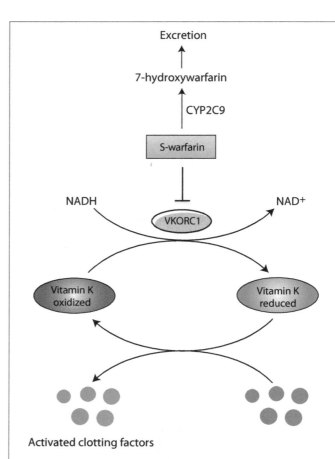

Figure 16.5 Metabolism of warfarin. The primary route of inactivation of warfarin is through metabolism by CYP2C9, which results in conversion of warfarin to 7-hydroxywarfarin. VKORC1 is the protein that reduces vitamin K, required for the activation of clotting factors. Warfarin inhibits VKORC1; polymorphisms in the *VKORC1* gene determine the sensitivity of the protein to inhibition by warfarin.

these two genes can enable a clinician to predict the dosage most likely to be safe and effective for an individual, potentially reducing the trial-and-error process, reducing costs, and improving outcomes.

In spite of this promise, there have been significant obstacles to overcome prior to wide-scale implementation. The decision to start a patient on warfarin is often made emergently, whereas standard genetic testing may take days to complete. It is feasible to return a result in hours instead of days, but this requires implementation of testing systems at the point of care, which is complex and expensive. There is a cost to testing, and it has not yet been determined that the costs of testing every patient who is started on warfarin are lower than the costs incurred from the trial-and-error dosing process, including the costs of managing side effects due to over- or under-dosing. Finally, physicians will need to be educated regarding how to adjust warfarin dosage based on pharmacogenetic testing. Efforts are underway to deal with these challenges, but this story underscores the point that a sound biological rationale is not sufficient reason to incorporate a new concept into routine medical practice.

Nevertheless, in the long run it is expected that pharmacogenetics will play a major role in the integration of genetics into routine medical practice; the use of genomic information to develop new drugs and identify new drug targets is called **pharmacogenomics**. Testing for drug metabolism polymor-phisms will permit individualization of drug dosing, avoiding side effects and increasing the likelihood of efficacy. Such testing need be done only once in a lifetime, and can serve as a guide for future therapy thereafter. As genetic and genomic studies further reveal the pathogenesis of disease and provide tools for disease stratification, there will be an increasing array of drugs that target relatively narrow subsets of patients. Some have predicted the routine use of genetic testing to provide a patient profile that will customize treatment, insuring the use of the correct medication at the correct dose in an individual patient. The day may be coming when virtually all treatment decisions are based on information obtained from genetic testing.

REFERENCE

Ali SZ, Taguchi A, Rosenberg H 2003, "Malignant hyperthermia", *Best Practice* and Research Clinical *Anaesthesiology*, vol. 17, pp. 519–33.

FURTHER READING

Evans WE, McLeod HL 2003, "Pharmacogenomics – drug disposition, drug targets, and side effects", *New England Journal of Medicine*, vol. 348, pp. 538–49.

Evans WE, Relling MV 2004, "Moving towards individualized medicine with pharmacogenomics", *Nature*, vol. 429, pp. 464–8.

Hopkins PM 2011, "Malignant hyperthermia: pharmacology of triggering", *British Journal of Anaesthesia*, vol. 107, pp. 48–56.

International Warfarin Pharmacogenetics Consortium 2009, "Estimation of the warfarin dose with clinical and pharmacogenetic data", *New England Journal of Medicine*, vol. 360, pp. 753–64.

Scott SA 2011, "Personalizing medicine with clinical pharmacogenetics", *Genetics in Medicine*, vol. 13, pp. 987–95.

Find interactive self-test questions and additional resources for this chapter at **www.korfgenetics.com**.

Self-Assessment

Review Questions

16.1   Why is genetic testing for the *RYR1* mutation not offered to all individuals as a prelude to surgery to avoid malignant hyperthermia?

16.2   What is the clinical utility of *TPMT* testing in individuals about to undergo chemotherapy with 6-mercaptopurine?

16.3   What is the value of *CYP2D6* testing in clinical practice?

16.4   What is the drug exposure risk associated with polymorphisms of sodium or potassium channel genes?

16.5   What is the principle behind disease stratification by genetic testing as a prelude to pharmacotherapy?

CHAPTER 17
Treatment of Genetic Disorders

Introduction

Understanding the molecular basis of genetic disease offers major hopes for diagnosis, prevention, and treatment. Treatment may take many forms, including surgery, pharmacological therapy, or in some cases actual repair of a genetic defect or replacement of a defective gene. Significant progress has been made in recent years toward developing therapeutic approaches, in many cases for conditions previously thought to be untreatable. In this chapter we will explore one disorder for which a mechanism-based treatment has been developed and tested, and now is available for clinical use. We will look at the approach to clinical trials of new treatments, and prospects for various therapeutic approaches that may emerge in the next few years.

Key points

- Understanding the pathogenesis of a genetic disorder may reveal targets for pharmacological-based therapies.
- Before a treatment is used on a routine clinical basis, clinical trials are conducted to demonstrate safety and efficacy and to continually monitor for adverse effects.
- A wide variety of approaches are being developed and applied to the treatment of genetic disorders, including approaches that may lead to correction of a genetic mutation.
- The therapeutic approach needs to be tailored to the particular genetic disorder and, in some cases, to the particular gene mutation.

PART I

👤 Though only 7 months old, Anna has already had an eventful life. She was born at term and seemed well as a newborn. She had an asymptomatic heart murmur, which has gradually disappeared. Recently, though, she began to develop episodes of staring and shaking that have concerned her mother. Anna's pediatrician has referred her to a child neurologist. The neurologist, Dr. Stevens, takes a history and, based on what he hears is concerned about seizures. He does a physician examination of Anna and finds her to be well, but notes several patches of hypopigmented skin (Figure 17.1). These are best seen with the Wood's lamp. He explains to Anna's parents that he is concerned about a possible seizure disorder, and also that Anna might have a condition called tuberous sclerosis. He arranges for an electroencephalogram (EEG) to be done, as well as a brain MRI (magnetic resonance imaging), renal ultrasound, echocardiogram, and eye exam.

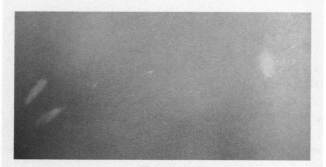

Figure 17.1 Multiple hypopigmented macules on back of child with tuberous sclerosis complex.

Tuberous sclerosis complex (TSC) (MIM 191100) is a dominantly inherited disorder that affects multiple systems of the body. It often presents in infancy with hypopigmented skin macules – flat patches of lightly pigmented skin. These are usually best seen with the Wood's lamp – an ultraviolet light used in an otherwise dark room. The spots are themselves harmless, but are an indication to look for other features of the disorder. One of the most concerning early signs involves the nervous system. Affected individuals are at risk of developing seizures, and, when these occur early in life there is often accompanying developmental impairment. Seizures can take many forms; the most worrisome are infantile spasms, which

are usually associated with severe developmental impairment. Developmental outcome can be improved by prompt diagnosis and treatment of the seizure disorder. The diagnosis of tuberous sclerosis complex is established clinically; criteria are listed in Table 17.1.

PART II

👤 The EEG does show evidence of seizure activity, and Dr. Stevens starts Anna on an anti-epileptic medication. The brain MRI also shows changes consistent with tuberous sclerosis complex (Figure 17.2). The echocardiogram shows a tiny spot that is interpreted as a probable cardiac rhabdomyoma, but it is not felt to be clinically significant. The renal ultrasound and eye exams are normal. He arranges for genetic testing, and Anna is found to have a mutation in the TSC2 gene. She is seen in the Genetics Clinic after the test results are available for genetic counseling. Family history reveals no known diagnosis of tuberous sclerosis in either parent or in any other family member.

A number of distinct lesions may be seen in the brains of individuals with tuberous sclerosis complex. The name of the disorder reflects swellings in the gyri that may be seen and were thought to resemble tubers. By MRI scanning one may see areas of abnormal cortical development as well as nodules in the subependymal region. The former are probably associated with the seizures and developmental impairment, but the latter, though useful diagnostic signs of the condition, do not in themselves cause neurological signs or symptoms. Infants with the disorder may have tumors in the myocardium, rhabdomyomas. Usually these are asymptomatic and tend to regress with time, though they can cause obstruction, heart failure, or cardiac arrhythmia. Renal lesions include cysts and tumors called angiomyolipomas (AML). AMLs can grow and lead to episodes of bleeding or can cause renal failure. Glial nodules may occur on the retina, which usually do not require treatment.

Tuberous sclerosis complex is a dominantly inherited condition with complete penetrance but variable expressivity. Either of two distinct genes may harbor pathogenic mutations; these are referred to as *TSC1* and *TSC2*. The protein products of these genes, named hamartin and tuberin, respectively, form a complex that regulates the activity of a protein involved in the control of cell growth and proliferation, referred to as mTOR (Figure 17.3). Mutation testing can be helpful to confirm a suspected diagnosis and can be used as a basis for genetic counseling.

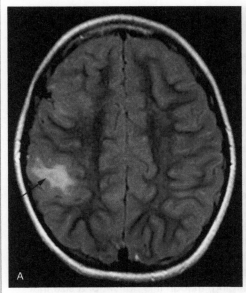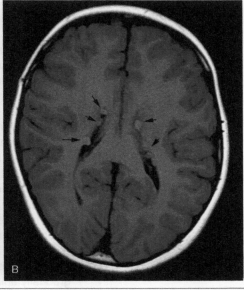

Figure 17.2 MRI scan showing typical brain lesions of tuberous sclerosis complex: (A) cortical dysplasia (arrow); and (B) multiple subependymal nodules (arrows).

Table 17.1 Diagnostic criteria for tuberous sclerosis complex.

Feature	Comments
Major features	
Facial angiofibroma or forehead plaque	Forehead plaque is collagenous deposition under skin.
Ungual or periungual fibromas	Nontraumatic soft tissue growths in or under nail beds on toes and fingers.
Hypomelanotic macules	Three or more; present at birth – best seen with Wood's lamp.
Shagreen patch	Connective tissue nevus, usually seen on back.
Retinal hamartoma	Multiple nodular hamartomas in retina.
Cortical tuber	Cerebral cortical dysplasia.
Subependymal nodule	Tend to calcify and are easily seen with CT scanning.
Subependymal giant cell astrocytoma	Located at foramen of Munro; may grow and cause hydrocephalus.
Cardiac rhabdomyoma	Usually congenital and tend to spontaneously regress.
Lymphangiomyomatosis	Usually present in adult females and are often associated with renal angiomyolipomas; may occur as sole feature, in which case they are not indicative of tuberous sclerosis complex.
Renal angiomyolipoma	Tumors of kidneys, as noted in this table, may occur in isolated cases in association with pulmonary lymphoangiomyomatosis; usually benign, but malignant change can occur.
Minor features	
Dental enamel pits	Multiple, randomly distributed pits in dental enamel.
Hamartomatous rectal polyps	Require histological confirmation.
Bone cysts	Confirmed Radiographically.
Cerebral white matter radial migration lines	Visible by MRI scanning or pathologically.
Gingival fibromas	Fibromas in gums.
Nonrenal hamartoma	Histological confirmation suggested.
Retinal achromic patch	Light or dark spots on retina.
Confetti skin lesions	Tiny white patches usually occurring in clusters.
Multiple renal cysts	Sometimes occur in association with deletion of *TSC2* gene and adjacent *PKD1* gene.

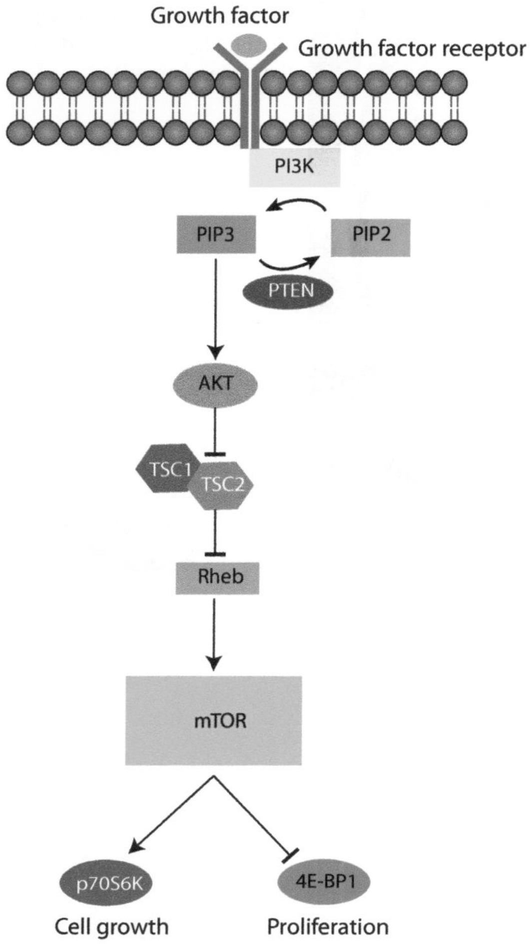

Growth factor

Growth factor receptor

PI3K

PIP3   PIP2

PTEN

AKT

TSC1 TSC2

Rheb

mTOR

p70S6K   4E-BP1

Cell growth   Proliferation

Figure 17.3 mTOR signaling pathway. Binding of ligand to membrane receptor activates PI3 kinase, which leads to phosphorylation of phosphatidylinositol biphosphase to triphosphate. This stimulates Akt, which inhibits the TSC1–TSC2 complex. This complex normally inhibits Rheb, which in turn stimulates mTOR. Activation of mTOR stimulates p70S6K and inhibits 4E-BP1, resulting in cell growth and proliferation. Mutation in the *TSC1* or *TSC2* genes leads to failure to inhibit Rheb, leading to increased mTOR activity, and ultimately increased protein synthesis, cell growth, and proliferation.

PART III

👤 Anna is now 7 years of age, and for the most part she has done well. Her seizures have been well controlled on medication, with very few episodes of recurrence. She has done well developmentally; she is a little behind in some cognitive skills, but attends regular classes and does well with extra help. Both of her parents had been evaluated by genetic testing, and neither was found to carry the TSC2 mutation.

They have had two other children since Anna was born, and both are well; neither has signs of tuberous sclerosis. Anna's parents have become involved in the local chapter of a patient support organization, and have helped many other families adjust to a new diagnosis. Anna has continued to have monitoring by brain MRI, renal ultrasound, and eye exam. She has not had any follow-up echocardiogram, and her cardiac function has been normal. Renal ultrasounds have shown some very small masses in the kidneys (Figure 17.4), but so far these have not required treatment. Her eye exams have also been normal. She has been found to have a mass in her brain, which Dr. Stevens has been monitoring by annual brain MRI. In this year's visit, he notes that the mass has been gradually enlarging, though it is not yet of a size that requires surgery (Figure 17.5A).

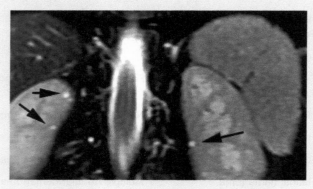

Figure 17.4 MRI of kidneys showing multiple small renal angiomyolipomas (arrows).

Approximately two-thirds of individuals with TSC are affected due to new mutation, with no signs of the condition in either parent. Parents can be offered genetic testing if the child's mutation is known, though negative testing does not rule out **germline mosaicism**. If the mutation is not known, parents can be examined for skin, eye, brain, and renal lesions by clinical assessment, MRI, and renal imaging. It is not unusual for a parent who is otherwise well to be diagnosed in this manner.

Affected individuals are offered surveillance for potential complications of the disorder. If cardiac rhabdomyoma is not symptomatic, it is unlikely to cause problems, as most regress in early childhood. Brain MRI is done to monitor for growth of a subependymal lesion, usually located at the foramen of Monro, that can obstruct cerebrospinal fluid (CSF) flow and lead to hydrocephalus. Although these are not malignant tumors, they are referred to as subependymal giant cell astrocytomas (SEGAs). Renal lesions are monitored by ultrasound or other imaging techniques such as computed tomography (CT) or MRI. Regular ophthalmological assessment is performed to monitor vision and the occurrence of retinal lesions. Adult women with TSC are at risk for lymphangiomyomatosis,

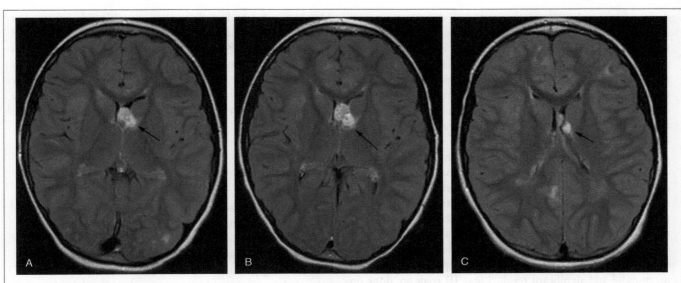

Figure 17.5 MRI showing subependymal giant cell astrocytoma (SEGA) at baseline (A), just prior to initiation of treatment (B), and after 1 year of treatment (C).

an infiltrative tumor of the lungs that can cause severe pulmonary disease.

PART IV

Two more years have passed, and Anna continues to do well overall. She has developed fairly noticeable facial angiofibroma (Figure 17.6), which has caused her to be quite self-conscious. She has recently had a brain MRI, and the mass has continued to grow (Figure 17.5B). Dr. Stevens has become increasingly concerned that she is likely to need surgery before she becomes symptomatic from the mass. Recently he has become aware that a medication has been developed that might be used to shrink the mass without surgery. He initially heard about this at an annual meeting of child neurologists, and subsequently he has read some of the literature on the topic. The medication is available by prescription, based on results of clinical trials that showed benefit of medication versus placebo. He discusses the possibility of treatment with Anna's parents, and they agree to go forward.

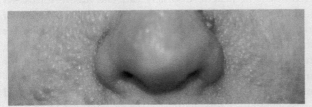

Figure 17.6 Facial angiofibroma in individual with tuberous sclerosis complex.

Aside from hypopigmented macules, skin lesions of TSC include angiofibroma, collagenous plaques, and periungual fibromas in the nail beds. The angiofibromas tend to occur in childhood and progress over the years; they can lead to significant cosmetic impairment and are not easy to treat.

SEGAs, as noted in this chapter, can cause ventricular obstruction and present with acute hydrocephalus. Lesions that are found to be growing and threaten this complication can be removed surgically. Given the invasive nature of this treatment, though, there has been major interest in finding nonsurgical approaches to management. The discovery of the *TSC1* and *TSC2* genes and the role of the hamartin–tuberin complex in control of mTOR signaling suggested a possible avenue of nonsurgical therapy. mTOR is so named because it is the mammalian form of a protein that is a "target of rapamycin." Rapamycin is a naturally occurring drug that has immunosuppressant effects, and is often used to prevent rejection of transplanted organs. Most lesions associated with tuberous sclerosis show loss of hamartin–tuberin due to mutation in both alleles of either *TSC1* or *TSC2*, indicating that these function as tumor suppressor genes. Consequent loss of function of the hamartin–tuberin complex leads to disinhibition of mTOR, resulting in hyperactivity of mTOR signaling. This raises the possibility that treatment of TSC patients with rapamycin might be useful in treatment of lesions associated with TSC.

Since rapamycin was available as a medication for immunosuppression, it was possible to treat some TSC patients with progressive SEGAs, and encouraging results were seen. This led to initiation of formal clinical trials using rapamycin (also called sirolimus), or an analog that tends to be better tolerated, everolimus.

A clinical trial is a formal study designed to test a medical intervention. A clinical trial involves the use of a carefully designed protocol to insure that testing is done in a rigorous and consistent manner. All participants must give their informed consent, and institutional ethics committees closely monitor the conduct of the trial. Treatment trials are designated as Phase 0, I, II, III, or IV. Phase 0 trials involve administration of an intervention (usually a drug) and determination of whether it is absorbed into the tissue intended to be treated; it may also explore whether the drug interacts with the tissue in the expected manner. Phase I trials are intended to determine safety of an intervention and, for a drug, the dosage that can be tolerated, any side effects, and the manner in which the drug is absorbed, metabolized, and excreted. Usually Phase I trials are done on a small number of patients, with no expectation of significant benefit. Phase II trials are intended to measure efficacy. They are done on larger numbers; the exact number who need to be treated depends on the outcome measures and statistical considerations required to achieve a meaningful and significant result. Phase III trials are done on larger numbers and compare results of treatment with the new approach to other conventional modes of treatment. Interventions that are deemed to be safe and effective may be approved in the United States by the US Food and Drug Administration (FDA), after which they may be marketed as a treatment. Phase IV involves surveillance of patients treated with the intervention to continue to monitor for adverse effects.

Clinical trials of everolimus were conducted for the treatment of SEGA in patients with tuberous sclerosis complex and did indicate both safety and efficacy. On this basis, the medication was registered with the FDA for use in patients with TSC for treatment of progressive SEGA.

PART V

👤 Dr. Stevens has reviewed the prescribing information for everolimus and discusses the risks and benefits with Anna's parents. He explains potential side effects, especially the possibility of suppression of the immune system and the occurrence of mouth sores. The plan is to start at an initial dosage based on Anna's body surface area, which he calculates from her height and weight. Anna is to be monitored by repeated blood level testing for a period of months until a therapeutic dosage level is attained, after which the frequency of monitoring can be reduced. She also has a number of blood tests done prior to treatment, including complete blood count, blood chemistries, liver and renal function tests, and blood lipid and cholesterol determination. All check out normal at the start, so the medication is begun.

The most common side effects of everolimus are mouth sores, immune suppression, and increases in lipids and cholesterol.

Monitoring is conducted for these possible side effects. The initial dosage is determined by body surface area, with blood levels guiding dosage changes. Mouth sores are managed with a mouthwash and might necessitate reduction of dosage if they become severe. The patient and doctor need to be vigilant for infection or kidney or respiratory problems. Patients may be treated with prophylactic antibiotics to prevent opportunistic infection.

PART VI

👤 Anna has been on everolimus for about a year and is doing very well. She has had intermittent problems with mouth sores, but has used a mouthwash to help manage these and they have not been a big problem. Her blood chemistries and lipid levels have remained in the normal range, though slightly elevated from baseline values. MRIs have shown measureable decrease in the size of the SEGA (Figure 17.5C). She is also doing well developmentally, and has not had any seizures in the past year. Finally, her skin has cleared significantly, to the point where the facial angiofibroma is barely visible. Anna and her parents are delighted with the results of treatment, and there is no plan to change the regimen.

Experience to date has indicated that everolimus can be effective in shrinking SEGAs. Although it has not yet been formally proven to be effective in treatment of other lesions such as angiofibromas, this is being investigated in the clinical trials. There are also studies ongoing to determine if clinical improvement in areas such as cognitive development and seizure control is seen. The necessary duration and long-term effects of treatment are also subjects of continuing study.

Therapy of Genetic Disorders

The idea of offering treatment for genetic disorders is not a new one; there is a long history of treatment of inborn errors of metabolism, for example based on dietary therapy. Advances at many levels, though, have significantly increased the scope of treatments that can be offered, with the prospect of expansion of treatment possibilities in the coming years.

Treatment of genetic disorders can take many forms. As noted in Chapter 11, dietary therapy for inborn errors of metabolism, such as restriction of phenylalanine intake for individuals with phenylketonuria, has been available for a long time. In some cases, enzyme activity can be stimulated for some inborn errors, for example by administration of a coenzyme (such as a vitamin). Some drugs have been developed that provide alternative pathways for excretion of toxic compounds, or reduction in the synthesis of substrates that might accumulate in some enzyme deficiency disorders. Some lysosomal storage disorders can be treated by enzyme replacement therapy. This involves intravenous infusion of a purified form of enzyme that contains exposed mannose-6-phosphate, enabling the enzyme to bind to membrane receptors and then be delivered to lysosomes through receptor-mediated endocytosis. Organ transplantation, such as transplantation of bone marrow or liver, has been used to correct some other enzyme deficiencies. In some cases, medications have been identified that can stabilize enzyme proteins in the cell that would otherwise be degraded due to an aberrant amino acid sequence due to mutation, at least partially restoring enzyme function.

The identification of genes that underlie various inherited disorders has helped to reveal the underlying cellular mechanisms that are disturbed when mutation alters the function of a critical protein. This has opened the door toward development of new approaches to treatment, using medications that modify the function of these pathways. This is the basis for treatment of tuberous sclerosis complex (described in this chapter), and also has been used in several other genetic disorders, including neurofibromatosis and Marfan syndrome, among others. Therapeutic compounds are usually identified in preclinical studies, first using cell culture systems and then using animal models of the condition. In some cases, a drug is identified that is already available for clinical use for other indications. This was the case with everolimus for TSC, and greatly accelerated the translation of therapy to clinical practice. If the drug is already available for other clinical indications, its safety profile may be known and physicians are able to prescribe it "off label" for patients with a problem that may be different from the one approved by the FDA. The pharmaceutical company cannot market the drug for off-label use, however. Only after the drug has passed appropriate clinical trials and been approved by the FDA can it be marketed for a new indication.

For many years, there has been hope that genetic disorders might be treatable directly at the genetic level. There has been a long history of experimental treatment using gene replacement approaches. These involve introduction of a normal version of a gene into target cells in a patient with the hope of restoring normal function. In most cases, the gene is intro-

duced by engineering a virus to include the genetic material and having the virus infect cells that would normally express the gene (Table 17.2). Although there has been major progress in the development of viral vectors and there have been some successes in treatment, gene therapy has been slow to develop and there have been significant setbacks along the way. It is extremely difficult to introduce a gene into a cell so that it will be expressed at physiologically normal levels in the right place and at the right time. There have also been concerns about side effects due to the inserted gene or the viral vector. Despite some setbacks, however, this remains an active area of clinical research.

Two other approaches to gene-level therapy have also been the subject of work in recent years. One involves efforts to restore function at the level of the gene itself. It has been found that aminoglycoside antibiotics and related chemical compounds can cause insertion of an amino acid at the site of a nonsense mutation that would otherwise cause premature termination of translation of a gene. This approach is being tested for disorders where nonsense mutations occur as a common type of mutation, for example Duchenne muscular dystrophy. The second approach is a form of gene replacement involving treatment of stem cells. It is possible to obtain cultured skin fibroblasts and convert them to stem cells by transfecting into these cells a set of genes that reprogram the cell to a more primitive, undifferentiated state. These cells are referred to as induced pleuripotent stem cells (iPS cells). Although it is not clear that they have the same plasticity as embryonic stem cells, it is clear that they can be differentiated into various cell types, such as blood cells or nerve cells. If a mutation can be corrected in these cells by introduction of a nonmutant form of the gene in cell culture, the cells can then be differentiated into the cell that needs to be corrected, for example blood cells, and then implanted back into the body. The approach offers the advantage that treatment can be done using cells from the individual being treated, avoiding risks of rejection as would occur in transplantation. Currently this approach is being tested in animal models, and, if successful in these systems, may eventually be tested in human clinical trials.

Table 17.2 Comparison of major vectors used in gene therapy.

System	Characteristics	Advantages	Disadvantages
Nonviral			
Naked DNA	Plasmid DNA exposed directly to target cells	Simplicity; lack of viral toxicity	Ex vivo Low efficiency of transfection
Cationic complexes	DNA complexed with cationic lipids or polylysine	Simplicity; lack of viral toxicity	Ex vivo Low efficiency of transfection
Gene gun	DNA forced into cells	Simplicity; lack of viral toxicity	Ex vivo
Viral			
Retrovirus	Single-stranded RNA vector that creates double-stranded DNA inside cell and integrates into chromosome	Stable integration of transfected DNA; wide range of susceptible cell types; relatively large capacity for inserted DNA	Insertional mutagenesis; only infects dividing cells
Adenovirus	Double-stranded DNA inserted into cell	Targets dividing and nondividing cells of many different types; relatively large capacity for inserted DNA; can be targeted to specific cell types	Lack of stable transfection; host immune response possible; possible toxicity of viral proteins
Adeno-associated virus	Single-stranded DNA with no viral genes; requires helper virus to package vector	Nonpathogenic; stable transfection as episome or integrated into chromosome; infects dividing and nondividing cells	Small capacity for inserted DNA; difficult to prepare
Herpes virus	Double-stranded DNA inserted into cell	Large capacity; tropism for nerve cells	Limited range of cells can be infected
Lentivirus	Retrovirus derived from HIV	Like retroviruses, but infects nondividing cells	Safety issues not clearly defined

FURTHER READING

Krueger DA, Care MM, Holland K, Agricola K, Tudor C, Mangeshkar P, Wilson KA, Myars A, Sahmoud T, Franz DN 2010, "Everolimus for subependymal giant-cell astrocytomas in tuberous sclerosis", *New England Journal of Medicine*, vol. 363, pp. 1801–11.

Roach ES, Gomez MR, Northrup H 1998, "Tuberous sclerosis complex consensus conference: revised clinical diag-nostic criteria", *Journal of Child Neurology*, vol. 13, pp. 624–8.

Staley BA, Vail EA, Thiele EA 2011, "Tuberous sclerosis complex: diagnostic challenges, presenting symptoms, and commonly missed signs", *Pediatrics*, vol. 127, pp. e117–25.

 Find interactive self-test questions and additional resources for this chapter at **www.korfgenetics.com**.

Self-Assessment

Review Questions

17.1 What is the biological rationale for use of mTOR inhibitors for the treatment of tuberous sclerosis complex?

17.2 What is the difference between a Phase I, Phase II, and a Phase III clinical trial?

17.3 A drug that has been approved for treatment of a specific disorder is discovered to also be effective in the treatment of a different genetic condition. What is required for the pharmaceutical company to market the drug for treatment of the genetic condition?

17.4 What is the difference between preclinical testing and a clinical trial?

17.5 What is the potential advantage of treatments based on use of iPS cells as compared with other methods of gene therapy or organ transplantation?

Answers to Review Questions

Chapter 1

1.1 The G–C base pairs have three hydrogen bonds rather than two for A–T pairs, making them more thermodynamically stable.

1.2 Transcription is required to synthesize short RNA primers that serve as a starting point for DNA synthesis.

1.3 RNA: AUG GUU GAU AGU CGU UGC CGC GGG CUG UGA

Peptide: met – val – asp – ser – arg – cys – arg – gly – leu

1.4 (1) Alternative promoters, leading to multiple, different proteins derived from the same gene; (2) alternative splicing, leading to different versions of a protein with or without various exons; (3) RNA editing may cause changes in the mRNA sequence after transcription; and (4) posttranslational modification of proteins.

1.5 Testing cultured fibroblasts in a heterozygous woman should produce two bands, but if clones of cells derived from a single cell are tested, only one of the two forms will be seen, due to X chromosome inactivation.

Chapter 2

2.1 A silent mutation might affect splicing, either by creating a new splice donor or acceptor sequence, or by affecting an exon splice enhancer. Such mutations would result in abnormal splicing. The hypothesis could be tested by looking at the RNA level, where one might see an abnormally spliced mRNA.

2.2 Stop mutation; frameshift mutation; splicing mutation that juxtaposes out of frame exons; and deletion of gene.

2.3 Nonsense-mediated decay might cause the degradation of RNA molecules with the stop mutation, leaving only wild-type molecules available for analysis.

2.4 If the mutation rate is 10^{-8} per nucleotide and there are 3×10^9 nucleotides per haploid genome, one might expect about 30 mutations per haploid germ cell.

2.5 A polymorphism can have phenotypic effects, including effects associated with medical problems. The term "polymorphism" conveys implications about frequency only, not the physiological effects of the change. Some common variants occur within genes and affect their function so that a disease phenotype results. Sickle cell anemia due to beta-globin mutation is an example.

Chapter 3

3.1 Bill and Zoe are not at risk of having a child with MELAS, since this is a mitochondrial disorder and Bill would not be at risk of passing it on. Zoe has a family history of developmental delay, however, in her maternal aunt's grandson. If this is an X-linked disorder, there is risk that Zoe could be a carrier and therefore might have an affected son.

3.2 It is possible that this is autosomal recessive, in which case the mutant allele must be relatively common, indicating that both partners of the father would be carriers. A more likely scenario, though, is autosomal dominant with either nonpenetrance in the father or germline mosaicism.

3.3 ½ × 0.75 = 0.375.

3.4 The disorder is expressed only in children who inherit the gene from their fathers. None of the children of an affected female is affected. The gene is probably expressed only in the paternal copy.

3.5 Anticipation is seen in conditions due to triplet repeat expansion. The larger the expansion, the earlier the age of onset and the more severe the disorder. Larger expansions are also prone to further expansion in the next generation. As a result, the expansion size increases from generation to generation, and severity increases accordingly.

Chapter 4

4.1 No; the bacteria would not be able to splice the introns out of the transcript to produce a functional mRNA. An insert derived from cDNA, where splicing has already occurred, would produce a functional product, provided that the insert is large enough.

4.2 Child c is recombinant. Allele 1 was inherited with the disease in the father of the sibship. The children who inherited 1 from the father are expected to have the disease and those who inherited 2 from the father are not affected. Child c inherited 1 from the father but is not affected. Assuming complete penetrance, this is best explained by recombination.

4.3 The lod score of −∞ implies that there was a recombination at $\theta = 0$ (i.e., the odds ratio at $\theta = 0$ was 0). This implies that the marker is not the actual disease gene.

4.4 In the past, after linkage was established it was necessary to "walk" along the chromosome to find an expressed sequence that corresponds with a gene of interest. Now, once linkage is established genes known to reside within the region can be directly tested for mutation in affected individuals.

4.5 This would cause mutation of the gene, probably associated with lack of expression of the gene product.

Chapter 5

5.1 This means that genes are not sufficient in themselves to determine the trait. There may be a genetic contribution, but

Human Genetics and Genomics, Fourth Edition. Bruce R. Korf and Mira B. Irons.
© 2013 John Wiley & Sons, Ltd. Published 2013 by John Wiley & Sons, Ltd.

something else, perhaps environmental factors or chance, also plays a role. There are also rare examples where identical twins will not share the same gene mutation, if the mutation arose somatically in just one twin.

5.2 For this trait it is always more likely that a female would be affected. The fact that their first child was of the less often affected sex implies that the recurrence risk is higher than if the affected child had been female.

5.3 The fact that the SNP is associated with the disease could be interpreted in many possible ways. It could be that the SNP itself alters function of the gene in such a way as to contribute to the disease. Alternatively, the SNP might be in linkage disequilibrium with another variant that is truly associated. The association also could be spurious, perhaps due to population stratification of the sample.

5.4 Much of the information that is provided through direct-to-consumer genetic testing is based on genetic association studies and should not be considered a diagnostic test. Since this type of testing does not either confirm or exclude the presence of disease, changes in medical management and therapy should not be based solely on these results. Your father should discuss this new information with his physician and determine how it might impact the management of his hypercholesterolemia

5.5 The haplotype map permits "tag SNPs" to be used as a marker for a haplotype block, which may be in the range of 10 kb in length. This reduces the number of SNPs that must be genotyped by an order of magnitude.

Chapter 6

6.1 The cell would normally pause before replicating DNA to either repair DNA damage or, if the damage is too severe, undergo apoptosis. Loss of TP53 causes the cell to continue to replicate DNA in spite of the presence of mutations, permitting the cell to accumulate mutations. Although most of such cells might not survive, some that do might become cancer cells.

6.2 Homologous centromeres separate during the first meiotic division. Not all homologous segments separate, since those that have undergone genetic recombination will not separate until the second meiotic prophase.

6.3 Nondisjunction occurred in his mother, since he received two chromosomes with alleles derived from his mother. The alleles are different, however, suggesting that nondisjunction occurred in meiosis I, such that he received both homologous chromosomes, with two different alleles.

6.4 The birth of a child with congenital anomalies is most likely for a pericentric inversion with a large inverted segment. Crossing over within the inversion loop gives rise to unbalanced products. If the inversion is paracentric, though, the products are dicentric or acentric, and are unlikely to be compatible with development. A pericentric inversion results in duplications and deficiencies of the chromosome, but chromosomes will be monocentric and therefore stable. If the inverted segment is large, there will be a higher chance for crossover

and the imbalance will be less severe and therefore more likely to be compatible with survival to birth.

6.5 (i) The copy number change is found in others with developmental impairment; (ii) if the child is sporadically affected, the change is *de novo* (i.e., not found in either parent), or if it is found in a parent, the child has an additional *de novo* change; or (iii) genes are located in the deleted region that may be associated with brain development.

Chapter 7

7.1 The woman has a two-thirds risk of being a carrier. The risk for her husband is derived from the Hardy–Weinberg equation:

$$q = 1/200; 2pq \sim 2(1/200) = 1/100$$

Therefore the risk of having an affected child is:

$$2/3 \times 1/100 \times 1/4 = 1/600$$

7.2 The carrier frequency is:

$$2 \times 1/20 = 1/10 \text{ (more precisely,}$$
$$2 \times 1/20 \times 19/20 = 19/200)$$

The risk of hemochromatosis in an offspring is:

$$1 \times 1/10 \times 1/2 = 1/20$$

Increased ability to absorb iron in heterozygotes might confer an advantage, maintaining this gene in the population.

7.3 $q^2 = 1/1600$. Therefore $q = 1/40$ and the carrier frequency $\approx 2q = 1/20$. This most likely represents a founder effect, in which a mutation becomes prevalent in a population that is small at the time when the mutation is introduced and in which the population remains relatively inbred.

7.4 Equilibrium is established in the first generation after migration, assuming that all the Hardy–Weinberg conditions are met. This would not be true for a sex-linked trait, however.

7.5 If [a] = p, [b] = q, and [c] = r, then the genotype frequencies can be calculated from:

$$(p + q + r)^2 = p^2 + q^2 + r^2 + 2pq + 2pr + 2qr$$

Therefore:

$$[bc] = 2pr = 2(0.3)(0.5) = 0.3$$

Chapter 8

8.1 It probably functions as a tumor suppressor gene. The lost allele would be the wild-type allele inherited from the mother. Radiation might stimulate loss of heterozygosity or acquisition of other genetic changes, contributing to tumor formation.

8.2 Such a mutation would lead to tumor formation in all cells of a susceptible tissue congenitally. It would likely be lethal.

8.3 The same two "hits" would occur in a tumor suppressor gene in a sporadic as in a familial cancer. It takes time for these two hits to accumulate in a cell to produce a sporadic cancer. If one hit is present in all cells, only a single additional hit needs to occur, which takes less time.

8.4 Chromosome translocation can activate a proto-oncogene by juxtaposing the gene with another gene that is actively transcribed. It is possible that a translocation could disrupt a tumor suppressor gene and thereby inactivate it.

8.5 Microsatellite instability indicates loss of function of one of the mismatch repair genes. It can be a sign of hereditary nonpolyposis colon cancer, which is a familial disorder inherited as a dominant trait.

Chapter 9

9.1 Interphase FISH may accurately diagnosis trisomy, but would not distinguish free trisomy 21 from trisomy due to a Robertsonian translocation. The latter would be important to identify because of the increased risk of recurrence in future pregnancies if one parent is a carrier.

9.2 The biochemical screen is not a diagnostic test. Depending on the components of the screen, sensitivity is between 60% and 80%. It is not 100% sensitive, however, and therefore some pregnancies at risk will not test positive.

9.3 The fetus would be at risk of uniparental disomy for chromosome 15, which could result in Prader–Willi or Angelman syndrome. Testing for UPD would be indicated.

9.4 Although a balanced reciprocal translocation generally does not cause gain or loss of genetic material, there can be exceptions. Sometimes there will be gains or losses at the site of translocation. In addition, a gene could be disrupted by the translocation, or there could be alteration of the expression of a gene due to "position effect." One way to further explore the significance of the translocation is to perform chromosome analysis on both parents. If the rearrangement is not present in either parent there is a greater likelihood that it is clinically significant, whereas if one parent has the same rearrangement it is less likely that it is the cause of the child's problems. Testing for uniparental disomy of the involved chromosomes also can be useful.

9.5 This individual has signs that could be compatible with chromosome 22 deletion syndrome, previously known as velo-cardiofacial syndrome (VCSF), associated with submicroscopic deletion of chromosome 22. A FISH or MLPA study should be done. If positive, there would be a 50% risk of transmission of the deleted chromosome to a child, who would also develop this condition.

Chapter 10

10.1 The fetus is at low risk of developing DMD. The two brothers received the 1–2 haplotype from their mother, who is an obligate carrier, and that haplotype was transmitted to the mother of the fetus, so she, too, is a carrier. The fetus, however, inherited the 3–4 haplotype, which is likely to be associated with a normal outcome.

10.2 There are many things that might help to determine whether the change is pathogenic. Has the change been seen before in affected individuals or in controls? If the disorder is present in the family, does the mutation track with the disease? If the child is the first family member affected, is the mutation present in either parent? Is the amino acid that is altered conserved in evolution? What is the predicted effect of the amino acid substitution on the function of the protein?

10.3 Sequencing the cDNA will reveal exon skips or insertions of intron sequence into the mRNA indicative of splicing mutations. These may be due to mutations within introns that would be difficult to detect with genomic DNA sequencing unless the entire genomic sequence, including introns, were studied.

10.4 His repeat size is in the range seen in affected individuals with Huntington disease (HD). HD displays age-dependent penetrance, though, so it is not guaranteed that he will become symptomatic before he might die of other causes.

10.5 Information about Noonan syndrome can be obtained at OMIM or GeneReviews. It is an autosomal dominant trait usually due to mutation of the gene *PTPN11*. Clinical molecular testing is available.

Chapter 11

11.1 Phenylalanine is cleared *in utero* through the placenta and begins to build up in the child only after birth. Mothers of children with PKU are heterozygous carriers, but their levels of phenylalanine hydroxylase are sufficient to metabolize both the mother's and fetus's phenylalanine.

11.2 Symptoms of lysosomal storage disorders occur due to the gradual buildup of undigested material within the lysosome. This requires time, typically months to years, to accumulate to the point where symptoms occur.

11.3 Mannose-6-phosphate enables the enzyme to bind to specific receptors in the cell membrane. Upon receptor-mediated endocytosis, the endocytic vesicles fuse with lysosomes, releasing enzyme into the organelle.

11.4 Assays such as the Guthrie bacterial inhibition test needed to be customized for each particular metabolic disorder to be tested. Tandem mass spectrometry provides data about a broad array of conditions in a single test based on mass spectra for a variety of metabolites.

11.5 (1) Substrate reduction; (2) removal of toxic metabolites; (3) enzyme replacement; (4) organ transplantation; (5) coenzyme supplementation; and (6) augmentation of enzyme action.

Chapter 12

12.1 A disruption involves the destruction of tissue during development, whereas deformation involves the alteration of shape without tissue destruction. Some teratogens are responsible for disruptions, based on tissue toxicity or interference with blood circulation.

12.2 Identification of a chromosome microdeletion that is associated with a specific pattern of malformations, such as the chromosome 22q11.2 deletion that causes the chromosome 22q11.2 deletion syndrome, allows investigators to identify the critical region of the deletion necessary for the clinical phenotype to be present. Once the critical region is identified, investigators can then study the gene(s) within the deleted segment in animal models to determine if mutation of one or more of the genes is responsible for the phenotype. Study of patients with the 22q11.2 deletion led to identification of the critical region for that condition that contained the *Tbx1* gene, which was subsequently shown to be responsible for abnormal cardiovascular development in mouse models.

12.3 Not necessarily. Some individuals with CHARGE syndrome have complete gene deletions detectable by microarray analysis or MLPA that are not detectable by sequencing. In addition, we may learn that another gene may cause the clinical features of CHARGE syndrome due to genetic heterogeneity.

12.4 Most of these disorders lead to early death or significant cognitive or physical impairment, any of which interferes with ability to reproduce. Parent-to-child transmission of a mutation will therefore be rare, except in cases of germline mosaicism. As a result, most cases arise by new mutation.

12.5 Hox genes are arranged in tandem arrays on the chromosome. The 3′ most genes are expressed in the most cephalad regions, with a progression of genes located in a 5′ direction being expressed more caudally.

Chapter 13

13.1 Yes. Both sickle cell anemia and beta thalassemia are seen in individuals of African descent, whereas beta thalassemia is common in the Mediterranean region. Compound heterozygotes with a beta thalassemia mutation and a sickle cell mutation do have a clinical hematological disorder (sickle–thalassemia).

13.2 Biochemical screening is offered if the biochemical test is less expensive and if it has higher sensitivity, which would be the case if there is a large diversity of mutations that can cause disease. DNA testing is used if the biochemical test does not accurately distinguish the carrier state or if it is difficult to do a biochemical test from readily available tissue such as blood.

13.3 The frequency of specific mutations differs in individuals of different ancestry. The residual risk to an individual who screens negative for mutation depends on the sensitivity of the mutation screen in that individual, which is largely dependent on ancestry.

13.4 Although complete sequencing will detect all mutations, there is also a possibility that variants will be found that are not pathogenic, or at least whose significance is unknown. Mutation screening panels are generally restricted to testing for mutations of known pathological significance.

13.5 There are many reasons to consider carrier screening aside from termination of an affected pregnancy. Other reproductive options can be considered, for example, such as use of a sperm or egg donor. Couples may also use screening for reassurance, or for planning for the medical needs of an affected child.

Chapter 14

14.1 Testing for Huntington disease may be done for a variety of reasons. Individuals may seek the reassurance of a negative test, recognizing that they may achieve the opposite if the test is positive. Test results may guide personal planning, such as arrangements for long-term care needs. Testing can also be done for reasons of family planning.

14.2 Presymptomatic genetic testing determines whether an individual at risk of inheriting a gene mutation has indeed inherited it, prior to onset of signs or symptoms of disease. Predispositional testing determines whether an individual is at increased risk of developing disease as compared with individuals in the general population.

14.3 An individual who is at risk of having inherited a gene mutation may wish to know if he or she has inherited it in order to be informed about risks of transmitting the trait to offspring. For a disorder with age-dependent penetrance, signs or symptoms may not be present at a time when reproductive decisions must be made.

14.4 The odds ratio compares his chance of developing the disease with that of the general population. This result indicates that the odds of his developing the disorder are 2.5 times higher than the population risk. If the disease is rare, however, there remains a high likelihood that he will not develop the disease.

14.5 It is possible that an individual who tests positive will be denied health, life, or disability insurance, or may be denied employment, although some of these risks should be avoided due to protection by laws. Although the individual is not affected by the disorder, if the test result were known, being at increased risk could trigger such responses. There is also concern that the individual may face a change in self-image, or in the way he or she is perceived by others.

Chapter 15

15.1 Breast cancer is rare in males, but occurs with increased frequency in *BRCA2* mutation heterozygotes. Testing of this man would be indicated, at least in part because of implications for his daughters, as well as other family members.

15.2 Testing for *BRCA1* or *BRCA2* mutations does not detect all possible mutations. Therefore, a negative test in the 30-year-old woman could mean either that she did not inherit a *BRCA* mutation, or that the mutation test did not detect it. Testing her affected relative offers a greater reliability. If her aunt is negative, it means that the mutation test would not pick up a mutation, or that a *BRCA* mutation is not responsible for the cancer in the family. If her aunt is found to have a mutation, the woman can be offered reliable testing to see if she inherited the mutation.

15.3 It is recommended that daughters of a BRCA gene mutation carrier be offered testing at an age when they can make an informed decision about being tested. Given that the cancers associated with BRCA mutation do not occur until adulthood, usually testing is offered beginning around 18 years of age.

15.4 It does substantially reduce the risk of cancer, but there could be residual tissue after surgery that could still result in occurrence of cancer.

15.5 It is important to carefully consider the risks of testing, in addition to the possible benefits. There is federal legislation that prohibits use of genetic information, including genetic testing, in decisions regarding health insurance or employment. It does not address disability or life insurance. Different states may offer additional protections.

Chapter 16

16.1 The RYR1 gene is large, and there is a wide diversity of mutations. DNA testing would not be cost effective, and there is a risk of missing some mutations. Testing of muscle requires invasive biopsy and is expensive and difficult to perform.

16.2 Those who have a polymorphism that renders them slow metabolizers are at risk of accumulation of toxic levels of the drug, which can cause bone marrow failure and may be lethal. In such individuals, the drug dosage would be adjusted to avoid toxicity.

16.3 Many drugs are metabolized by the CYP2D6 enzyme. Knowledge of genotype can provide a basis for adjustment of drug dosage to avoid toxic side effects or to insure therapeutic levels.

16.4 Individuals who carry specific sodium or potassium channel polymorphisms are at risk of cardiac arrhythmia upon exposure to certain drugs.

16.5 Disease stratification involves discernment of genetic differences in pathogenesis of disease that occur among individuals with what seems to be the same disorder. This permits precise matching of treatments with specific individual needs.

Chapter 17

17.1 The products of the TSC1 and TSC2 genes function to inhibit mTOR activation. Mutation of either gene is therefore associated with hyperactive mTOR. Drugs that reduce mTOR activity are therefore potential therapeutic candidates.

17.2 A phase I trial is intended to determine the safety and maximum tolerated dosage of a drug. A phase II trial is designed to test efficacy. A phase III trial is intended to compare the efficacy of the treatment to established modes of treatment in large populations.

17.3 In order to market the drug for this new indication, separate clinical trials must be done so that the drug can be registered for this indication by the FDA.

17.4 Preclinical testing involves study of a drug in a model system, such as cell culture or an animal model, whereas a clinical trial is done in humans. The goal of preclinical testing is to screen a drug for safety and efficacy prior to launching clinical trials.

17.5 Induced pleuripotent stem cells (iPS cells) are derived from the individual to be treated and then differentiated into cells that are needed to treat the disorder. As such, they are not "foreign" transplanted cells and therefore should not induce an immune reaction.

Glossary

acrocentric   placement of centromere near one end of a chromosome

adenine   one of four bases of DNA; abbreviated "A"; pairs with thymine or uracil

age-dependent penetrance   increasing likelihood of manifesting signs or symptoms of a genetic disorder with increasing age

allele   specific form of a gene

alpha-fetoprotein (AFP)   protein secreted during fetal life; high AFP is indicative of congenital anomalies such as open neural tube defects; low AFP can be a sign of Down syndrome

alpha-satellite DNA   repeated DNA sequence enriched at chromosome centromeres

alternative splicing   different patterns of exon splicing of a transcript, resulting in production of peptides that differ in amino acid sequence

Alu sequence   one of a class of intermediate repeated DNA sequences, concentrated within coding regions of the genome

amino acid   chemical building block of a protein, consisting of an amine group, a carboxyl group, and one of 20 specific functional groups

amino acid substitution   mutation that leads to production of a peptide with a different amino acid at one site

amniocentesis   method of prenatal diagnostic testing in which a sample of amniotic fluid is withdrawn for analysis

amniotic fluid   fluid that bathes the fetus within the amniotic cavity, consisting largely of fetal urine with skin, bladder, and amnion cells

anaphase   the stage of mitosis in which the two chromatids separate and move toward the poles

aneuploidy   nonintegral multiple of the haploid chromosome set due to one or more missing or extra chromosomes

A site   site in ribosome that will accept next amino acyl tRNA to bind to growing peptide

anticipation   phenomenon whereby a genetic disorder becomes more severe from one generation to the next; characteristics of triplet repeat expansion disorders

anticodon   tRNA sequence that recognizes codon in mRNA to insert appropriate amino acid into the growing peptide

antisense oligonucleotide   sequence of DNA that is complementary to part of an mRNA, used to specifically inhibit expression of that gene

apoptosis   programmed cell death

autocrine growth control   production of growth factor by the same cell that responds to that factor

autosomal dominant   mode of genetic transmission wherein a single mutant allele is sufficient to produce a phenotype, carried on a non-sex chromosome

autosome   non-sex chromosome

bacterial artificial chromosome (BAC)   cloning vector that allows replication of inserted DNA in bacteria cells, allowing cloning of very large segments

bacteriophage   virus that infects bacterial cells

balanced polymorphism   genetic variant that is maintained at relatively high frequency in a population due to selection against homozygotes for the wild-type or variant sequence, with fitness being highest in heterozygotes

balanced translocation   exchange of segments between chromosomes so that no genetic material is lost or gained

Barr body   condensed chromatin representing inactivated X chromosome in interphase cell

bioinformatics   use of computers to catalog and analyze large sets of biological data

blastomere   pluripotent embryonic cell during the first few divisions following fertilization

branch point   point within intron to which splice acceptor sequence binds during splicing process

Human Genetics and Genomics, Fourth Edition. Bruce R. Korf and Mira B. Irons.
© 2013 John Wiley & Sons, Ltd. Published 2013 by John Wiley & Sons, Ltd.

candidate gene   gene thought to be involved in a specific genetic trait or disorder on the basis of mapping information or physiologic evidence

carboxyl terminal   last amino acid in a protein (in order of assembly)

carrier   individual who has a mutant gene (usually used to describe individual who does not manifest signs of the trait)

case–control study   study of genetic association in which one compares the frequency of an allele in a cohort of affected individuals with a control cohort

C banding   chromosome-staining technique that produces dark staining at centromeres

centimorgan   unit of genetic distance corresponding with 1% recombination

centromere   site of attachment of spindle fibers to the chromosome representing the last point of separation of replicated chromatids

centromeric heterochromatin   highly condensed chromatin near the centromere consisting of repeated DNA

checkpoint protein   protein involved in pausing cell cycle to repair DNA damage

chorionic villus sampling (CVS)   method of prenatal diagnosis in which fetal placenta is sampled either transabdominally or transcervically

chromatid   one of two replicated arms of a chromosome

chromatin   DNA with associated proteins

chromosomal rearrangement   changes of chromosome structure that can involve single chromosomes or an exchange of material between chromosomes

chromosome   structure in cell on which genes are located, consisting of a highly compacted stretch of DNA with associated proteins

chromosome abnormality   clinically significant change of chromosome number or structure

chromosome banding   means of staining chromosomes to elicit characteristic and specific patterns to aid chromosome identification

chromosome painting   means of staining a chromosome based on hybridization with fluorescent-labeled DNA sequences specific to that chromosome

clone   group of cells derived from a common progenitor; in recombinant DNA denotes a purified sequence of DNA

coactivator   protein that interacts with transcription factor to activate transcription

codon   triplet of bases that encode a specific amino acid

cofactor   substance that participates, along with an enzyme, in a chemical reaction

colchicine   chemical that disrupts the mitotic spindle; used to collect cells at metaphase for chromosome analysis

comparative genomic hybridization   method in which a control and reference DNA sample are competitively hybridized to a reference sequence used to detect deletions or duplications

complementarity   occurrence of sequence of bases in DNA or RNA that will form stable double helix by pairing of A to T (or U) and G to C

complementary DNA (cDNA)   DNA copy of RNA made using enzyme reverse transcriptase

complementary DNA (cDNA) library   collection of cloned DNA sequences, representing portion of sequences transcribed in the cells or tissue of origin

complex segregation analysis   analysis of pattern of genetic transmission that tests various models to explain dataset, establishing a best-fit model

compound heterozygote   individual with two different mutant alleles at a locus

conditional knockout   mouse model in which a target sequence is flanked by repeated sequences that undergo recombinational excision when another element, referred to as *cre*, is activated by a tissue-specific promoter

congenital anomaly   structural abnormality present at birth

consanguinity   blood relationship between a couple

conservative change   substitution of one amino acid for another with similar chemical properties, with little or no effect on the structure and function of the protein

consultand   individual seeking genetic counseling

contig   set of overlapping clones of DNA covering a large region

corepressor   protein that interacts with transcription factor to repress transcription

cosmid   cloning vector consisting of plasmid with sequences that allow packaging in a lambda phage head; used for cloning large segments of DNA

CpG dinucleotides   adjacent pair of nucleotides, with 5′-C-G-3′; the C in this location may be methylated

CpG islands — region in which there are many CpG dinucleotides, often near the 5′ end of a gene

crossover — consequence of genetic recombination

cryptic donor or acceptor — sequence within an intron that can serve as a splice donor or acceptor if the usual site is disrupted by mutation

CVS — acronym for chorionic villus sampling

cyclin — protein involved in control of cell cycle

cyclin-dependent kinase (CDK protein) — enzyme involved in phosphorylation of proteins involved in cell cycle

cytogenetic — pertaining to chromosomes

cytogenomics — use of genomic technologies to detect copy number changes in chromosomes

cytokinesis — process of separation of two daughter cells at end of mitosis

cytosine — one of four bases of DNA; abbreviated "C"; pairs with guanine

deformation — alteration of developing structure in embryo or fetus due to extrinsic pressure

deletion — mode of mutation due to loss of large chromosomal region

denaturation — separation of double-stranded nucleic acid into single strands

dideoxy sequencing — mode of DNA sequencing using 2′ deoxynucleotides

digenic inheritance — mode of inheritance in which heterozygosity at two separate loci lead to phenotype

dinucleotide repeat — stretch of DNA containing a pair of bases (often C–A) repeated many times; repeat number may by polymorphic

diploid — having two copies of each chromosome (except sex chromosomes)

disomic — having two copies of a specific chromosome

disruption — alteration of developing structure in embryo or fetus due to destruction of tissue

dizygotic twins — twins resulting from separate fertilization events

DNA — acronym for deoxyribonucleic acid, the chemical basis of heredity

DNA polymerase — enzyme responsible for replication of DNA

DNA transposon — form of repeated sequence similar to transposable genetic elements in bacteria

dominant — allele that exerts its phenotypic effect whether present in heterozygous or homozygous state

dominant negative — mutation in which the gene product of one allele exerts an inhibitory effect on the function of the system

dosage compensation — mechanism of equalizing X-linked gene expression in males and females by suppression of most genes on one X in females

Down syndrome — complex of congenital anomalies resulting from an extra copy of chromosome 21

duplication — mode of mutation due to repetition of one or more bases of DNA, or of a chromosomal region

dysmorphology — study of structural abnormalities of human development

electrophoresis — separation of chemical substances by differential migration in an electric field

elongation factor — protein involved in process of translation in ribosome

endoplasmic reticulum — subcellular structure representing site of protein synthesis

enhancer element — sequence that binds to proteins that "open" the DNA in the region of the promoter

enzyme — protein that catalyzes a specific chemical reaction

ethidium bromide — fluorescent dye that intercalates into DNA; used to stain DNA

exome — component of genome consisting of protein-encoding sequences (exons)

exon — segment of gene that encodes amino acid sequence of protein; adjacent exons are separated by introns, which are spliced out during RNA processing

exon junctional complex — ribonucleoprotein complex remnant of splicing apparatus at junctional between exons in spliced mRNA

exon skipping — mutation that alters pattern of splicing and results in splicing out of an exon

expressivity — range of phenotypic variability of a genetic trait in a population

extinction — elimination of a genetic trait from a population due to selection or genetic drift

fertilization — union of sperm and egg leading to initiation of embryonic development

fibroblast — cell type prevalent in connective tissue

FISH — acronym for fluorescence *in situ* hybridization

fixation — establishment of an allele as the sole allele at a given locus in a population due to extinction of other alleles

fluorescence in situ hybridization (FISH)
means of localization of cloned segment of DNA on chromosome by binding of complementary DNA and visualization by fluorescence microscopy

founder effect
prevalence of a specific allele in a population due to its presence in one of the original members of the population and tendency of members of the population to be relatively inbred

fragile X syndrome
genetic disorder associated with the expansion of a triplet repeat at the FMR 1 locus; associated with X-linked mental retardation

frameshift
mutation that disrupts the sequence so that the reading frame is altered

fraternal twins
nonidentical twins

G1 phase
portion of cell cycle after mitosis prior to next round of cell division

G2 phase
portion of cell cycle between DNA synthesis and mitosis

G-banding
mode of chromosome staining by Giemsa resulting in characteristic patterns of light and dark bands along chromosome

gene walking
cloning overlapping segments of DNA to isolate large region starting from single cloned site

genetic counseling
means of communication by medical professionals to an individual or family to educate them about natural history and genetics of a clinical disorder, along with available options for testing and treatment

genetic determinism
concept that genetic factors are completely determinant of phenotypic characteristics

genetic drift
fluctuation of frequency of an allele in a small population from generation to generation due to statistical variation

genetic heterogeneity
occurrence of multiple alleles at a gene locus or multiple loci that result in a similar phenotype

genetic linkage
proximity of a set of gene loci on the same chromosome

genetic modifier
gene that alters the phenotype associated with another gene

genome
collection of genes in an organism

genome-wide association study (GWAS)
study used to identify genetic markers associated with common disorders

genomic library
collection of cloned DNA fragments from random sites in the genome

genomics
the study of large sets of genes, or gene products, including the entire genome or the entire set of transcripts or proteins

genotype
set of specific alleles at a gene locus in an individual

germ cell
sperm or egg cell

germline mosaicism
occurrence of two or more cell lines derived from a single fertilization event but differing by presence or absence of one or more mutant alleles

guanine
one of four bases of DNA; abbreviated "G"; pairs with cytosine

GWAS
acronym for genome-wide association study

haploid
having only one complete set of chromosomes

haploinsufficiency
presence of only a single functional copy of a gene due to mutational loss of the other allele

haplotype
set of alleles at a group of linked genes together on a specific chromosome

HapMap
map of haplotypes of single-nucleotide polymorphisms that have been co-inherited through human evolution

Hardy–Weinberg equilibrium
mathematical statement of the relation between allele frequencies and frequencies of corresponding genotypes in a population

helicase
enzyme that unwinds DNA double helix at site of DNA replication

hemizygosity
presence of one copy of a gene at a given locus instead of two; applies to X-linked genes in males, or any gene whose homologous copy has been deleted

heritability
statistical measure of the contribution of genetics to a multifactorial trait

heterochromatin
chromatin that remains highly condensed during interphase and usually contains DNA that is genetically inactive

heteroduplex
double-stranded molecule derived from two similar, but not identical, DNA or RNA sequences

heteroplasmy
occurrence of two or more populations of genetically distinct mitochondrial DNAs in a cell

heterozygote advantage
selective advantage of heterozygous individuals over homozygotes; results in balanced polymorphism

heterozygous
having two different alleles at a gene locus

histones
basic proteins that form a complex with DNA in chromosome

HLA
acronym for human lymphocyte antigen region on chromosome 6

homeobox (Hox)	DNA sequence that encodes a 60 amino acid region that is common to homeotic genes	**isochromosome**	abnormal chromosome formed from duplication of either the short or long arms
homeotic genes	genes involved in the control of development, discovered originally in *Drosophilia* mutants, that lead to alteration in structures forming in specific body segments	**kb**	abbreviation for kilobase
		kilobase	one thousand bases
homologous chromosomes	pair of chromosomes, one inherited from each parent	**lagging strand**	strand of DNA synthesized in a set of smaller fragments (Okazaki fragments) at a DNA replication fork
homozygous	having a pair of identical alleles for a particular gene	**large-scale variation**	polymorphism of copy number of segmental duplications
housekeeping genes	genes that are expressed in a wide variety of cell types and are involved in common, basic mechanisms of cell physiology	**LCR**	abbreviation for low-copy repeat (synonymous with segmental duplication)
Hox	abbreviation for homeobox	**leading strand**	strand of DNA synthesized in a continuous fragment from a DNA replication fork
hybridization	formation of double helix from complementary strands of DNA or RNA derived from different sources	**lethal trait**	genetic trait that renders an individual unable to reproduce
hypermutability	genetic trait that leads to high rate of mutation during DNA replication; characteristic of some neoplastic cells	**liability**	tendency toward expression of a multifactorial trait, consisting of a combination of genetic and nongenetic factors
identical twins	monozygotic twins	**library**	set of cloned nucleic acid segments (genomic or cDNA)
imprinting	differential expression of maternally and paternally derived genes	**LINE sequence**	type of repeated DNA, concentrated in noncoding segments
in situ **hybridization**	technique of identifying chromosome region that contains sequence complementary with a cloned segment of DNA	**linkage**	proximity of a set of gene loci on the same chromosome
		linkage disequilibrium	nonrandom association of alleles at linked loci
indel	mutation consisting of insertion and deletion of bases of DNA	**linkage equilibrium**	random association of alleles at linked loci
informative mating	mating in which one partner is heterozygous such that the polymorphic marker and alleles can be distinguished from those contributed by partner to offspring; used in genetic linkage analysis	**locus**	site of specific DNA sequence on chromosome
		lod score	logarithm of odds ratio of likelihood of data given specified value of recombination compared with random segregation; often abbreviated z
informativeness	likelihood of informative mating for particular genetic polymorphism	**long interspersed element (LINE)**	form of repeated sequence >400 base pairs in length
initiation complex	set of transcription factors and RNA polymerase that bind to promoter to initiate transcription	**loss of heterozygosity**	phenomenon wherein a polymorphic marker that is heterozygous in somatic cells is homozygous or hemizygous in tumor cells due to loss of one allele
insertional mutation	mutation resulting from insertion of one or more bases into DNA	**LTR retroposon**	form of repeated sequences derived from retrovirus-like elements
interspersed repeated sequences	set of repeated sequences interspersed at multiple sites within genome	**Lyon hypothesis**	scheme of dosage compensation involving inactivation of one X chromosome in every cell in females; formulated by Mary Lyon
intron	segment of noncoding DNA between exons, spliced out during RNA processing	**lysosomal storage disease**	clinical disorder due to absence of activity of a specific lysosomal enzyme, leading to buildup of substrate in lysosome
inversion	mutation due to reverse orientation of a segment of DNA		

M phase   *See* mitosis

malformation   abnormality of the formation of a fetal structure

marker gene   polymorphic DNA sequence used in linkage mapping

massively parallel sequencing   approach to simultaneous sequencing of large populations of DNA fragments

maternal transmission   characteristic of mitochondrial genetic traits, passed from a mother to all her offspring

maximum likelihood estimate   value of recombination fracture (θ) at which peak lod score is obtained

Mb   abbreviation for megabase

megabase   one million bases

meiosis   process of reduction division in germline, leading to formation of haploid germ cells

Mendelian trait   genetic trait that follows patterns of simple Mendelian inheritance

messenger RNA (mRNA)   processed gene transcript ready for translation into protein

metacentric   presence of centromere at center of chromosome

metaphase   stage of cell division when chromosomes are aligned at the center of the cell prior to separation

metastasis   spread of neoplastic cells from their site or origin to remote sites

methylation   addition of methyl groups to cytosine bases (usually at CpG dinucleotides)

microarray   grid of multiple DNA fragments fixed to a glass slide for hybridization to test sequence

microRNAs (miRNAs)   RNAs that do not encode protein

microsatellite polymorphisms   DNA sequence variants due to different numbers of repeats of a simple sequence

misattributed parentage   finding that the stated father or mother is not the biological parent of the child

missense mutation   base change in the coding sequence of a protein that leads to amino acid substitution

mitochondrial DNA   circular double-stranded DNA within mitochondrion that encodes 13 mitochondrial proteins, and transfer and ribosomal RNAs

mitochondrion   organelle in cell involved in aerobic metabolism

mitosis   process of cell division

mitotic spindle   structure in dividing cells that pulls chromatids to opposite poles to make daughter cells

molecular diagnostic testing   identification of specific nucleic acid sequences for medical diagnosis

monosomy   presence of one rather than two copies of a specific chromosome in an individual

monozygotic twins   genetically identical twins resulting from a single fertilization event

mosaicism   occurrence of two or more genetically distinct cell lines derived from a common progenitor

Müllerian duct   embryonic structure that gives rise to uterus and fallopian tubes

multifactorial inheritance   traits determined by a combination of multiple genetic and/or nongenetic factors

multiplex PCR   simultaneous amplification of multiple sequences in a single reaction using multiple sets of primers

mutation   change in the sequence of DNA at a genetic locus

neoplasm   clone of cells released from normal controls of growth

next-generation sequencing   new DNA-sequencing technologies that permit rapid and high-throughput DNA sequencing

nondirective counseling   approach to genetic counseling in which the counselor provides information and encourages the consult and to make an individual decision without influence by the counselor's views

nondisjunction   failure of proper chromosome segregation, leading to both copies of a chromosome (or both chromatids) going to the same daughter cell

nonhistone protein   protein associated with DNA, not one of the basic histone proteins

nonpenetrance   the absence of phenotype in a person known to carry a specific mutant gene

nonsense mutation   mutation that changes a codon for an amino acid to a stop codon

nonsense-mediated decay   process whereby mRNA carrying a nonsense mutation is degraded in cell

nucleolus organizer regions   sites on acrocentric chromosomes containing ribosomal DNA

nucleosome   knoblike structure consisting of approximately 140 base pairs of DNA and associated histones, forming a structural unit of chromatin

nucleotide	base of DNA or RNA
Okazaki fragments	short segments of newly synthesized DNA on lagging strand at replication fork
oligonucleotide	segment of several bases of DNA or RNA
oncogene	gene that confers some neoplastic properties on a cell, usually derived by activation of a proto-oncogene
oogonial cell	immature egg cell, prior to meiosis
open reading frame	region of cDNA sequence starting with an AUG codon that initiates protein synthesis and including a region that encodes protein, ending at a stop codon
p arm	short arm of a chromosome
paired box (Pax)	DNA-binding domain of set of gene products involved in development, consisting of 128 amino acids
paracentric inversion	inversion of chromosome region not involving centromere
pathogenic mutation	mutation responsible for a genetic disorder
Pax	abbreviation for paired box
pedigree	diagram of family using standard symbols
penetrance	expression of genetic trait in an individual with mutant genotype
peptidyl transferase	enzyme involved in formation of peptide bond in translation
pericentric inversion	inversion of chromosome region involving centromere
phage lambda	bacterial virus used as a cloning vector
pharmacogenetics	genetic traits that influence the way drugs are absorbed, distributed, excreted, or reacted to physiologically
pharmacogenomics	use of genomic information to develop new drugs and identify new drug targets
phenotype	physical manifestations resulting from a specific genotype
phytohemagglutinin	substance derived from kidney beans that stimulates division of T cells; used to culture cells for chromosomal analysis
plasmid	circular double-stranded DNA capable of autonomous replication in bacterial cells; used as a cloning vector
pleiotropy	diverse physical characteristics resulting from a single genetic trait
point mutation	single base change of DNA sequence
polyacrylamide gel electrophoresis	method for high-resolution separation of nucleic acids or proteins

polygenic inheritance	traits determined by two or more separate genes
polymerase chain reaction (PCR)	means of amplification of a DNA sequence by multiple cycles of replication starting from the pair of primers that flank the sequence
polymorphism	occurrence of at least two alleles at a locus each having a frequency of at least 1%
polyploidy	the occurrence of one or more entire extra sets of chromosomes
population genetics	study of the factors that influence the frequency of genetic traits in a population
positional cloning	means of cloning a gene based on its location in the genome
predispositional test	genetic test used to determine if an individual is at increased risk of disease
preimplantation diagnosis	genetic diagnosis from early embryo, prior to implantation in uterus
premutation	sequence variation that predisposes to mutation; usually moderate expansion of a triplet that leads to further expansion, such as in fragile X syndrome
prenatal diagnosis	diagnosis of a medical problem in embryo or fetus
presymptomatic test	genetic test to determine if an individual carries a gene mutation to determine risk of disease prior to onset of symptoms
primer	oligonucleotide used as the point of initiation of DNA synthesis
proband	individual in family who brings family to medical attention
probe	cloned nucleic acid sequence used to identify homologous sequence by nucleic acid hybridization
prokaryote	microorganism lacking cell nucleus promoter region site of initiation of transcription at which RNA polymerase and regulatory factors bind
prophase	stage of mitosis when nuclear membrane disappears and chromosomes condense
proteome	entire set of gene proteins
proto-oncogene	cellular gene that, when appropriately altered, becomes an oncogene
pseudoautosomal	gene located on both the X and Y chromosomes, and hence segregating as an autosomal locus
pseudodominant	pattern of transmission of a recessive trait in which one partner is homozygous and one is heterozygous, leading to apparent vertical transmission of the trait

pseudogene — DNA sequence with substantial homology to a gene, but not encoding protein

P site — site in ribosome that carries the growing peptide chain

purine — chemical structure of adenine and guanosine

pyrimidine — chemical structure of thymine, cytosine, and uracil

q arm — long arm of a chromosome

random segregation — independent segregation of nonlinked genes to gametes

reading frame — set of triplet codons in a gene that encode the protein

recessive — allele that exerts its phenotypic effect only if present in homozygous state

reciprocal translocation — exchange of segments between two or more chromosomes

recombination — association of new set of alleles in coupling on a given chromosome due to crossing over in meiosis

recombination fraction (θ) — probability of recombination between two genetic loci

release factors — proteins involved in release of complete peptide from ribosome during protein translation

renaturation — re-annealing of separated single strands of nucleic acid into a double helix

reproductive fitness — relative ability of individuals with a specified genotype to reproduce

response element — sequence in promoter region that binds transcription factors

restriction endonuclease — enzyme that cuts DNA at a defined sequence, usually consisting of 4–8 bases

reverse transcriptase — enzyme present in retroviruses that copies RNA into DNA

ribosomal RNA (rRNA) — RNA component of ribosome

ribosome — cellular structure involved in translation of mRNA into protein

ring chromosome — chromosome abnormality in which ring forms following breakage of both long and short arms

RNA — acronym for ribonucleic acid, a single-stranded nucleic acid involved in protein synthesis

RNA interference — process whereby small single-stranded RNA molecule binds to mRNA and inhibits translation

RNA-seq — method of detection of RNA molecules expressed by cells or in a tissue based on massively parallel sequencing of cDNA copies of the RNA

Robertsonian translocation — translocation involving fusion of the long arms of a pair of acrocentric chromosomes

S phase — part of cell cycle when DNA synthesis occurs

segmental duplication — blocks of 10–300 kb of homologous DNA sequence repeated at multiple sites in the genome

selection — impairment of reproductive fitness of individuals with a specific genotype

semiconservative replication — mode of DNA replication in a parent strand is used as template to copy a complementary daughter strand

senescence — phenomenon wherein a cell can undergo a limited number of rounds of division

sex chromosome — X or Y chromosome involved in sex determination

sex-linked gene — gene present on X or Y chromosome

short interspersed element (SINE) — form of repeated sequence 100–400 base pairs in length

short tandem repeat — DNA sequence of tens to hundreds of bases tandemly repeated multiple times

simple sequence repeat — stretch of di-, tri-, or tetranucleotide repeated multiple times

single-nucleotide polymorphism (SNP) — polymorphic single base change

small nuclear RNA (snRNA) — RNA molecules shorter than 200 base pairs in length, having a role in the splicing process

somatic mosaicism — presence of two or more genetically distinct cell lines in an individual, derived from a common progenitor

splice acceptor — sequence at 3′ border of intron

splice donor — sequence at 5′ border of intron

splice enhancer — sequence that increases likelihood that an intron will be spliced out of mRNA

splice silencer — sequence that reduces likelihood that an intron will be spliced out of mRNA

splicing — process of removal of introns and ligation of exons during processing of RNA

splicing mutations — mutations that change the patterns of RNA splicing, usually by altering splice donor or acceptor sites

SR proteins — proteins involved in selecting sites for initiation of splicing

SRY — gene on Y chromosome required for differentiation of the testes

stop codon — codon that leads to termination of translation

submetacentric — location of a centromere between the middle of the chromosome and one end, producing a short and long arm

synaptonemal complex protein–DNA complex involved in pairing of homologous chromosomes during meiosis

syndrome set of reproducible clinical features due to a common underlying mechanism

systems biology integrated approach to study of complex biological phenomena

telomere specific DNA structure at the ends of chromosomes

telophase the final stage of mitosis, involving the formation of two new nuclear membranes, and daughter cells separating by a process of cytokinesis

teratogen substance that interferes with normal embryonic development

tetraploidy four complete chromosome sets

theta (θ) abbreviation for recombination fraction

threshold model theory of multifactorial inheritance stating that a trait occurs when liability exceeds a threshold

thymine one of four bases of DNA; abbreviated "T"; pairs with adenine

transcription factor protein that binds to DNA and either activates or represses transcription

transcriptome entire set of gene transcripts

transfection introduction of segment of foreign DNA into a cell

transfer RNA (tRNA) RNA molecule that carries a specific amino acid and recognizes the corresponding codon in mRNA, inserting that amino acid into a growing peptide

transformed cell cell capable of unlimited number of rounds of replication

transgene cloned gene inserted into foreign genome

transgenic mouse mouse into which a foreign gene has been inserted into germline

transition mutation that substitutes a pyrimidine for a pyrimidine (e.g., G to A or A to G), or a purine for a purine (e.g., T to C or C to T)

translation process of production of protein from mRNA

translocase enzyme involved in moving ribosome along mRNA to next codon in protein translation

translocation exchange of segments between chromosomes

transposon-derived repeats repeated sequences derived from integration of transposable genetic elements at various sites in genome

transversion mutation that substitutes a purine for a pyrimidine (e.g., T to G) or vice versa

triplet repeat expansion type of mutation in which a gene segment containing multiple copies of a triplet of bases is expanded in length

triploidy three complete chromosome sets

trisomy presence of three copies of a chromosome rather than two

tumor suppressor gene gene that, when both alleles are mutated, leads to transformation of a cell toward a neoplastic phenotype

two-hit hypothesis hypothesis formulated by A. Knudson, postulating that malignant transformation occurs following a two-step process

ultrasound mode of imaging using high-frequency sound waves, used to visualize a developing fetus for prenatal diagnosis

uniparental disomy inheritance of both copies of a chromosome from the same parent

uracil base that substitutes for thymine in RNA; abbreviated "U"; pairs with adenine

vector DNA sequence that conveys an inserted segment into a cell

wild type most common allele in a population at a particular gene locus

Wolffian duct embryonic structure that gives rise to epididymis vas deferens and seminal vesicle

X chromosome one of the sex chromosomes

X-inactivation center (Xic) region on X chromosome at which X inactivation is initiated

Xist gene on X chromosomes believed to be involved in the initiation of X inactivation

Y chromosome one of the sex chromosomes

yeast artificial chromosome (YAC) cloning vector that allows replication of inserted DNA in yeast cells, allowing cloning of very large segments

zygote sperm or egg cell

Index

A
achondroplasia, 47, 48f
acrocentric, 104
adenine
   in DNA, 4
albinism, 40
alkaptonuria, 40
allele(s), 40
alpha-satellite DNA, 105
Alzheimer disease, 92, 94, 94f
   testing for risk of, 219
amino acid sequence
   of proteins, 9
amniocentesis, 163, 164f
anaphase
   in mitosis, 102, 103f, 104f
anemia(s)
   sickle cell, 130, 131, 131f
aneuploidy, 107, 110–12, 110f, 111t, 112f,
      113f
Angelman syndrome, 54, 55f, 118, 122f
angiofibroma
   facial
      in TSC, 243, 243f
animal models of human disease, 75–6, 76f,
      77f
ankylosing spondylitis, 92
anticipation
   in myotonic dystrophy, 57, 58f
   triplet repeat disorders and, 54–7,
      55f–8f
anaphase
   in mitosis, 102, 103f, 104f
ApoE testing, 219
apoptosis, 101
Ashkenazi Jewish carrier screening panel
   conditions included in, 208, 208t
Ashkenazi Jews
   background of, 204
   breast cancer in, 225–6
   Tay–Sachs disease in, 204
ataxia(s)
   Friedreich, 57
autosomal dominant inheritance, 45–7,
      46f–8f
autosomal recessive congenital deafness, 45,
      45f

autosomal recessive inheritance, 40–5,
      41f–4f
autosome(s), 103

B
bacterial artificial chromosomes, 65
balanced polymorphism
   in population genetics, 128
Bardet–Biedl syndrome, 51–2
Barr body, 16
basal cell nevus syndrome, 201
bioinformatics
   in Human Genome Project, 81
   in systems biology, 81
bone marrow transplantation
   for inborn errors of metabolism, 191
branch point, 12f, 13
BRCA gene(s)
   testing for
      breast cancer–related, 226
BRCA1 gene
   breast cancer related to, 224–7, 225t
BRCA2 gene
   breast cancer related to, 224–7, 225t
breast cancer, 222–9
   in Ashkenazi Jews, 225–6
   BRCA1 and BRCA2 genes related to,
      224–7, 225t
   BRCA testing for, 226
   epithelial cells in, 223
   genetics in, 224–6, 225t
   infiltrating ductal carcinoma, 223–4
   mammography in detection of, 223,
      223f
   prevalence of, 223
   risk factors for, 224–6, 225t
   risk-to-benefit analysis testing for,
      226
   treatment of, 223–4
breast-conserving surgery, 223–4
breast masses
   causes of, 223

C
CACAN1S gene
   in malignant hyperthermia, 233–4
café-au-lait macules, 172–4, 172f

caffeine
   metabolism of
      by CYP1A2 genes, 217, 218f
Canavan disease, 208, 208t
cancer(s)
   breast, 222–9. see also breast cancer
   chromosomal basis of, 138, 138f, 139f
   colon
      hereditary nonpolyposis, 146
   diagnosis of, 148, 149
   epigenetics in, 147
   familial clustering of, 138
   familial predisposition to, 227–8
   as genetic disorder, 138–40, 138f, 139f
   genetic testing for, 148
      in children, 227
   genetics of, 137–53
   miRNAs in, 147
   oncogenes, 142–4, 144f, 145f
   oncogenesis in
      molecular basis of, 147–8, 149f, 150f
   prevalence of, 227
   risk factors for
      genetic testing for, 222–9
   treatment of
      new methods, 148–52, 151f
   tumor suppressor genes in, 140–2, 141f,
      142f, 143t
cancer genome sequencing, 149
candidate genes, 92–3
carrier screening, 203–12
   in Ashkenazi Jews, 204
   for cystic fibrosis, 206–8, 206t, 207f
   described, 204
   disorders subject to, 206t
   programs related to, 210
   for Tay–Sachs disease, 204–6, 205f,
      206t
   for thalassemia, 205, 205f, 206t
carrier testing, 135
CdK proteins. see cyclin-dependent kinases
      (Cdk) proteins
cDNA. see complementary DNA (cDNA)
cell cycle, 101, 102f
cell division, 101–3, 102f–4f
centromere, 102, 103f
CF. see cystic fibrosis (CF)

Human Genetics and Genomics, Fourth Edition. Bruce R. Korf and Mira B. Irons.
© 2013 John Wiley & Sons, Ltd. Published 2013 by John Wiley & Sons, Ltd.